IMPRC DIAGNOSIS IN HEALTH CARE

Committee on Diagnostic Error in Health Care

Erin P. Balogh, Bryan T. Miller, and John R. Ball, *Editors*

Board on Health Care Services

Institute of Medicine

The National Academies of
SCIENCES · ENGINEERING · MEDICINE

THE NATIONAL ACADEMIES PRESS
Washington, DC
www.nap.edu

THE NATIONAL ACADEMIES PRESS   500 Fifth Street, NW   Washington, DC 20001

This activity was supported by Contracts HHSH25034020T and 200-2011-38807, TO#20 between the National Academy of Sciences and the Agency for Healthcare Research and Quality and the Centers for Disease Control and Prevention, respectively. This study was also supported by the American College of Radiology, American Society for Clinical Pathology, Cautious Patient Foundation, College of American Pathologists, The Doctors Company Foundation, Janet and Barry Lang, Kaiser Permanente National Community Benefit Fund at the East Bay Community Foundation, and Robert Wood Johnson Foundation. Any opinions, findings, conclusions, or recommendations expressed in this publication do not necessarily reflect the views of any organization or agency that provided support for the project.

Library of Congress Cataloging-in-Publication Data

Names: Balogh, Erin, editor. | Miller, Bryan T., editor. | Ball, John, 1944- ,
  editor. | Institute of Medicine (U.S.). Committee on Diagnostic Error in
  Health Care, issuing body.
Title: Improving diagnosis in health care / Committee on Diagnostic Error in
  Health Care ; Erin P. Balogh, Bryan T. Miller, and John R. Ball, editors ;
  Board on Health Care Services, Institute of Medicine, The National
  Academies of Sciences, Engineering, and Medicine.
Description: Washington, DC : The National Academies Press, [2015] | Includes
  bibliographical references.
Identifiers: LCCN 2015041708 | ISBN 9780309377690 (pbk.) | ISBN
9780309377706 (pdf)
Subjects: | MESH: Diagnostic Errors—prevention & control—United States. |
  Diagnostic Techniques and Procedures—United States.
Classification: LCC RC71.5 | NLM WB 141 | DDC 616.07/50289—dc23 LC
record available at
http://lccn.loc.gov/2015041708

Additional copies of this report are available for sale from the National Academies Press, 500 Fifth Street, NW, Keck 360, Washington, DC 20001; (800) 624-6242 or (202) 334-3313; http://www.nap.edu.

Cover credit: LeAnn Locher & Associates.

Suggested citation: National Academies of Sciences, Engineering, and Medicine. 2015. *Improving diagnosis in health care.* Washington, DC: The National Academies Press.

MICHELLE ROGERS, Associate Professor, College of Computing and Informatics, Drexel University
URMIMALA SARKAR, Associate Professor of Medicine, University of California, San Francisco
GEORGE E. THIBAULT, President, Josiah Macy Jr. Foundation
JOHN B. WONG, Chief, Division of Clinical Decision Making, Tufts Medical Center

Study Staff

ERIN BALOGH, Study Director
BRYAN MILLER, Research Associate (from August 2014)
SARAH NAYLOR, Research Associate (until August 2014)
KATHRYN GARNHAM ELLETT, Research Associate (from April 2015 to July 2015)
CELYNNE BALATBAT, Research Assistant (until June 2015)
PATRICK ROSS, Research Assistant (from April 2015)
LAURA ROSEMA, Christine Mirzayan Science and Technology Policy Graduate Fellow (from January to April 2014)
BEATRICE KALISCH, Nurse Scholar in Residence (until August 2014)
PATRICK BURKE, Financial Associate
ROGER HERDMAN, Director, Board on Health Care Services (until June 2014)
SHARYL NASS, Director, Board on Health Care Services (from June 2014); Director, National Cancer Policy Forum

Reviewers

This report has been reviewed in draft form by individuals chosen for their diverse perspectives and technical expertise. The purpose of this independent review is to provide candid and critical comments that will assist the institution in making its published report as sound as possible and to ensure that the report meets institutional standards for objectivity, evidence, and responsiveness to the study charge. The review comments and draft manuscript remain confidential to protect the integrity of the deliberative process. We wish to thank the following individuals for their review of this report:

SUZANNE BAKKEN, Columbia University
DONALD BERWICK, Institute for Healthcare Improvement
PAUL CHANG, University of Chicago Hospitals
JAMES J. CIMINO, University of Alabama at Birmingham
SARA J. CZAJA, University of Miami Miller School of Medicine
GURPREET DHALIWAL, University of California, San Francisco, and San Francisco Veterans Affairs Medical Center
TEJAL GANDHI, National Patient Safety Foundation
HELEN HASKELL, Mothers Against Medical Error
JOHN M. HICKNER, University of Illinois at Chicago
MICHELLE MELLO, Stanford Law School
JEFFREY MEYERS, University of Michigan
MARGARET E. O'KANE, National Committee for Quality Assurance

GORDON SCHIFF, Brigham and Women's Hospital and Harvard
 Medical School
SUSAN SHERIDAN, Patient-Centered Outcomes Research Institute
HARDEEP SINGH, Houston Veterans Affairs Health Services
 Research Center for Innovations, Michael E. DeBakey Veterans
 Affairs Medical Center, and Baylor College of Medicine
BRIAN R. SMITH, Yale University School of Medicine
LAURA ZWAAN, Erasmus Medical Center

Although the reviewers listed above have provided many constructive comments and suggestions, they were not asked to endorse the conclusions or recommendations nor did they see the final draft of the report before its release. The review of this report was overseen by **BRADFORD H. GRAY,** Editor Emeritus, *The Milbank Quarterly*, Senior Fellow, Urban Institute, and **KRISTINE GEBBIE,** Flinders University School of Nursing and Midwifery, Adelaide, South Australia. They were responsible for making certain that an independent examination of this report was carried out in accordance with institutional procedures and that all review comments were carefully considered. Responsibility for the final content of this report rests entirely with the authoring committee and the institution.

Acknowledgments

We thank the following individuals who spoke at the committee's meetings:

Bibb Allen, *American College of Radiology*
Leonard Berlin, *Skokie Hospital, Rush Medical College, University of Illinois*
Barbara Brandt, *National Center for Interprofessional Practice and Education, University of Minnesota*
David Classen, *Pascal Metrics and University of Utah School of Medicine*
Gurpreet Dhaliwal, *University of California, San Francisco,* and *San Francisco Veterans Affairs Medical Center*
Paul Epner, *Society to Improve Diagnosis in Medicine*
Tejal Gandhi, *National Patient Safety Foundation*
Emmy Ganos, *Robert Wood Johnson Foundation*
David Gross, *College of American Pathologists*
Kerm Henriksen, *Agency for Healthcare Research and Quality*
Devery Howerton, *Centers for Disease Control and Prevention*
Heidi Julavits, *Columbia University*
Allen Kachalia, *Brigham and Women's Hospital, Harvard Medical School,* and *Harvard School of Public Health*
Michael Kanter, *Kaiser Permanente*
Jerome Kassirer, *Tufts University School of Medicine*
Steven Kroft, *American Society for Clinical Pathology*
Michael Millenson, *Cautious Patient Foundation*
Elizabeth Montgomery, *Cautious Patient Foundation*
Jeffrey Myers, *University of Michigan*

David E. Newman-Toker, *Johns Hopkins University School of Medicine*
Harold Pincus, *New York–Presbyterian Hospital, Columbia University,* and
    RAND Corporation
Donald Redelmeier, *University of Toronto*
Eduardo Salas, *University of Central Florida*
Nadine Sarter, *University of Michigan*
Gordon Schiff, *Brigham and Women's Hospital* and *Harvard Medical School*
Hardeep Singh, *Houston Veterans Affairs Health Services Research Center
    for Innovations, Michael E. DeBakey Veterans Affairs Medical Center,*
    and *Baylor College of Medicine*
Stephen Teret, *Johns Hopkins University*
Eric Thomas, *University of Texas Houston Medical School*
Robert Trowbridge, *Maine Medical Center* and *Tufts University School of
    Medicine*
David Troxel, *The Doctors Company Foundation*

We would also like to thank a number of individuals who submitted
written input or provided public comments at the committee meetings
that informed the committee's deliberations. These individuals included:

Melissa Anselmo, *OpenNotes*
Signall Bell, *OpenNotes*
Ann Bisantz, *University at Buffalo*
Dennis Boyle, *COPIC*
John E. Brush, Jr., *Eastern Virginia Medical School* and *Sentara Healthcare,
    Norfolk, Virginia*
Tom Delbanco, *OpenNotes*
Gerri Donohue, *Physicians' Reciprocal Insurers*
Steven J. Durning, *Uniformed Services University of the Health Sciences*
Gary Klein, *MacroCognition*
Alan Lembitz, *COPIC*
George Lundberg, *Medscape*
David L. Meyers, *American College of Emergency Physicians*
Harold Miller, *Center for Healthcare Quality and Payment Reform*
Geoff Norman, *McMaster University*
Carolyn Oliver, *Cautious Patient Foundation*
Frank Papa, *University of North Texas Health Science Center*
P. Divya Parikh, *PIAA*
W. Scott Richardson, *GRU/UGA Medical Partnership Campus*
Meredith Rosenthal, *Harvard School of Public Health*
Alan Schwartz, *University of Illinois, Chicago*
Dana Siegal, *CRICO*
Olle ten Cate, *University Medical Center Utrecht*

Bill Thatcher, *Cautious Patient Foundation*
Bill Thorwarth, *American College of Radiology*
David Troxel, *The Doctors Company*
Jan Walker, *OpenNotes*
Saul Weiner, *University of Illinois, Chicago, Jesse Brown Veterans Affairs Medical Center*
David Wennberg, *Northern New England Accountable Care Collaborative*

Funding for the study was provided by the Agency for Healthcare Research and Quality, the American College of Radiology, the American Society for Clinical Pathology, the Cautious Patient Foundation, the Centers for Disease Control and Prevention, the College of American Pathologists, The Doctors Company Foundation, Janet and Barry Lang, Kaiser Permanente National Community Benefit Fund at the East Bay Community Foundation, and the Robert Wood Johnson Foundation. The committee appreciates the support extended by these sponsors for the development of this report.

We would also like to thank the individuals who shared their experiences with diagnosis in the dissemination video: Sue, Jeff, and Carolyn.

Finally, many within the National Academies of Sciences, Engineering, and Medicine were helpful to the study staff. We would like to thank Clyde Behney, Chelsea Frakes, Greta Gorman, Laurie Graig, Julie Ische, Nicole Joy, Ellen Kimmel, Katye Magee, Fariha Mahmud, Abbey Meltzer, Jonathan Phillips, and Jennifer Walsh.

Preface

Fifteen years ago, in its landmark report *To Err Is Human: Building a Safer Health System,* the Institute of Medicine (IOM) dramatically exposed the issue of patient safety in health care. Stating the obvious—that human beings make errors—but highlighting the theretofore rarely discussed fact that those of us in health care also make errors, the report began a quiet revolution in the way in which health care organizations address the safety and quality of care. This report, *Improving Diagnosis in Health Care,* is a follow-up to the earlier report and the most recent in the IOM's Quality Chasm Series. This report has three major themes.

First, *Improving Diagnosis in Health Care* exposes a critical type of error in health care—diagnostic error—that has received relatively little attention since the release of *To Err Is Human.* There are several reasons why diagnostic error has been underappreciated, even though the correct diagnosis is a critical aspect of health care. The data on diagnostic error are sparse, few reliable measures exist, and often the error is identified only in retrospect. Yet the best estimates indicate that all of us will likely experience a meaningful diagnostic error in our lifetime. Perhaps the most significant contribution of this report is to highlight the importance of the issue and to direct discussion among patients and health care professionals and organizations on what should be done about this complex challenge.

Second, patients are central to the solution. The report defines diagnostic error from the patient's viewpoint as "the failure to (a) establish an accurate and timely explanation of *the patient's* health problem(s) or (b) communicate that explanation to *the patient.*" The report's first goal centers on the need to establish partnerships with patients and their families to improve diagnosis, and several recommendations aim to facilitate and enhance such partnerships.

Third, diagnosis is a collaborative effort. The stereotype of a single physician contemplating a patient case and discerning a diagnosis is not always true; the diagnostic process often involves intra- and inter-professional teamwork. Nor is diagnostic error always due to human error; often, it occurs because of errors in the health care system. The complexity of health and disease and the increasing complexity of health care demands collaboration and teamwork among and between health care professionals, as well as with patients and their families.

In addition to these major themes, the report highlights several key issues that must be addressed if diagnostic errors are to be reduced:

- Health care professional education and training does not take fully into account advances in the learning sciences. The report emphasizes training in clinical reasoning, teamwork, and communication.
- Health information technology, while potentially a boon to quality health care, is often a barrier to effective clinical care in its current form. The report makes several recommendations to improve the utility of health information technology in the diagnostic process specifically and the clinical process more generally.
- There are few data on diagnostic error. The report recommends, in addition to specified research, the development of approaches to monitor the diagnostic process and to identify, learn from, and reduce diagnostic error.
- The health care work system and culture do not sufficiently support the diagnostic process. Echoing previous IOM work, the report also recommends the development of an organizational culture that values open discussion and feedback on diagnostic performance.
- In addition, the report highlights the increasingly important role of radiologists and pathologists as integral members of the diagnostic team.

There were also areas where the committee that developed the report wished we could go further but found that there are insufficient data currently to support strong recommendations. One of those areas is the payment system, now evolving from fee-for-service to more value- and population-based. Research on the effects of novel payment systems on diagnosis is sorely needed. Another area is that of medical liability. The report recommends the adoption of communication and resolution programs as a key lever to improve the disclosure of diagnostic errors to patients and to facilitate improved organizational learning from these events. However, other approaches for the resolution of medical injuries, such as safe harbors for the adherence to evidence-based clinical practice guidelines and administrative health courts, hold promise. More needs to be known of their effect on the diagnostic process, and the report recommends demonstration projects to expand the knowledge base in these areas.

A final area of potential controversy is the measurement of diagnostic errors for public reporting and accountability purposes. The committee believed that, given the lack of an agreement on what constitutes a diagnostic error, the paucity of hard data, and the lack of valid measurement approaches, the time was simply not ripe to call for mandatory reporting. Instead, it is appropriate at this time to leverage the intrinsic motivation of health care professionals to improve diagnostic performance and to treat diagnostic error as a key component of quality improvement efforts by health care organizations. Better identification, analysis, and implementation of approaches to improve diagnosis and reduce diagnostic error are needed throughout all settings of care.

As chair of the committee, I thank all of the members of the committee for their individual and group contributions. I am grateful for the time, energy, and diligence, as well as the diversity of experience and expertise, they all brought to the process. When a diverse group of good people with good intent come together for a common purpose, the process is richer and more enjoyable, and the product more likely to be worthwhile. None of the work of the committee would have been possible without the professional IOM staff, led by the study director, Erin Balogh. Both personally and on behalf of the committee, I thank them for a truly collaborative, incredibly responsive, and productive process.

John R. Ball
Chair
Committee on Diagnostic Error in Health Care

Contents

Boxes, Figures, and Tables

BOXES

FIGURES

TABLES

Acronyms and Abbrevations

AAFP	American Academy of Family Physicians
ABMS	American Board of Medical Specialties
ACGME	Accreditation Council for Graduate Medical Education
ACO	accountable care organization
ACR	American College of Radiology
AHRQ	Agency for Healthcare Research and Quality
AMA	American Medical Association
ANTS	Anesthetists' Non-Technical Skills
AOA	American Osteopathic Association
APN	advanced practice nurse
ASCP	American Society for Clinical Pathology
CAD	computer-aided detection
CAP	College of American Pathologists
CBE	competency-based evaluation
CCNE	Commission on Collegiate Nursing Education
CDC	Centers for Disease Control and Prevention
CDS	clinical decision support
CEO	chief executive officer
CLIA	Clinical Laboratory Improvement Amendments
CLIAC	Clinical Laboratory Improvement Advisory Committee
CMS	Centers for Medicare & Medicaid Services
CPG	clinical practice guideline
CPT	current procedural terminology
CRP	communication and resolution program

CT	computed tomography

DMT	diagnostic management team
DOD	Department of Defense
DRG	diagnosis-related group
DSM	*Diagnostic and Statistical Manual of Mental Disorders*

E&M	evaluation and management
ED	emergency department
EHR	electronic health record
EKG	electrocardiogram

FDA	Food and Drug Administration
FFS	fee-for-service
FMEA	failure mode and effects analysis

| GABHS | Group A β-hemolytic streptococcus |
| GME | graduate medical education |

health IT	health information technology
HFAP	Healthcare Facilities Accreditation Program
HHS	Department of Health and Human Services
HIMSS	Healthcare Information Management Systems Society
HIV	human immunodeficiency virus
HRO	high reliability organization

ICD	*International Classification of Diseases*
IOM	Institute of Medicine
IPU	integrated practice unit
IVD	in vitro diagnostic test

LCME	Liaison Committee on Medical Education
LDT	laboratory developed test
LOINC	Logical Observation Identifiers Names and Codes

M&M	morbidity and mortality
MACRMI	Massachusetts Alliance for Communication and Resolution following Medical Injury
MCAT	Medical College Aptitude Test
mHealth	mobile health
MI	myocardial infarction
MIPPA	Medicare Improvements for Patients and Providers Act

MOC	maintenance of certification
MQSA	Mammography Quality Standards Act
MRI	magnetic resonance imaging
NCQA	National Committee for Quality Assurance
NDC	National Drug Code
NIH	National Institutes of Health
NLM	National Library of Medicine
NLNAC	National League for Nursing Accrediting Commission
NPDB	National Practitioner Data Bank
NPSD	Network of Patient Safety Databases
ONC	Office of the National Coordinator for Health Information Technology
PA	physician assistant
PCMH	patient-centered medical home
PCORI	Patient-Centered Outcomes Research Institute
PET	positron emission tomography
PRI	Physician Reciprocal Insurers
PSO	patient safety organization
PSO PPC	PSO Privacy Protection Center
PSQIA	Patient Safety and Quality Improvement Act
PT	proficiency testing
RSNA	Radiological Society of North America
TeamSTEPPS	Team Strategies and Tools to Enhance Performance and Patient Safety
UDP	Undiagnosed Diseases Program
UMHS	University of Michigan Health System
VA	Department of Veterans Affairs

Summary

The delivery of health care has proceeded for decades with a blind spot: Diagnostic errors—inaccurate or delayed diagnoses—persist throughout all settings of care and continue to harm an unacceptable number of patients. For example:

- A conservative estimate found that 5 percent of U.S. adults who seek outpatient care each year experience a diagnostic error.
- Postmortem examination research spanning decades has shown that diagnostic errors contribute to approximately 10 percent of patient deaths.
- Medical record reviews suggest that diagnostic errors account for 6 to 17 percent of hospital adverse events.
- Diagnostic errors are the leading type of paid medical malpractice claims, are almost twice as likely to have resulted in the patient's death compared to other claims, and represent the highest proportion of total payments.

In reviewing the evidence, the committee concluded that most people will experience at least one diagnostic error in their lifetime, sometimes with devastating consequences. Despite the pervasiveness of diagnostic errors and the risk for serious patient harm, diagnostic errors have been largely unappreciated within the quality and patient safety movements in health care. Without a dedicated focus on improving diagnosis, these errors will likely worsen as the delivery of health care and the diagnostic process continue to increase in complexity.

Getting the right diagnosis is a key aspect of health care—it provides an explanation of a patient's health problem and informs subsequent health care decisions. Diagnostic errors stem from a wide variety of causes, including: inadequate collaboration and communication among clinicians, patients, and their families;[1] a health care work system that is not well designed to support the diagnostic process; limited feedback to clinicians about diagnostic performance; and a culture that discourages transparency and disclosure of diagnostic errors—impeding attempts to learn from these events and improve diagnosis. Diagnostic errors may result in different outcomes, and as evidence accrues, these outcomes will be better characterized. For example, if there is a diagnostic error, a patient may or may not experience harm. Errors can be harmful because they can prevent or delay appropriate treatment, lead to unnecessary or harmful treatment, or result in psychological or financial repercussions. Harm may not result, for example, if a patient's symptoms resolve even with an incorrect diagnosis.

Improving the diagnostic process is not only possible, but also represents a moral, professional, and public health imperative. Achieving that goal will require a significant reenvisioning of the diagnostic process and a widespread commitment to change among health care professionals, health care organizations, patients and their families, researchers, and policy makers.

DEFINITION AND CONCEPTUAL MODEL

The committee concluded that a sole focus on diagnostic error reduction will not achieve the extensive change necessary; a broader focus on *improving diagnosis* is warranted. To provide a framework for this dual focus, the committee developed a conceptual model to articulate the diagnostic process (see Figure S-1), describe work system factors that influence this process (see Figure S-2), and identify opportunities to improve the diagnostic process and outcomes (see Figure S-3).

The diagnostic process is a complex and collaborative activity that unfolds over time and occurs within the context of a health care work system. The diagnostic process is iterative, and as information gathering continues, the goal is to reduce diagnostic uncertainty, narrow down the diagnostic possibilities, and develop a more precise and complete understanding of a patient's health problem.

The committee sought to develop a definition of diagnostic error that reflects the iterative and complex nature of the diagnostic process, as

---

[1] The term "family" is used for simplicity, but the term is meant to encompass all individuals who provide support or informal caregiving to patients in the diagnostic process.

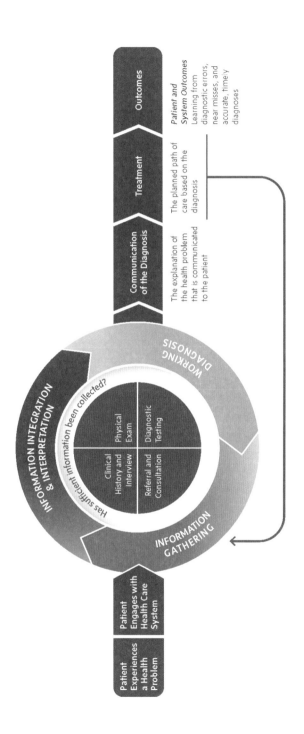

FIGURE S-1 The diagnostic process.

TIME

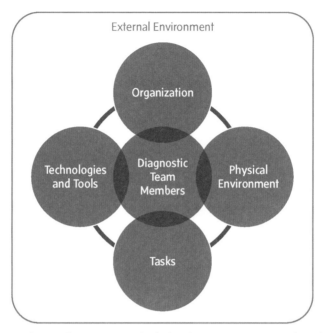

FIGURE S-2 The work system in which the diagnostic process takes place.

well as the need for a diagnosis to convey more than simply a label of a disease. The term "health problem" is used in the definition because it is a patient-centered and inclusive term to describe a patient's overall health condition. The committee's definition of diagnostic error is *the failure to (a) establish an accurate and timely explanation of the patient's health problem(s) or (b) communicate that explanation to the patient.* The definition employs a patient-centered perspective because patients bear the ultimate risk of harm from diagnostic errors. A diagnosis is not accurate if it differs from the true condition a patient has (or does not have) or if it is imprecise and incomplete. Timeliness means that the diagnosis was not meaningfully delayed; however, timeliness is context-dependent. While some diagnoses may take days, weeks, or even months to establish, timely may mean quite quickly (minutes to hours) for other urgent diagnoses. The inclusion of communication is distinct from previous definitions, in recognition that communication is a key responsibility throughout the diagnostic process. From a patient's perspective, an accurate and timely explanation of the health problem is meaningless unless this information

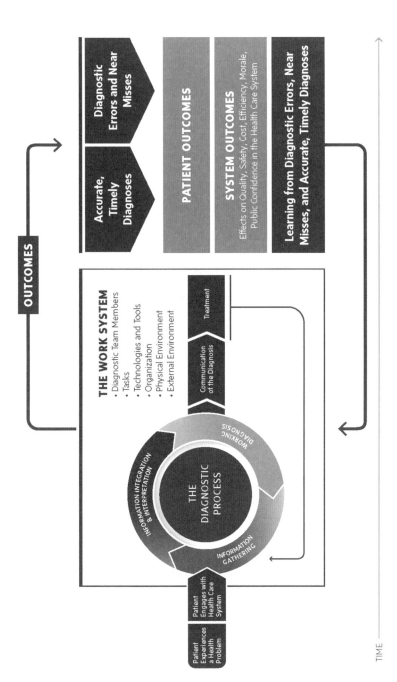

FIGURE S-3 The outcomes from the diagnostic process.

TIME

reaches the patient so that a patient and health care professionals can act on the explanation.[2]

In addition to defining and identifying diagnostic errors in clinical practice, the report places a broader emphasis on improving the diagnostic process. Analyzing failures in the diagnostic process can provide important opportunities for learning and continued improvement. Some failures in the diagnostic process will lead to diagnostic errors; however, other failures in the diagnostic process will not ultimately lead to a diagnostic error, because subsequent steps in the process compensate for the initial failure. In this report, the committee describes "failures in the diagnostic process that do not lead to diagnostic errors" as near misses.

A related but distinct concept to diagnostic error is overdiagnosis, defined as when a condition is diagnosed that is unlikely to affect the individual's health and well-being. While overdiagnosis represents a true challenge to health care quality, it is not a diagnostic error. Overdiagnosis is only detectable in population-based analyses—it is virtually impossible to assess whether overdiagnosis has occurred for an individual patient. However, improving the diagnostic process—such as reducing unnecessary diagnostic testing—may help avert overdiagnosis.

RECOMMENDATIONS

The committee's recommendations address eight goals to improve diagnosis and reduce diagnostic error (see Box S-1). These recommendations apply to all diagnostic team members and settings of care. Given the early state of the field, the evidence base for some of the recommendations stems from the broader patient safety and quality improvement literature. Patients and patient advocates have much to offer on how to implement the committee's recommendations; leveraging the expertise, power, and influence of the patient community will help spur progress.

Facilitate More Effective Teamwork in the Diagnostic Process Among Health Care Professionals, Patients, and Their Families

The diagnostic process requires collaboration among health care professionals, patients, and their families. Patients and their families are critical partners in the diagnostic process; they contribute valuable input that facilitates the diagnostic process and ensures shared decision mak-

---

[2] Because not all patients will be able to participate in the communication process, in some instances communication would be between the health care professionals and a patient's family or designated health care proxy.

BOX S-1
Goals for Improving Diagnosis and Reducing Diagnostic Error

- Facilitate more effective teamwork in the diagnostic process among health care professionals, patients, and their families
- Enhance health care professional education and training in the diagnostic process
- Ensure that health information technologies support patients and health care professionals in the diagnostic process
- Develop and deploy approaches to identify, learn from, and reduce diagnostic errors and near misses in clinical practice
- Establish a work system and culture that supports the diagnostic process and improvements in diagnostic performance
- Develop a reporting environment and medical liability system that facilitates improved diagnosis by learning from diagnostic errors and near misses
- Design a payment and care delivery environment that supports the diagnostic process
- Provide dedicated funding for research on the diagnostic process and diagnostic errors

---

ing about the path of care. Health care professionals and organizations[3] are responsible for creating environments in which patients and their families can learn about and engage in the diagnostic process and provide feedback about their experiences. One strategy is to promote the use of health information technology (health IT) tools that make a patient's health information more accessible to patients. Involving patients and their families in efforts to improve diagnosis is also critical because they have unique insights into the diagnostic process and the occurrence of diagnostic errors.

The diagnostic process hinges on successful intra- and interprofessional collaboration among health care professionals, including primary care clinicians, physicians in various specialties, nurses, pharmacists, technologists, therapists, social workers, patient navigators, and many others. Thus, all health care professionals need to be well prepared and supported to engage in diagnostic teamwork. The roles of some health care professionals who participate in the diagnostic process have been insufficiently recognized. The fields of pathology and radiology are criti-

---

[3] The term "health care organization" is used for simplicity, but is meant to encompass all settings in which the diagnostic process takes place, including integrated care delivery settings, hospitals, clinician practices, retail clinics, and long-term care settings.

cal to diagnosis, but professionals in these fields are not always engaged as full members of the diagnostic team. Enhanced collaboration among pathologists, radiologists, other diagnosticians, and treating health care professionals[4] has the potential to improve diagnostic testing.[5] In addition, nurses are often not recognized as collaborators in the diagnostic process, despite their critical roles in ensuring communication, care coordination, and patient education; monitoring a patient's condition; and identifying and preventing potential diagnostic errors.

Goal 1: Facilitate more effective teamwork in the diagnostic process among health care professionals, patients, and their families

> **Recommendation 1a: In recognition that the diagnostic process is a dynamic team-based activity, health care organizations should ensure that health care professionals have the appropriate knowledge, skills, resources, and support to engage in teamwork in the diagnostic process. To accomplish this, they should facilitate and support:**
> * **Intra- and interprofessional teamwork in the diagnostic process.**
> * **Collaboration among pathologists, radiologists, other diagnosticians, and treating health care professionals to improve diagnostic testing processes.**
>
> **Recommendation 1b: Health care professionals and organizations should partner with patients and their families as diagnostic team members and facilitate patient and family engagement in the diagnostic process, aligned with their needs, values, and preferences. To accomplish this, they should:**
> * **Provide patients with opportunities to learn about the diagnostic process.**
> * **Create environments in which patients and their families are comfortable engaging in the diagnostic process and sharing feedback and concerns about diagnostic errors and near misses.**
> * **Ensure patient access to electronic health records (EHRs), including clinical notes and diagnostic testing results, to facili-**

---

[4] Treating health care professionals are clinicians who directly interact with patients.

[5] The term "diagnostic testing" is broadly inclusive of all types of testing, including medical imaging, anatomic pathology and laboratory medicine, as well as other types of testing, such as mental health assessments, vision and hearing testing, and neurocognitive testing.

tate patient engagement in the diagnostic process and patient
review of health records for accuracy.
- Identify opportunities to include patients and their families
  in efforts to improve the diagnostic process by learning from
  diagnostic errors and near misses.

Enhance Health Care Professional Education and Training in the Diagnostic Process

Getting the right diagnosis depends on all health care professionals
involved in the diagnostic process receiving appropriate education and
training. The learning sciences, which study how people learn, can be
used to improve education and training. For example, feedback—or information about the accuracy of a clinician's diagnosis—is essential for
improved diagnostic performance. The authenticity of the learning environment can affect the acquisition of diagnostic skills; better alignment
of training environments with clinical practice promotes development of
diagnostic skills.

Opportunities to improve education and training in the diagnostic
process include: greater emphasis on teamwork and communication with
patients, their families, and other health care professionals; appropriate
use of diagnostic testing and the application of test results to subsequent
decision making; and the use of health IT. In addition, the lack of focus on
developing clinical reasoning and understanding the cognitive contributions to decision making represents a major gap in education within all
health care professions. Proposed strategies to improve clinical reasoning
include instruction and practice on generating and refining a differential
diagnosis, generating illness scripts, developing an appreciation of how
diagnostic errors occur and strategies to mitigate them, and engaging in
metacognition and debiasing strategies.

Oversight processes play a critical role in promoting competency in
the diagnostic process. Many accreditation organizations already require
skills important for diagnostic performance, but diagnostic competencies
need to be a larger priority within these requirements. Organizations responsible for licensure and certification can also help ensure that health
care professionals have achieved and maintain competency in the skills
essential for the diagnostic process.

*Goal 2: Enhance health care professional education and training in the
diagnostic process*

**Recommendation 2a: Educators should ensure that curricula and
training programs across the career trajectory:**

- Address performance in the diagnostic process, including areas such as clinical reasoning; teamwork; communication with patients, their families, and other health care professionals; appropriate use of diagnostic tests and the application of these results on subsequent decision making; and use of health information technology.
- Employ educational approaches that are aligned with evidence from the learning sciences.

Recommendation 2b: Health care professional certification and accreditation organizations should ensure that health care professionals have and maintain the competencies needed for effective performance in the diagnostic process, including the areas listed above.

Ensure That Health Information Technologies Support Patients and Health Care Professionals in the Diagnostic Process

Health IT has the potential to improve diagnosis and reduce diagnostic errors by facilitating timely and easy access to information; communication among health care professionals, patients, and their families; clinical reasoning; and feedback and follow-up in the diagnostic process. However, many experts are concerned that health IT currently is not effectively facilitating the diagnostic process and may even be contributing to diagnostic errors. Challenges include problems with usability, poor integration into clinical workflow, difficulty sharing a patient's health information, and a limited ability to support clinical reasoning and identification of diagnostic errors in clinical practice. Better alignment of health IT with the diagnostic process is warranted.

Because the diagnostic process occurs over time and can involve multiple health care professionals across different care settings, the free flow of information is critical. Improved interoperability across health care organizations and across laboratory and radiology information systems is needed to achieve this information flow.

Although there may be patient safety risks in the diagnostic process related to the use of health IT, it is difficult to determine the extent of the problem. Health IT vendors often limit the sharing of information about these risks. A previous IOM report recommended that the Department of Health and Human Services (HHS) ensure insofar as possible that health IT vendors support the free exchange of information about patient safety and not prohibit sharing of such information. The present committee endorses this recommendation and highlights the need for shared information about user experiences with health IT used in the diagnostic process. Independent evaluations of health IT products could also identify potential adverse consequences that contribute to diagnostic errors.

Goal 3: Ensure that health information technologies support patients and health care professionals in the diagnostic process

> **Recommendation 3a: Health information technology (health IT) vendors and the Office of the National Coordinator for Health Information Technology (ONC) should work together with users to ensure that health IT used in the diagnostic process demonstrates usability, incorporates human factors knowledge, integrates measurement capability, fits well within clinical workflow, provides clinical decision support, and facilitates the timely flow of information among patients and health care professionals involved in the diagnostic process.**

> **Recommendation 3b: ONC should require health IT vendors to meet standards for interoperability among different health IT systems to support effective, efficient, and structured flow of patient information across care settings to facilitate the diagnostic process by 2018.**

> **Recommendation 3c: The Secretary of Health and Human Services should require health IT vendors to:**
> - **Routinely submit their products for independent evaluation and notify users about potential adverse effects on the diagnostic process related to the use of their products.**
> - **Permit and support the free exchange of information about real-time user experiences with health IT design and implementation that adversely affect the diagnostic process.**

Develop and Deploy Approaches to Identify, Learn from, and Reduce Diagnostic Errors and Near Misses in Clinical Practice

Due to the difficulty in identifying diagnostic errors and competing demands from existing quality and safety improvement priorities, very few health care organizations have processes in place to identify diagnostic errors and near misses. Nonetheless, identifying these experiences, learning from them, and implementing changes will improve diagnosis and reduce diagnostic errors. Health care organizations can also ensure that systematic feedback on diagnostic performance reaches individuals, care teams, and organizational leadership.

Postmortem examinations are a critical source of information on the epidemiology of diagnostic errors, but the number of postmortem examinations has declined precipitously. A greater emphasis on postmortem examination research—including more limited approaches to postmortem examinations—is warranted to better understand the incidence of diagnostic errors and the role of postmortem examinations in modern clinical practice.

Health care professional societies can be engaged to identify high-priority areas to improve diagnosis, similar to the Choosing Wisely initiative on avoiding unnecessary care. Early efforts could focus on identifying the most common diagnostic errors, "don't miss" health conditions that may result in patient harm, or diagnostic errors that are relatively easy to address.

Goal 4: Develop and deploy approaches to identify, learn from, and reduce diagnostic errors and near misses in clinical practice

> **Recommendation 4a: Accreditation organizations and the Medicare conditions of participation should require that health care organizations have programs in place to monitor the diagnostic process and identify, learn from, and reduce diagnostic errors and near misses in a timely fashion. Proven approaches should be incorporated into updates of these requirements.**
>
> **Recommendation 4b: Health care organizations should:**
> - **Monitor the diagnostic process and identify, learn from, and reduce diagnostic errors and near misses as a component of their research, quality improvement, and patient safety programs.**
> - **Implement procedures and practices to provide systematic feedback on diagnostic performance to individual health care professionals, care teams, and clinical and organizational leaders.**
>
> **Recommendation 4c: The Department of Health and Human Services should provide funding for a designated subset of health care systems to conduct routine postmortem examinations on a representative sample of patient deaths.**
>
> **Recommendation 4d: Health care professional societies should identify opportunities to improve accurate and timely diagnoses and reduce diagnostic errors in their specialties.**

Establish a Work System and Culture That Supports the Diagnostic Process and Improvements in Diagnostic Performance

Health care organizations influence the work system in which diagnosis occurs and play a role in implementing change. The work systems of many health care organizations could better support the diagnostic process, for example, by integrating mechanisms to improve error recovery and resiliency in the diagnostic process.

The culture and leadership of health care organizations are key factors in ensuring continuous learning in the diagnostic process. Organizations need to promote a nonpunitive culture in which clinicians can identify and learn from diagnostic errors. Organizational leadership can facilitate this culture, provide resources, and set priorities for achieving progress in diagnostic performance and reducing diagnostic errors.

Health care organizations can also work to address diagnostic challenges related to fragmentation of the broader health care system. Although improved teamwork and interoperability will help with fragmentation in health care, organizations need to recognize that patients cross organizational boundaries and that this has the potential to contribute to diagnostic errors and failures to learn from them. Strengthening communication and reliable diagnostic test reporting is one area where this can be addressed.

Goal 5: Establish a work system and culture that supports the diagnostic process and improvements in diagnostic performance

Recommendation 5: Health care organizations should:
- Adopt policies and practices that promote a nonpunitive culture that values open discussion and feedback on diagnostic performance.
- Design the work system in which the diagnostic process occurs to support the work and activities of patients, their families, and health care professionals and to facilitate accurate and timely diagnoses.
- Develop and implement processes to ensure effective and timely communication between diagnostic testing health care professionals and treating health care professionals across all health care delivery settings.

Develop a Reporting Environment and Medical Liability System That Facilitates Improved Diagnosis by Learning from Diagnostic Errors and Near Misses

Reporting

Conducting analyses of diagnostic errors, near misses, and adverse events presents the best opportunity to learn from such experiences and implement changes to improve diagnosis. There is a need for safe environments, without the threat of legal discovery or disciplinary action, to analyze and learn from these events. Previously, the IOM recommended that Congress extend peer review protections to data that are collected for improving the safety and quality of care. Subsequent legislation established the Agency for Healthcare Research and Quality (AHRQ)-administered Patient Safety Organization (PSO) program which conferred privilege and confidentiality protections to patient safety information that is shared with PSOs.

The PSO program is an important national lever to increase voluntary error reporting and analysis, but progress has been impeded by several challenges. For example, AHRQ developed Common Formats to encourage standardized event reporting, but the use of these formats is voluntary, and there is no Common Format specific to diagnostic error. Concern that the federal privilege protections do not protect organizations from state reporting requirements could also prevent voluntary submissions to PSOs and decrease the potential for improved learning. Given the PSO program's potential to improve learning about diagnostic errors and near misses, it is important to evaluate the program.

Medical Liability

The core functions of medical liability are to compensate negligently injured patients and to promote quality by encouraging clinicians and organizations to avoid medical errors. The current approach for resolving medical liability claims sets up barriers to improvements in quality and patient safety. In addition, patients and their families are poorly served by the current system. While medical liability is broader than diagnosis, diagnostic errors are the leading type of paid medical malpractice claims.

Traditional medical liability reforms have not been effective in compensating negligently injured patients or deterring unsafe care. Alternative approaches are needed that enable patients and clinicians to become allies in making health care safer by encouraging transparency and disclosure of medical errors. These reforms can enable prompt and fair compensation for avoidable injuries, while turning errors into opportunities for learning and improvement.

Communication and resolution programs (CRPs) provide a pragmatic approach for changing medical liability in that they are the most likely to be implemented. Safe harbors for adherence to evidence-based clinical practice guidelines could also help facilitate improvements in diagnostic accuracy by incentivizing the use of evidence-based diagnostic approaches; however, there are few clinical practice guidelines available for diagnosis, and implementation is complex. Administrative health courts offer a fundamental change that would promote a more open environment for identifying, studying, and learning from errors, but implementation is very challenging because of their operational complexity and resistance from stakeholders who are strongly committed to preserving the current tort-based system.

Risk Management

Professional liability insurance carriers and health care organizations that participate in captive or other self-insurance arrangements have an inherent interest and expertise in improving diagnosis. Improved collaboration between health professional liability insurance carriers and health care professionals and organizations could support education, training, and practice improvement strategies focused on improving diagnosis and minimizing diagnostic errors.

Goal 6: Develop a reporting environment and medical liability system that facilitates improved diagnosis by learning from diagnostic errors and near misses

Recommendation 6a: The Agency for Healthcare Research and Quality (AHRQ) or other appropriate agencies or independent entities should encourage and facilitate the voluntary reporting of diagnostic errors and near misses.

Recommendation 6b: AHRQ should evaluate the effectiveness of patient safety organizations (PSOs) as a major mechanism for voluntary reporting and learning from these events and modify the PSO Common Formats for reporting of patient safety events to include diagnostic errors and near misses.

Recommendation 6c: States, in collaboration with other stakeholders (health care organizations, professional liability insurance carriers, state and federal policy makers, patient advocacy groups,

and medical malpractice plaintiff and defense attorneys), should promote a legal environment that facilitates the timely identification, disclosure, and learning from diagnostic errors. Specifically, they should:

- Encourage the adoption of communication and resolution programs with legal protections for disclosures and apologies under state laws.
- Conduct demonstration projects of alternative approaches to the resolution of medical injuries, including administrative health courts and safe harbors for adherence to evidence-based clinical practice guidelines.

Recommendation 6d: Professional liability insurance carriers and captive insurers should collaborate with health care professionals on opportunities to improve diagnostic performance through education, training, and practice improvement approaches and increase participation in such programs.

Design a Payment and Care Delivery Environment That Supports the Diagnostic Process

Fee-for-service (FFS) payment has long been recognized for its inability to incentivize well-coordinated, high-quality, and efficient health care. There is limited information about the impact of payment and care delivery models on diagnosis, but it likely influences the diagnostic process and the occurrence of diagnostic errors. For example, FFS payment lacks financial incentives to coordinate care among clinicians involved in the diagnostic process, such as the communication among treating clinicians, pathologists, and radiologists about diagnostic test ordering, interpretation, and subsequent decision making.

For all medical specialties, there are well-documented fee schedule distortions that result in more generous payments for procedures and diagnostic testing interpretations than for evaluation and management (E&M) services. E&M services reflect the cognitive expertise and skills that all clinicians use in the diagnostic process, and these distortions may be diverting attention and time from important tasks in the diagnostic process. Realigning relative value fees to better compensate clinicians for cognitive work in the diagnostic process has the potential to improve diagnosis while reducing incentives that drive inappropriate diagnostic testing utilization.

E&M documentation guidelines have been criticized as onerous, often irrelevant to patient care, and preventing clinical reasoning in the diagnostic process. Payment and liability concerns, facilitated by the growth in EHRs, have resulted in extensive clinical documentation that obscures key information in patients' medical records, results in inaccuracies in patients' EHRs, and can contribute to diagnostic errors.

Due to the limitations in FFS payment, a number of alternative payment and care delivery models are under evaluation; for example, half of Medicare payments are expected to be based on alternative models by 2018. There is limited evidence concerning the impact of payment and care delivery models—including FFS—on the diagnostic process and the accuracy of diagnosis, and this represents a fundamental research need. Even when alternative approaches to FFS are employed, they are often influenced by FFS. Thus, the current challenges with FFS will need to be addressed, even with the implementation of alternative payment and care delivery models.

Goal 7: Design a payment and care delivery environment that supports the diagnostic process

Recommendation 7a: As long as fee schedules remain a predominant mechanism for determining clinician payment, the Centers for Medicare & Medicaid Services (CMS) and other payers should:
- **Create current procedural terminology codes and provide coverage for additional evaluation and management activities not currently coded or covered, including time spent by pathologists, radiologists, and other clinicians in advising ordering clinicians on the selection, use, and interpretation of diagnostic testing for specific patients.**
- **Reorient relative value fees to more appropriately value the time spent with patients in evaluation and management activities.**
- **Modify documentation guidelines for evaluation and management services to improve the accuracy of information in the electronic health record and to support decision making in the diagnostic process.**

Recommendation 7b: CMS and other payers should assess the impact of payment and care delivery models on the diagnostic process, the occurrence of diagnostic errors, and learning from these errors.

Provide Dedicated Funding for Research on the Diagnostic Process and Diagnostic Errors

The diagnostic process and diagnostic errors have been neglected areas within the national research agenda; federal resources devoted to diagnostic research are overshadowed by those devoted to treatment. A major barrier to research is the organization and funding of the National Institutes of Health by disease or organ systems, which facilitates the study of these specific areas but impedes research efforts that seek to provide a more comprehensive understanding of diagnosis as a distinct research area. Given the potential for federal research on diagnosis and diagnostic error to fall between institutional missions, collaboration among agencies is needed to develop a national research agenda on these topics. Because overall federal investment in biomedical and health services research is declining, funding for diagnosis and diagnostic error will draw federal resources away from other priorities. However, given the consistent lack of resources for research on diagnosis, and the potential for diagnostic errors to contribute to patient harm and health care costs, funding for this research is necessary for broader improvements to the quality and safety of health care. In addition, improving diagnosis could potentially lead to cost savings by preventing diagnostic errors, inappropriate treatment, and related adverse events.

In addition to federal-level research, there is an important role for public–private collaboration and coordination among the federal government, foundations, industry, and other stakeholders. Collaborative funding efforts extend the existing financial resources and reduce duplications in research efforts. Parties can unite around areas of mutual interest and spearhead progress.

Goal 8: Provide dedicated funding for research on the diagnostic process and diagnostic errors

> **Recommendation 8a: Federal agencies, including the Department of Health and Human Services, the Department of Veterans Affairs, and the Department of Defense, should:**
> - **Develop a coordinated research agenda on the diagnostic process and diagnostic errors by the end of 2016.**
> - **Commit dedicated funding to implementing this research agenda.**
>
> **Recommendation 8b: The federal government should pursue and encourage opportunities for public–private partnerships among a broad range of stakeholders, such as the Patient-Centered Outcomes Research Institute, foundations, the diagnostic testing and health information technology industries, health care organizations, and professional liability insurers to support research on the diagnostic process and diagnostic errors.**

1

Introduction

For decades, the delivery of health care has proceeded with a blind spot: Diagnostic errors—inaccurate or delayed diagnoses—persist throughout all care settings and harm an unacceptable number of patients. Getting the right diagnosis is a key aspect of health care, as it provides an explanation of a patient's health problem and informs subsequent health care decisions (Holmboe and Durning, 2014). Diagnostic errors can lead to negative health outcomes, psychological distress, and financial costs. If a diagnostic error occurs, inappropriate or unnecessary treatment may be given to a patient, or appropriate—and potentially lifesaving—treatment may be withheld or delayed. However, efforts to identify and mitigate diagnostic errors have so far been quite limited. Absent a spotlight to illuminate this critical challenge, diagnostic errors have been largely unappreciated within the quality and patient safety movements. The result of this inattention is significant: It is likely that most people will experience at least one diagnostic error in their lifetime, sometimes with devastating consequences.

The topic of diagnosis raises a number of clinical, personal, cultural, ethical, and even political issues that commonly capture public interest. Members of the public are concerned about diagnosis and many have reported experiencing diagnostic errors. For example, a survey by Isabel Healthcare found that 55 percent of adults indicated that their main concern when visiting a family practitioner was being correctly diagnosed (Isabel Healthcare, 2006). A poll commissioned by the National Patient Safety Foundation found that approximately one in six of those surveyed had experience with diagnostic error, either personally or through a close friend or relative (Golodner, 1997). More recently, 23 percent of people surveyed in Massachusetts stated that they or someone close to them had experienced a medical error, and approximately half of these errors were diagnostic errors (Betsy Lehman Center for Patient Safety and Medical Error Reduction, 2014). In the United Kingdom, the country's National Health Service concluded that diagnosis—including diagnostic error— was the most common reason individuals complained about their health care, accounting for approximately 35 percent of complaints (Parliamentary and Health Service Ombudsman, 2014).

In addition to diagnostic errors, the public is concerned about other aspects of diagnosis, such as the value of making and communicating diagnoses at early stages in conditions such as Alzheimer's disease and amyotrophic lateral sclerosis (Lou Gehrig's disease) for which there is currently no known cure (Hamilton, 2015). There is also a growing concern about overdiagnosis, such as the assignment of diagnostic labels to conditions that are unlikely to affect the individual's health and well-being (Welch et al., 2011); the focus of clinical attention on making new diagnoses in older patients while ignoring limitations to their daily living that need immediate attention (Gawande, 2014; Mechanic, 2014); and the elevation of common behavioral traits to the level of formal diagnoses, with the attendant treatment and confidentiality implications (Hazen et al., 2013; Kavan and Barone, 2014; NHS, 2013). The Institute of Medicine (IOM) report *Beyond Myalgic Encephalomyelitis/Chronic Fatigue Syndrome: Redefining an Illness* brought attention to the problem that individuals with debilitating but previously non-recognized symptom complexes may be given inadequate attention by clinicians or ignored altogether because a diagnosis is lacking (IOM, 2015; Rehmeyer, 2015). Diagnoses also affect the health care that patients receive, eligibility for social security and veterans disability benefits, as well as health care research and education priorities.

The widespread challenge of diagnostic errors frequently rises to broad public attention, whether the widely reported diagnostic error of Ebola virus infection in a Dallas hospital emergency department or in the occasional report of an extraordinarily high malpractice award for failure to make a timely diagnosis of cancer or some other life threatening disease (Pfeifer, 2015; Upadhyay et al., 2014; Wachter, 2014). The subjects of diagnosis and diagnostic error have captured media interest, as indicated by television shows and columns about perplexing diagnoses and coverage of patient experiences with diagnosis (Dwyer, 2012; Genzlinger, 2012; Gubar, 2014; *New York Times*, 2014; *Washington Post*, 2014). For example, *Harper's Magazine* featured an essay that chronicled one patient's diagnostic journey and experience with diagnostic error through multiple clinicians, Internet searches, conversations with friends and family, and decision support tools (Julavits, 2014). Books featuring patients' experiences with diagnosis and the health care system have also been published (Cahalan, 2012; Groopman, 2007; Sanders, 2010).

Given the importance of diagnosis to patients and to health care decision making, as well as the pervasiveness of diagnostic errors in practice, it is surprising that this issue has been neglected within the quality improvement and patient safety movement (Gandhi et al., 2006; Graber et al., 2012; Newman-Toker and Pronovost, 2009; Singh, 2014). There are a number of reasons for the lack of attention to diagnostic errors. Major contributors are the lack of effective measurement of diagnostic error and the difficulty in detecting these errors in clinical practice (Graber et al., 2012; Singh, 2013). Even if they can be measured or identified, diagnostic errors may not be recognized, for example, when the error is identified by a second clinician and feedback about the error is not provided to the original clinician. There may also be debate about what constitutes a diagnostic error; even after an extensive review of a patient's chart, expert reviewers often disagree about whether or not an error has occurred (Wachter, 2010; Zwaan and Singh, 2015). Diagnostic errors may also be perceived as too difficult to address because the reasons for their occurrence are often complex and multifaceted (Berenson et al., 2014; Croskerry, 2003; Graber et al., 2005; Schiff et al., 2005; Zwaan et al., 2009). This difficulty in identifying the etiology of errors, combined with a lack of feedback on diagnostic performance in many health care settings, limits understanding and makes it more difficult to prioritize improving diagnosis and reducing diagnostic errors. Other factors that contribute to the limited focus on diagnostic error include a lack of awareness of the problem, attitudes and culture that encourage inaction and tolerance of errors, poorly understood characteristics of the diagnostic and clinical reasoning processes, and the need for financial and other resources to address the problem (Berenson et al., 2014; Croskerry, 2012).

Although diagnostic error has been largely underappreciated in efforts to improve the quality and safety of health care, this issue has garnered national attention, and there is growing momentum for change (Graber et al., 2012; Schiff and Leape, 2012; Wachter, 2010). Emerging research has found new opportunities for the identification of diagnostic errors and has led to a better understanding of the epidemiology and etiology of these errors and of potential interventions to improve diagnosis (Singh et al., 2014; Tehrani et al., 2013; Trowbridge et al., 2013; Zwaan and Singh, 2015; Zwaan et al., 2010). Patients and families who have experienced diagnostic error have become increasingly vocal about their desire to share their unique insights to help identify patterns and improve the diagnostic process for future patients (Haskell, 2014; McDonald et al., 2013).

Efforts to accelerate progress toward improving diagnosis can leverage four important movements in health care: the movements to improve patient safety, to increase patient engagement, to foster professionalism, and to encourage collaboration. Diagnostic error has been called the next frontier in patient safety, even though the challenge of diagnostic error will have benefits beyond the realm of patient safety, as such errors are a major challenge to the quality of patient care (Newman-Toker and Pronovost, 2009). Patient engagement and the importance of shared decision making are recognized as critical aspects of improving health care quality (IOM, 2001). The current focus on professionalism emphasizes health care professionals' intrinsic motivation and commitment to provide patients with high-quality, patient-centered care (Berwick, 2015; Chassin and Baker, 2015; Madara and Burkhart, 2015). The growing recognition of health care as a team-based activity has led to greater collaboration among health care professionals, both intra- and interprofessionally (IOM, 2001; Josiah Macy Jr. Foundation and Carnegie Foundation for the Advancement of Teaching, 2010). These four movements have collectively transformed the way that health care is provided in the United States, and progress toward improving diagnosis and reducing diagnostic errors is a natural outgrowth of these movements. This report by the Committee on Diagnostic Error in Health Care synthesizes current knowledge about diagnostic error and makes recommendations on how to reduce diagnostic errors and improve diagnosis.

CONTEXT OF THE STUDY

This study is a continuation of the IOM Quality Chasm Series, which focuses on assessing and improving the quality and safety of health care. It includes the IOM reports *To Err Is Human: Building a Safer Health System* and *Crossing the Quality Chasm: A New Health System for the 21st Century*. The first report was a call to action: The committee concluded that the care patients receive is not as safe as it should be (IOM, 2000). Estimating that tens of thousands of lives are lost each year because of medical errors, the report catalyzed a movement to improve the safety of health care in America. The second report defined high-quality care broadly and set out a vision to close the chasm between what was known to be high-quality care and what patients received in practice (IOM, 2001). Together these reports stimulated widespread scrutiny of the health care system and brought about large-scale efforts to improve the quality and safety of care.

However, these reports focused primarily on the quality and safety of medical treatment rather than on the diagnostic process. The majority of quality improvement and patient safety efforts that have since followed have been focused on improving the delivery of evidence-based care and preventing the adverse outcomes of treatment, such as medication and surgical errors, and health care–associated infections.

ORIGIN OF TASK AND COMMITTEE CHARGE

In the summer of 2013, the Society to Improve Diagnosis in Medicine requested that the IOM Board on Health Care Services undertake a study on diagnostic error as a continuation of the IOM's Quality Chasm Series. With support from a broad coalition of sponsors—the Agency for Healthcare Research and Quality, the American College of Radiology, the American Society for Clinical Pathology, the Cautious Patient Foundation, the Centers for Disease Control and Prevention, the College of American Pathologists, The Doctors Company Foundation, Janet and Barry Lang, Kaiser Permanente National Community Benefit Fund at the East Bay Community Foundation, and the Robert Wood Johnson Foundation—the study began in January 2014.

An independent committee was appointed with a broad range of expertise, including diagnostic error, patient safety, health care quality and measurement, patient engagement, health policy, health care professional education, cognitive psychology, health disparities, human factors and ergonomics, health information technology (health IT), decision analysis, nursing, radiology, pathology, law, and health economics. Brief biographies of the 21 members of this Committee on Diagnostic Error in Health Care are presented in Appendix B. The charge to the committee was to synthesize what is known about diagnostic error as a quality of care challenge and to propose recommendations for improving diagnosis (see Box 1-1).

METHODS OF THE STUDY

The committee deliberated during five in-person meetings and numerous conference calls between April 2014 and April 2015. At three of the meetings, the committee invited a number of speakers to inform its deliberations. These speakers provided invaluable input to the committee on a broad range of topics, including patient experiences with diagnostic error; the measurement, reporting, and feedback of diagnostic error; health IT design and decision support; diagnostic errors in pathology and radiology; patient safety culture; teams in diagnosis; psychiatry and diagnostic error; legal issues in diagnosis; and the prioritization of diagnostic error. The committee also held a webinar with experts in cognition and health care professional education. A number of experts and organizations provided written input to the committee on a broad array of topics. In addition to receiving this expert input, the committee reviewed an extensive body of literature to inform its deliberations.

BOX 1-1
Charge to the Committee on Diagnostic Error in Health Care

An ad hoc committee of the Institute of Medicine will evaluate the existing knowledge about diagnostic error as a quality of care challenge; current definitions of diagnostic error and illustrative examples; and areas where additional research is needed. The committee will examine topics such as the epidemiology of diagnostic error, the burden of harm and economic costs associated with diagnostic error, and current efforts to address the problem.

The committee will propose solutions to the problem of diagnostic error, which may include: clarifying definitions and boundaries; integrating educational approaches; addressing behavioral/cognitive processes and cultural change; teamwork and systems engineering; measures and measurement approaches; research; changes in payment; approaches to medical liability; and health information technology and other technology changes.

The committee will devise conclusions and recommendations that will propose action items for key stakeholders, such as patients/advocates, health care providers, health care organizations, federal and state policy makers, purchasers and payers, credentialing organizations, educators, researchers, and the diagnostic testing and health information technology industries to achieve desired goals.

CONCEPTUAL MODEL

To help frame and organize its work, the committee developed a conceptual model that defined diagnostic error and also illustrated the diagnostic process, the work system in which the diagnostic process occurs, and the outcomes that result from this process (see Chapters 2 and 3 for detailed information on the conceptual model). The committee developed a patient-centered definition of diagnostic error: *the failure to (a) establish an accurate and timely explanation of the patient's health problem(s) or (b) communicate that explanation to the patient.*

EXAMPLES OF DIAGNOSIS AND DIAGNOSTIC ERRORS

To illustrate the complexity of the diagnostic process and the range of diagnostic errors that can occur, the committee has included a variety of examples of experiences with diagnosis and diagnostic error. The committee was honored to hear patients' and family members' experiences with diagnosis, both positive and negative; three of these experiences are described in Box 1-2. During the committee's deliberations, the United States experienced its first case of Ebola virus infection; because the diagnosis was initially missed in the emergency department, it illustrated a

BOX 1-2
Patient and Family Experiences with Diagnosis

Jeff

Jeff was driving home from work when he started experiencing sharp chest pains. Because he was close to the local hospital, he decided to drive directly to the emergency department (ED). Jeff entered the ED stating that he believed he was having a heart attack. He was immediately provided aspirin and nitroglycerin. An electrocardiogram (EKG) was performed, with normal results. Jeff continued to have chest pain. Because of his ongoing symptoms, the clinicians told Jeff that they would ready the hospital's helicopter in case he needed to be quickly transported to another hospital for heart surgery. Jeff then started complaining of pain in his leg to his wife, who had by then arrived at the hospital, and she told the nurse that something must really be wrong because Jeff rarely complained of pain. Upon further examination, clinicians found that Jeff's left foot and leg were swollen, and a computed tomography (CT) scan of Jeff's chest was performed. The CT scan showed that Jeff had an aortic dissection, "a serious condition in which there is a tear in the wall of the major artery carrying blood out of the heart" (MedlinePlus, 2015). His clinicians immediately put him in a helicopter and flew him to another hospital, where he underwent an extensive surgery to repair the aortic dissection and repair damage to his leg.

Jeff cited the willingness of his clinicians to listen to him and his wife and to continue investigating his symptoms despite his normal EKG results as major contributors to his rapid diagnosis. Because aortic dissections are life-threatening events that require urgent treatment, the quick action of the ED to get Jeff to surgery also contributed to the successful outcome.

Before his aortic dissection, Jeff was in good health. He now has several ongoing medical conditions as well as continued surveillance and treatment related to the dissection. He sees a number of health care professionals on a regular basis. Jeff's experience has taught him the importance of communicating with one's health care professionals. He now proactively educates himself on his health conditions, speaks up when he has a concern, prepares questions in advance when he has an appointment, and continues to seek answers to questions that he feels are not adequately addressed.

Carolyn

Carolyn came to the ED with chest pain, nausea, sweating, and radiating pain through her left arm, which are often considered classic symptoms of a heart attack. The ED clinicians ordered an EKG, blood tests, a chest X-ray, and a treadmill stress test; all of these tests came back normal. Her ED clinician diagnosed her as having acid reflux, noting she was in the right demographic for this condition. When she asked the ED doctor about the pain in her arm, he was dismissive of the symptom. Privately, a nurse in the ED asked Carolyn to stop asking questions of the doctor, noting that he was a very good doctor and didn't like to be questioned. Carolyn was released from the hospital less than 5 hours after the onset of her symptoms, feeling embarrassed about making a "big fuss"

continued

BOX 1-2 Continued

over a relatively common condition. Over the next 2 weeks, she developed increasingly debilitating symptoms, which prompted her return to the ED where she received a diagnosis of significant heart disease. Carolyn had a myocardial infarction caused by 99 percent blocked artery—what clinicians still call the "widow maker" heart attack.

Sue and Her Family

Sue's son, Cal, was born healthy in a large hospital, but jaundice appeared soon afterward. Jaundice, or yellowing of the skin, occurs when many red blood cells break down and release a chemical called bilirubin into the bloodstream. Cal's father, Pat, and Sue were informed that treatment for such newborn jaundice isn't usually necessary. Unfortunately, because of an incorrect entry of the family blood types into Cal's medical record, the hospital's clinicians had not recognized that a common blood incompatibility existed and could lead to serious elevations in Cal's bilirubin levels. Within 36 hours, Cal's jaundice had deepened and spread from head to toe. Nevertheless, without measuring his bilirubin level, the hospital discharged Cal to home and provided Pat and Sue with reassuring information about jaundice, never mentioning that high levels of bilirubin in the blood can cause damage to the brain (Mayo Clinic, 2015). Four days later, Cal was more yellow, lethargic, and feeding poorly. His parents took him to a pediatrician, who noted the jaundice, still did not do a bilirubin test, and advised them to wait 24 more hours to see if Cal improved. The next day, at the request of his parents, Cal was admitted to the hospital, and a blood test showed that the bilirubin level in Cal's blood was dangerously high. Over the next few days while Cal was in the hospital, Pat and Sue reported to staff that he was exhibiting worrisome new behaviors, such as a high-pitched cry, respiratory distress, increased muscle tone, and arching of the neck and back. They were told not to worry. Later it became clear that Cal was experiencing kernicterus, a preventable form of brain damage caused by high bilirubin levels in the blood of newborns. As a result, at age 20, Cal now has significant cerebral palsy, with spasticity of his trunk and limbs, marked impairment of his speech, difficulty aligning his eyes, and other difficulties.

high-profile example of diagnostic error with important public health implications (Upadhyay et al., 2014) (see Chapter 5). Appendix D includes additional examples of diagnostic error in order to convey a broader sense of the types of diagnostic errors that can occur.

ORGANIZATION OF THE REPORT

The report is organized into three major sections. Section I consists of Chapters 2 and 3 and provides an overview of the diagnostic process

Several years after Cal's birth, Pat experienced progressively severe neck pain, and a scan showed a mass on his cervical spine. While removing the mass, the neurosurgeon sent a tissue sample to a hospital pathologist, who examined the sample and called back to the operating room to report that it was an atypical spindle cell neoplasm. Assuming that this meant a benign mass, the surgical team completed the operation and declared Pat cured. Following the operation, however, the hospital pathologist performed additional stains and examinations of Pat's tissue, eventually determining that the tumor was actually a malignant synovial cell sarcoma. Twenty-one days after the surgery, the pathologist's final report of a malignant tumor was sent to the neurosurgeon's office, but it was somehow lost, misplaced, or filed without the neurosurgeon seeing it. The revised diagnosis of malignancy was not communicated to Pat or to his referring clinician. Six months later, when his neck pain recurred, Pat returned to his neurosurgeon. A scan revealed a recurrent mass that had invaded his spinal column. This mass was removed and diagnosed to be a recurrent invasive malignant synovial cell sarcoma. Despite seven additional operations and numerous rounds of chemotherapy and radiation, Pat died 2 years later, at 45 years old, with a 4-year-old daughter and a 6-year-old son.

Cal's and Pat's (and Sue's) experiences are examples of diagnostic errors that led to inadequate treatment with major adverse consequences—all enabled by poor communication and uncoordinated care by multiple health care providers. Based on her family's experiences, Sue believes that health care systems, providers, patient advocates, payers, and regulators have a responsibility to collaborate to reduce diagnostic errors by:

- Improving the processes of—and the accountability for—secure intra- and interprofessional communication of patients' clinical information.
- Engaging patients more actively as true partners with their health care providers—with improved information sharing, joint decision making, and self-monitoring and reporting of health conditions and symptoms.

SOURCE: Personal communications with Jeff, Carolyn, and Sue (last names are not provided for anonymity).

and diagnostic error in health care. Section II, or Chapters 4 through 8, describes the challenges of diagnosis and is organized by the elements of the work system: Chapter 4 discusses the diagnostic team members and the tasks they perform in the diagnostic process; Chapter 5 discusses the technologies and tools (specifically health IT) used in the diagnostic process; Chapter 6 focuses on health care organizations and their impact on the diagnostic process and diagnostic error; Chapter 7 describes the external elements that influence diagnosis, including payment and care delivery, reporting, and medical liability; and Chapter 8 highlights the research needs concerning the diagnostic process and diagnostic errors, as drawn from the previous Chapters. Section III (Chapter 9) synthesizes the committee's main conclusions and recommendations for improving diagnosis and reducing diagnostic error.

REFERENCES

Berenson, R. A., D. K. Upadhyay, and D. R. Kaye. 2014. *Placing diagnosis errors on the policy agenda.* Washington, DC: Urban Institute. www.urban.org/research/publication/placing-diagnosis-errors-policy-agenda (accessed May 22, 2015).

Berwick, D. M. 2015. Postgraduate education of physicians: Professional self-regulation and external accountability. *JAMA* 313(18):1803–1804.

Betsy Lehman Center for Patient Safety and Medical Error Reduction. 2014. *The public's views on medical error in Massachusetts.* Cambridge, MA: Harvard School of Public Health.

Cahalan, S. 2012. *Brain on fire.* New York: Simon & Schuster.

Chassin, M. R., and D. W. Baker. 2015. Aiming higher to enhance professionalism: Beyond accreditation and certification. *JAMA* 313(18):1795–1796.

Croskerry, P. 2003. The importance of cognitive errors in diagnosis and strategies to minimize them. *Academic Medicine* 78(8):775–780.

Croskerry, P. 2012. Perspectives on diagnostic failure and patient safety. *Healthcare Quarterly* 15(Special issue) April:50–56.

Dwyer, J. 2012. An infection, unnoticed, turns unstoppable. *The New York Times*, July 11. www.nytimes.com/2012/07/12/nyregion/in-rory-stauntons-fight-for-his-life-signs-that-went-unheeded.html?pagewanted=all&_r=0 (accessed December 5, 2014).

Gandhi, T. K., A. Kachalia, E. J. Thomas, A. L. Puopolo, C. Yoon, T. A. Brennan, and D. M. Studdert. 2006. Missed and delayed diagnoses in the ambulatory setting: A study of closed malpractice claims. *Annals of Internal Medicine* 145(7):488–496.

Gawande, A. 2014. *Being mortal: Medicine and what matters in the end.* New York: Metropolitan Books.

Genzlinger, N. 2012. A medical guessing game, with life as the ultimate prize. *The New York Times*, June 24. www.nytimes.com/2012/06/25/arts/television/diagnosis-dead-or-alive-on-discovery-fit-health.html (accessed August 5, 2014).

Golodner, L. 1997. How the public perceives patient safety. *Newsletter of the National Patient Safety Foundation* 1(1):1–4.

Graber, M. L., N. Franklin, and R. Gordon. 2005. Diagnostic error in internal medicine. *Archives of Internal Medicine* 165(13):1493–1499.

Graber, M., R. Wachter, and C. Cassel. 2012. Bringing diagnosis into the quality and safety equations. *JAMA* 308(12):1211–1212.

Groopman, J. 2007. *How doctors think,* 2nd ed. New York: Mariner Books.

Gubar, S. 2014. Missing a cancer diagnosis. *The New York Times*, January 2. http://well.blogs.nytimes.com/2014/01/02/missing-a-cancer-diagnosis/?_php=true&_type=blogs&_r=0 (accessed December 5, 2014).

Hamilton, J. 2015. Many doctors who diagnose Alzheimer's fail to tell the patient. *NPR*, March 24. www.npr.org/sections/health-shots/2015/03/24/394927484/many-doctors-who-diagnose-alzheimers-fail-to-tell-the-patient (accessed August 5, 2015).

Haskell, H. W. 2014. What's in a story? Lessons from patients who have suffered diagnostic failure. *Diagnosis* 1(1):53–54.

Hazen, E. P., C. J. McDougle, and F. R. Volkmar. 2013. Changes in the diagnostic criteria for autism in DSM-5: Controversies and concerns. *Journal of Clinical Psychiatry* 74(7):739–740.

Holmboe, E. S., and S. J. Durning. 2014. Assessing clinical reasoning: Moving from in vitro to in vivo. *Diagnosis* 1(1):111–117.

IOM (Institute of Medicine). 2000. *To err is human: Building a safer health system.* Washington, DC: National Academy Press.

IOM. 2001. *Crossing the quality chasm: A new health system for the 21st century.* Washington, DC: National Academy Press.

IOM. 2015. *Beyond myalgic encephalomyelitis/chronic fatigue syndrome: Redefining an illness.* Washington, DC: The National Academies Press.

Isabel Healthcare. 2006. Misdiagnosis is an overlooked and growing patient safety issue and core mission of isabel healthcare. www.isabelhealthcare.com/home/uspressrelease (accessed December 4, 2014).

Josiah Macy Jr. Foundation and Carnegie Foundation for the Advancement of Teaching. 2010. *Educating nurses and physicians: Towards new horizons. Advancing inter-professional education in academic health centers, Conference summary.* New York: Josiah Macy Jr. Foundation. www.macyfoundation.org/docs/macy_pubs/JMF_Carnegie_Summary_Web-Version_%283%29.pdf (accessed June 5, 2015).

Julavits, H. 2014. Diagnose this! How to be your own best doctor. *Harper's Magazine* April:25–35.

Kavan, M. G., and E. J. Barone. 2014. Grief and major depression—Controversy over changes in DSM-5 diagnostic criteria. *American Family Physician* 90(10):690–694.

Madara, J. L., and J. Burkhart. 2015. Professionalism, self-regulation, and motivation: How did health care get this so wrong? *JAMA* 313(18):1793–1794.

Mayo Clinic. 2015. Infant jaundice: Definition. www.mayoclinic.org/diseases-conditions/infant-jaundice/basics/definition/con-20019637 (accessed May 8, 2015).

McDonald, K. M., C. L. Bryce, and M. L. Graber. 2013. The patient is in: Patient involvement strategies for diagnostic error mitigation. *BMJ Quality & Safety* 22(Suppl 2):ii33–ii39.

Mechanic, M. 2014. Atul Gawande: "We have medicalized aging, and that experiment is failing us." *Mother Jones*, October 7. www.motherjones.com/media/2014/10/atul-gawande-being-mortal-interview-assisted-living (accessed August 5, 2015).

MedlinePlus. 2015. Aortic dissection. www.nlm.nih.gov/medlineplus/ency/article/000181.htm (accessed May 8, 2015).

New York Times. 2014. Diagnosis: A collection of "diagnosis" columns published in the New York Times. http://topics.nytimes.com/top/news/health/columns/diagnosis/index.html (accessed December 5, 2014).

Newman-Toker, D., and P. J. Pronovost. 2009. Diagnostic errors—The next frontier for patient safety. *JAMA* 301(10):1060–1062.

NHS (National Health Service). 2013. News analysis: Controversial mental health guide DSM-5. www.nhs.uk/news/2013/08august/pages/controversy-mental-health-diagnosis-and-treatment-dsm5.aspx#two (accessed May 13, 2015).

Parliamentary and Health Service Ombudsman. 2014. *Complaints about acute trusts 2013–14 and Q1, Q2 2014–15* United Kingdom: Parliamentary and Health Service Ombudsman.

Pfeifer, S. 2015. Kaiser ordered to pay woman more than $28 million. *LA Times*, March 26. www.latimes.com/business/la-fi-jury-awards-kaiser-cancer-patient-20150326-story.html (accessed August 5, 2015).

Rehmeyer, J. 2015. A disease doctors refuse to see. *New York Times*, February 25. www.nytimes.com/2015/02/25/opinion/understanding-chronic-fatigue.html (accessed August 5, 2015).

Sanders, L. 2010. *Every patient tells a story: Medical mysteries and the art of diagnosis.* New York: Harmony.

Schiff, G. D., and L. L. Leape. 2012. Commentary: How can we make diagnosis safer? *Academic Medicine* 87(2):135–138.

Schiff, G. D., S. Kim, R. Abrams, K. Cosby, B. Lambert, A. S. Elstein, S. Hasler, N. Krosnjar, R. Odwazny, M. F. Wisniewski, and R. A. McNutt. 2005. Diagnosing diagnosis errors: Lessons from a multi-institutional collaborative project. In K. Henriksen, J. B. Battles, E. S. Marks, and D. I. Lewin (eds.), *Advances in patient safety: From research to implementation (Volume 2: Concepts and methodolgy)* (pp. 255–278). AHRQ Publication No: 05-0021-1. Rockville, MD: Agency for Healthcare Research and Quality.

Singh, H. 2013. Diagnostic errors: Moving beyond "no respect" and getting ready for prime time. *BMJ Quality & Safety* 22(10):789–792.

Singh, H. 2014. Editorial: Helping health care organizations to define diagnostic errors as missed opportunities in diagnosis. *Joint Commission Journal on Quality and Patient Safety* 40(3):99–101.

Singh, H., A. N. Meyer, and E. J. Thomas. 2014. The frequency of diagnostic errors in outpatient care: Estimations from three large observational studies involving U.S. adult populations. *BMJ Quality & Safety* 23(9):727–731.

Tehrani, A. S., H. Lee, S. C. Mathews, A. Shore, M. A. Makary, P. J. Pronovost, and D. E. Newman-Toker. 2013. 25-year summary of U.S. malpractice claims for diagnostic errors, 1986–2010: An analysis from the National Practitioner Data Bank. *BMJ Quality & Safety* 22(8):672–680.

Trowbridge, R. L., G. Dhaliwal, and K. S. Cosby. 2013. Educational agenda for diagnostic error reduction. *BMJ Quality & Safety* 22(Suppl 2):ii28–ii32.

Upadhyay, D. K., D. F. Sittig, and H. Singh. 2014. Ebola U.S. Patient Zero: Lessons on misdiagnosis and effective use of electronic health records. *Diagnosis* 10.1515/dx-2014-0064.

Wachter, R. M. 2010. Why diagnostic errors don't get any respect—and what can be done about them. *Health Affairs (Millwood)* 29(9):1605–1610.

Wachter, R. M. 2014. What Ebola error in Dallas shows. USA Today, October 13. www.usatoday.com/story/opinion/2014/10/12/what-ebola-error-in-dallas-shows-column/17159839 (accessed December 5, 2014).

Washington Post. 2014. Medical mysteries. www.washingtonpost.com/sf/national/collection/medical-mysteries (accessed December 5, 2014).

Welch, H. G., L. Schwartz, and S. Woloshin. 2011. *Overdiagnosed: Making people sick in the pursuit of health.* Boston, MA: Beacon Press.

Zwaan, L., and H. Singh. 2015. The challenges in defining and measuring diagnostic error. *Diagnosis.* Epub ahead of print. www.degruyter.com/view/j/dx.2015.2.issue-2/dx-2014-0069/dx-2014-0069.xml (accessed June 1, 2015).

Zwaan, L., A. Thijs, C. Wagner, G. van der Wal, and D. R. Timmermans. 2009. Design of a study on suboptimal cognitive acts in the diagnostic process, the effect on patient outcomes and the influence of workload, fatigue and experience of physician. *BMC Health Services Research* 9:65.

Zwaan, L., M. de Bruijne, C. Wagner, A. Thijs, M. Smits, G. van der Wal, and D. R. Timmermans. 2010. Patient record review of the incidence, consequences, and causes of diagnostic adverse events. *Archives of Internal Medicine* 170(12):1015–1021.

2

The Diagnostic Process

This chapter provides an overview of diagnosis in health care, including the committee's conceptual model of the diagnostic process and a review of clinical reasoning. Diagnosis has important implications for patient care, research, and policy. Diagnosis has been described as both a process and a classification scheme, or a "pre-existing set of categories agreed upon by the medical profession to designate a specific condition" (Jutel, 2009).[1] When a diagnosis is accurate and made in a timely manner, a patient has the best opportunity for a positive health outcome because clinical decision making will be tailored to a correct understanding of the patient's health problem (Holmboe and Durning, 2014). In addition, public policy decisions are often influenced by diagnostic information, such as setting payment policies, resource allocation decisions, and research priorities (Jutel, 2009; Rosenberg, 2002; WHO, 2012).

The chapter describes important considerations in the diagnostic process, such as the roles of diagnostic uncertainty and time. It also highlights the mounting complexity of health care, due to the ever-increasing options for diagnostic testing[2] and treatment, the rapidly rising levels of biomedical and clinical evidence to inform clinical practice, and the frequent comorbidities among patients due to the aging of the popula-

---

[1] In this report, the committee employs the terminology "the diagnostic process" to convey diagnosis as a process.

[2] The committee uses the term "diagnostic testing" to be inclusive of all types of testing, including medical imaging, anatomic pathology, and laboratory medicine, as well as other types of testing, such as mental health assessments, vision and hearing testing, and neurocognitive testing.

tion (IOM, 2008, 2013b). The rising complexity of health care and the sheer volume of advances, coupled with clinician time constraints and cognitive limitations, have outstripped human capacity to apply this new knowledge. To help manage this complexity, the chapter concludes with a discussion of the role of clinical practice guidelines in informing decision making in the diagnostic process.

OVERVIEW OF THE DIAGNOSTIC PROCESS

To help frame and organize its work, the committee developed a conceptual model to illustrate the diagnostic process (see Figure 2-1). The committee concluded that the diagnostic process is a complex, patient-centered, collaborative activity that involves information gathering and clinical reasoning with the goal of determining a patient's health problem. This process occurs over time, within the context of a larger health care work system that influences the diagnostic process (see Box 2-1). The committee's depiction of the diagnostic process draws on an adaptation of a decision-making model that describes the cyclical process of information gathering, information integration and interpretation, and forming a working diagnosis (Parasuraman et al., 2000; Sarter, 2014).

The diagnostic process proceeds as follows: First, a patient experiences a health problem. The patient is likely the first person to consider his or her symptoms and may choose at this point to engage with the health care system. Once a patient seeks health care, there is an iterative process of information gathering, information integration and interpretation, and determining a working diagnosis. Performing a clinical history and interview, conducting a physical exam, performing diagnostic testing, and referring or consulting with other clinicians are all ways of accumulating information that may be relevant to understanding a patient's health problem. The information-gathering approaches can be employed at different times, and diagnostic information can be obtained in different orders. The continuous process of information gathering, integration, and interpretation involves hypothesis generation and updating prior probabilities as more information is learned. Communication among health care professionals, the patient, and the patient's family members is critical in this cycle of information gathering, integration, and interpretation.

The working diagnosis may be either a list of potential diagnoses (a differential diagnosis) or a single potential diagnosis. Typically, clinicians will consider more than one diagnostic hypothesis or possibility as an explanation of the patient's symptoms and will refine this list as further information is obtained in the diagnostic process. The working diagnosis should be shared with the patient, including an explanation of the degree of uncertainty associated with a working diagnosis. Each time there is a

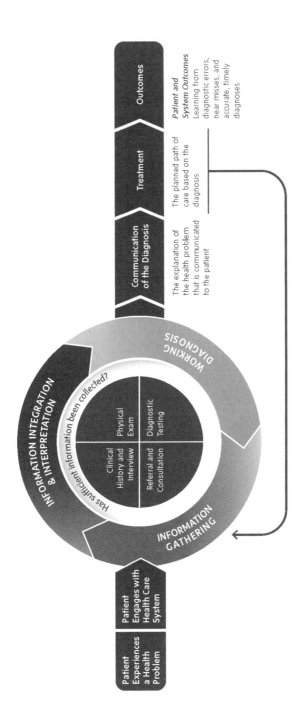

FIGURE 2-1 The committee's conceptualization of the diagnostic process.

TIME

BOX 2-1
The Work System

The diagnostic process occurs within a work system that is composed of diagnostic team members, tasks, technologies and tools, organizational factors, the physical environment, and the external environment (see figure on opposite page) (Carayon et al., 2006, 2014; Smith and Sainfort, 1989):

- Diagnostic team members include patients and their families and all health care professionals involved in their care.
- Tasks are goal-oriented actions that occur within the diagnostic process.
- Technologies and tools include health information technology (health IT) used in the diagnostic process.
- Organizational characteristics include culture, rules and procedures, and leadership and management considerations.
- The physical environment includes elements such as layout, distractions, lighting, and noise.
- The external environment includes factors such as the payment and care delivery system, the legal environment, and the reporting environment.

All components of the work system interact, and each component can affect the diagnostic process (e.g., a change in the physical environment may affect the usefulness and accessibility of health IT, and a change in the diagnostic team may affect the assignment of tasks). The work system provides the context in which the diagnostic process occurs (Carayon et al., 2006, 2014). There is a range of settings (i.e., work systems) in which the diagnostic process can occur—for example, outpatient primary or specialty care office settings, emergency departments, inpatient hospital settings, long-term care facilities, and retail clinics. Each of these includes the six components of a work system—diagnostic team members and tasks, technologies and tools, organizational factors, the physical environment, and the external environment—although the nature of the components may differ among and between settings. The six components of the work system and how they are related to diagnosis and diagnostic error are described in detail in Chapters 4–7.

---

revision to the working diagnosis, this information should be communicated to the patient. As the diagnostic process proceeds, a fairly broad list of potential diagnoses may be narrowed into fewer potential options, a process referred to as diagnostic modification and refinement (Kassirer et al., 2010). As the list becomes narrowed to one or two possibilities, diagnostic refinement of the working diagnosis becomes diagnostic verification, in which the lead diagnosis is checked for its adequacy in explaining the signs and symptoms, its coherency with the patient's context (physiology, risk factors), and whether a single diagnosis is appropriate. When considering invasive or risky diagnostic testing or treatment options, the

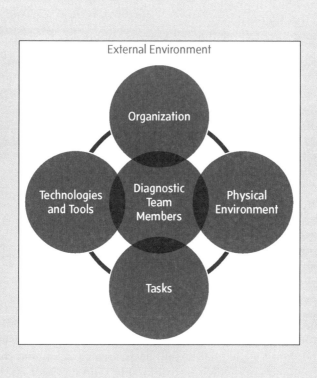

diagnostic verification step is particularly important so that a patient is not exposed to these risks without a reasonable chance that the testing or treatment options will be informative and will likely improve patient outcomes.

Throughout the diagnostic process, there is an ongoing assessment of whether sufficient information has been collected. If the diagnostic team members are not satisfied that the necessary information has been collected to explain the patient's health problem or that the information available is not consistent with a diagnosis, then the process of information gathering, information integration and interpretation, and developing a working diagnosis continues. When the diagnostic team members judge that they have arrived at an accurate and timely explanation of the patient's health problem, they communicate that explanation to the patient as the diagnosis.

It is important to note that clinicians do not need to obtain diagnostic certainty prior to initiating treatment; the goal of information gathering in the diagnostic process is to reduce diagnostic uncertainty enough to make optimal decisions for subsequent care (Kassirer, 1989; see section on diagnostic uncertainty). In addition, the provision of treatment can also inform and refine a working diagnosis, which is indicated by the feedback loop from treatment into the information-gathering step of the diagnostic process. This also illustrates the need for clinicians to diagnose health problems that may arise during treatment.

The committee identified four types of information-gathering activities in the diagnostic process: taking a clinical history and interview; performing a physical exam; obtaining diagnostic testing; and sending a patient for referrals or consultations. The diagnostic process is intended to be broadly applicable, including the provision of mental health care. These information-gathering processes are discussed in further detail below.

Clinical History and Interview

Acquiring a clinical history and interviewing a patient provides important information for determining a diagnosis and also establishes a solid foundation for the relationship between a clinician and the patient. A common maxim in medicine attributed to William Osler is: "Just listen to your patient, he is telling you the diagnosis" (Gandhi, 2000, p. 1087). An appointment begins with an interview of the patient, when a clinician compiles a patient's medical history or verifies that the details of the patient's history already contained in the patient's medical record are accurate. A patient's clinical history includes documentation of the current concern, past medical history, family history, social history, and other relevant information, such as current medications (prescription and over-the-counter) and dietary supplements.

The process of acquiring a clinical history and interviewing a patient requires effective communication, active listening skills, and tailoring communication to the patient based on the patient's needs, values, and preferences. The National Institute on Aging, in guidance for conducting a clinical history and interview, suggests that clinicians should avoid interrupting, demonstrate empathy, and establish a rapport with patients (NIA, 2008). Clinicians need to know when to ask more detailed questions and how to create a safe environment for patients to share sensitive information about their health and symptoms. Obtaining a history can be challenging in some cases: For example, in working with older adults with memory loss, with children, or with individuals whose health problems limit communication or reliable self-reporting. In these cases it may be necessary to include family members or caregivers in the history-taking process. The time pressures often involved in clinical appointments also contribute to challenges in the clinical history and interview. Limited time for clinical visits, partially attributed to payment policies (see Chapter 7), may lead to an incomplete picture of a patient's relevant history and current signs and symptoms.

There are growing concerns that traditional "bedside evaluation" skills (history, interview, and physical exam) have received less attention due the large growth in diagnostic testing in medicine. Verghese and colleagues noted that these methods were once the primary tools for diagnosis and clinical evaluation, but "the recent explosion of imaging and laboratory testing has inverted the diagnostic paradigm. [Clinicians] often bypass the bedside evaluation for immediate testing" (Verghese et al., 2011, p. 550). The interview has been called a clinician's most versatile diagnostic and therapeutic tool, and the clinical history provides direction for subsequent information-gathering activities in the diagnostic process (Lichstein, 1990). An accurate history facilitates a more productive and efficient physical exam and the appropriate utilization of diagnostic testing (Lichstein, 1990). Indeed, Kassirer concluded: "Diagnosis remains fundamentally dependent on a personal interaction of a [clinician] with a patient, the sufficiency of communication between them, the accuracy of the patient's history and physical examination, and the cognitive energy necessary to synthesize a vast array of information" (Kassirer, 2014, p. 12).

Physical Exam

The physical exam is a hands-on observational examination of the patient. First, a clinician observes a patient's demeanor, complexion, posture, level of distress, and other signs that may contribute to an understanding of the health problem (Davies and Rees, 2010). If the clinician has seen the patient before, these observations can be weighed against previous interactions with the patient. A physical exam may include an analysis of many parts of the body, not just those suspected to be involved in the patient's current complaint. A careful physical exam can help a clinician refine the next steps in the diagnostic process, can prevent unnecessary diagnostic testing, and can aid in building trust with the patient (Verghese, 2011). There is no universally agreed upon physical examination checklist; myriad versions exist online and in textbooks.

Due to the growing emphasis on diagnostic testing, there are concerns that physical exam skills have been underemphasized in current health care professional education and training (Kassirer, 2014; Kugler and Verghese, 2010). For example, Kugler and Verghese have asserted that there is a high degree in variability in the way that trainees elicit physical signs and that residency programs have not done enough to evaluate and improve physical exam techniques. Physicians at Stanford have developed the "Stanford 25," a list of physical diagnostic maneuvers that are very technique-dependent (Verghese and Horwitz, 2009). Educators observe students and residents performing these 25 maneuvers to ensure that trainees are able to elicit the physical signs reliably (Stanford Medicine 25 Team, 2015).

Diagnostic Testing

Over the past 100 years, diagnostic testing has become a critical feature of standard medical practice (Berger, 1999; European Society

---

BOX 2-2
Laboratory Medicine, Anatomic
Pathology, and Medical Imaging

Pathology is usually separated into two disciplines: laboratory medicine and anatomic pathology. Laboratory medicine, also referred to as clinical pathology, focuses on the testing of fluid specimens, such as blood or urine. Anatomic pathology addresses the microscopic examination of tissues, cells, or other solid specimens.

Laboratory medicine is a medical subspecialty concerned with the examination of specific analytes in body fluids (e.g., cholesterol in serum, protein in urine, or glucose in cerebrospinal fluid), the specific identification of microorganisms (e.g., disease-causing bacteria in sputum, human immunodeficiency virus in blood, or parasites in stool), the analysis of bone marrow specimens (e.g., the identification of a specific of type of leukemia), and the management of transfusion therapy (e.g., cross-matching blood products, or plasmapheresis). Generally, clinical pathologists, except those with blood banking and coagulation expertise, do not interact directly with patients.

Anatomic pathology is a medical subspecialty concerned with the testing of tissue specimens or bodily fluids, typically by specialists referred to as anatomic pathologists, to interpret results and diagnose diseases or health conditions. Some anatomic pathologists perform postmortem examinations (autopsies). Typically, anatomic pathologists do not interact directly with patients, with the notable exception of the performance of fine needle aspiration biopsies.

Laboratory scientists, historically referred to as medical technologists, may contribute to this process by preparing and collecting samples and performing tests. Especially for laboratory medicine, the ordering of diagnostic tests and the

of Radiology, 2010). Diagnostic testing may occur in successive rounds of information gathering, integration, and interpretation, as each round of information refines the working diagnosis. In many cases, diagnostic testing can identify a condition before it is clinically apparent; for example, coronary artery disease can be identified by an imaging study indicating the presence of coronary artery blockage even in the absence of symptoms.

The primary emphasis of this section focuses on laboratory medicine, anatomic pathology, and medical imaging (see Box 2-2). However, there are many important forms of diagnostic testing that extend beyond these fields, and the committee's conceptual model is intended to be broadly applicable. Aditional forms of diagnostic testing include, for example, screening tools used in making mental health diagnoses (SAMHSA and HRSA, 2015), sleep apnea testing, neurocognitive assessment, and vision and hearing testing.

interpretation of results are usually performed by the patient's treating clinician, although pathologists have much to offer in these areas.

It is worth mentioning that with the advent of precision medicine, molecular diagnostic testing is not specifically aligned with either clinical or anatomic pathology (see Box 2-3).

Medical imaging, also known as radiology, is a medical specialty that uses imaging technologies (such as X-ray, ultrasound, computed tomography [CT], magnetic resonance imaging [MRI], and positron emission tomography [PET]) to diagnose diseases and health conditions. For many conditions, it is also used to select and plan treatments, monitor treatment effectiveness, and provide long-term follow-up. Image interpretation is typically performed by radiologists or, for selected tests involving radioactive nuclides, nuclear medicine physicians. Technologists support the process by carrying out the imaging protocols. Most radiologists today have subspecialty training (e.g., in pediatric radiology or neuro-radiology), while the remainder (about 18 percent) are generalists (Bluth et al., 2014). Specialists in other clinical disciplines, such as emergency medicine physicians and cardiologists, may be trained and credentialed to perform and interpret certain types of medical imaging. This can include imaging (such as ultrasound) to localize tissue targets during biopsy.

A new subspecialty in radiology is molecular imaging, which involves the use of functional MRI techniques as well as MRI, PET/CT, or PET/MRI with molecular imaging probes. Several new molecular imaging probes have recently been approved for clinical use, and a growing number are entering clinical trials. The field of radiology also includes interventional radiology, which offers image-guided biopsy and diagnostic procedures as well as image-guided, minimally invasive treatments.

Although it was developed specifically for laboratory medicine, the brain-to-brain loop model is useful for describing the general process of diagnostic testing (Lundberg, 1981; Plebani et al., 2011). The model includes nine steps: test selection and ordering, sample collection, patient identification, sample transportation, sample preparation, sample analysis, result reporting, result interpretation, and clinical action (Lundberg, 1981). These steps occur during five phases of diagnostic testing: pre-pre-analytic, pre-analytic, analytic, post-analytic, and post-post-analytic phases. Errors related to diagnostic testing can occur in any of these five phases, but the analytic phase is the least susceptible to errors (Eichbaum et al., 2012; Epner et al., 2013; Laposata, 2010; Nichols and Rauch, 2013; Stratton, 2011) (see Chapter 3).

The pre-pre-analytic phase, which involves clinician test selection and ordering, has been identified as a key point of vulnerability in the work process due to the large number and variety of available tests, which makes it difficult for nonspecialist clinicians to accurately select the correct test or series of tests (Hickner et al., 2014; Laposata and Dighe, 2007). The pre-analytic phase involves sample collection, patient identification, sample transportation, and sample preparation. During the analytic phase, the specimen is tested, examined, or both. Adequate performance in this phase depends on the correct execution of a chemical analysis or morphological examination (Hollensead et al., 2004), and the contribution to diagnostic errors at this step is small. The post-analytic phase includes the generation of results, reporting, interpretation, and follow-up. Ensuring accurate and timely reporting from the laboratory to the ordering clinician and patient is central to this phase. During the post-post-analytic phase, the ordering clinician, sometimes in consultation with pathologists, incorporates the test results into the patient's clinical context, considers the probability of a particular diagnosis in light of the test results, and considers the harms and benefits of future tests and treatments, given the newly acquired information. Possible factors contributing to failure in this phase include an incorrect interpretation of the test result by the ordering clinician or pathologist and the failure by the ordering clinician to act on the test results: for example, not ordering a follow-up test or not providing treatment consistent with the test results (Hickner et al., 2014; Laposata and Dighe, 2007; Plebani and Lippi, 2011).

The medical imaging work process parallels the work process described for pathology. There is a pre-pre-analytic phase (the selection and ordering of medical imaging), a pre-analytic phase (preparing the patient for imaging), an analytic phase (image acquisition and analysis), a post-analytic phase (the imaging results are interpreted and reported to the ordering clinician or the patient), and a post-post-analytic phase (the integration of results into the patient context and further action). The relevant differences between the medical imaging and pathology processes include the nature of the examination and the methods and technology used to interpret the results.

Laboratory Medicine and Anatomic Pathology

In 2008 a Centers for Disease Control and Prevention (CDC) report described pathology as an "essential element of the health care system," stating that pathology is "integral to many clinical decisions, providing physicians, nurses, and other health care providers with often pivotal information for the prevention, diagnosis, treatment, and management of disease" (CDC, 2008, p. 19). Primary care clinicians order laboratory tests in slightly less than one third of patient visits (CDC, 2010; Hickner et al., 2014), and direct-to-patient testing is becoming increasingly prevalent (CDC, 2008). There are now thousands of molecular diagnostic tests available, and this number is expected to increase as the mechanisms of disease at the molecular level are better understood (CDC, 2008; Johansen Taber et al., 2014) (see Box 2-3).

The task of selecting the appropriate diagnostic testing is challenging for clinicians, in part because of the sheer volume of choices. For example, Hickner and colleagues (2014) found that primary care clinicians report uncertainty in ordering laboratory medicine tests in approximately 15 percent of diagnostic encounters. Choosing the appropriate test requires understanding the patient's history and current signs and symptoms, as well as having a sufficient suspicion or pre-test probability of a disease or condition (see section on probabilistic reasoning) (Pauker and Kassirer, 1975, 1980; Sox, 1986). The likelihood of disease is inherently uncertain in this step; for instance, the clinician's patient population may not reflect epidemiological data, and the patient's history can be incomplete or otherwise complicated. Advances in molecular diagnostic technologies and new diagnostic tests have introduced another layer of complexity. Many clinicians are struggling to keep up with the growing availability of such tests and have uncertainty about the best application of these tests in screening, diagnosis, and treatment (IOM, 2015a; Johansen Taber et al., 2014).

Diagnostic tests have "operating parameters," including sensitivity and specificity that are particular to the diagnostic test for a specific disorder (see section on probabilistic reasoning). Even if a test is performed correctly, there is a chance for a false positive or false negative result. Test interpretation involves reviewing numerical or qualitative (yes or no) results and combining those results with patient history, symptoms, and pretest disease likelihood. Test interpretation needs to be patient-specific and to consider information learned during the physical exam and the clinical history and interview. Several studies have highlighted test inter-

---

BOX 2-3
Molecular Diagnostics

The President's Precision Medicine Initiative highlights the growing interest in taking individual variability into account when defining disease, tailoring treatment, and improving prevention (NIH, 2015). This initiative hinges on recent advances in molecular and cellular biology, which have provided insights into the mechanisms of disease at the molecular level. These advances have contributed to the development of molecular diagnostic testing, which analyzes a patient's biomarkers in the genome or proteome. Concurrently, the role of pathology has expanded from morphologic observations into comprehensive analyses using combined histological, immunohistochemical, and molecular evaluations.

The use of molecular diagnostics is a rapidly developing area. Molecular diagnostic tests are being developed and used to diagnose and monitor disease, assess risk, inform whether a particular therapy is likely to be effective in a specific patient, and predict a patient's response to therapy (AvaMedDx, 2013). Molecular diagnostic testing can identify a variety of specific genetic alterations relevant to diagnosis and treatment; molecular diagnostic techniques are also used to detect the genetic material of organisms causing infection. Panels of biomarkers are being developed into molecular diagnostic tests (omics-based tests) that are used to assess risk and inform treatment decisions, such as Oncotype DX and MammaPrint in breast cancer (IOM, 2012).

Molecular diagnostic testing is expected to improve patient management and outcomes. The potential advantages of molecular diagnostics include (1) providing earlier and more accurate diagnostic methods; (2) offering information about disease that will better tailor treatments to patients; (3) reducing the occurrence

---

pretation errors, such as the misinterpretation of a false positive human immunodeficiency virus (HIV) screening test for a low-risk patient as indicative of HIV infection (Gigerenzer, 2013; Kleinman et al., 1998). In addition, test performance may only be characterized in a limited patient population, leading to challenges with generalizability (Whiting et al., 2004).

The laboratories that conduct diagnostic testing are some of the most regulated and inspected areas in health care (see Table 2-1). Some of the relevant entities include The Joint Commission and other accreditors, the federal government, and various other organizations, such as the College of American Pathologists (CAP) and the American Society for Clinical Pathology. There are many ways in which quality is assessed. Examples include proficiency testing of clinical laboratory assays and pathologists (e.g., Pap smear proficiency testing), many of which are regulated under the Clinical Laboratory Improvement Amendments, and inter-laboratory

of side effects from unnecessary treatments; (4) providing better tools to for the monitoring of patients for treatment success or disease recurrence; and (5) improving patient outcomes and quality of life.

However, the translation of molecular diagnostic technologies into clinical practice has been a complex and challenging endeavor. One major challenge is the development and rigorous evaluation of molecular diagnostic tests before their implementation in clinical practice. The development pathway is often time-consuming, expensive, and uncertain. In addition, there are underdeveloped and inconsistent standards of evidence for evaluating the scientific validity of tests and a lack of appropriate study designs and analytical methods for these analyses (IOM, 2007, 2010, 2012). Ensuring that diagnostic tests have adequate analytical and clinical validity is critical to preventing diagnostic errors. For example, in 2005 the Centers for Disease Control and Prevention and the Food and Drug Administration issued a warning about potential diagnostic errors related to false positives caused by contamination in a Lyme disease test (Nelson et al., 2014). As molecular diagnostic testing becomes increasingly complex (such as the movement from single biomarker tests to omics-based tests that rely on high-dimensional data and complex algorithms), there is considerable interest in ensuring their appropriate development and use (IOM, 2012). Molecular diagnostic testing presents many regulatory, clinical practice, and reimbursement challenges; an Institute of Medicine study is looking into these issues and is expected to release a report in 2016 (IOM, 2015b). For example, one regulatory issue is the oversight of laboratory-developed tests, an area that has been met with considerable controversy (see Table 2-1) (Evans and Watson, 2015; Sharfstein, 2015). A clinical practice issue is next generation sequencing, which may frequently identify new genetic variants with unknown implications for health outcomes (ACMG Board of Directors, 2012).

comparison programs (e.g., CAP's Q-Probes, Q-Monitors, and Q-Tracks programs).

Medical Imaging

Medical imaging plays a critical role in establishing the diagnoses for innumerable conditions and it is used routinely in nearly every branch of medicine. The advancement of imaging technologies has improved the ability of clinicians to detect, diagnose, and treat conditions while also allowing patients to avoid more invasive procedures (European Society of Radiology, 2010; Gunderman, 2005). For many conditions (e.g., brain tumors), imaging is the only noninvasive diagnostic method available. The appropriate choice of imaging modality depends on the disease, organ, and specific clinical questions to be addressed. Computed tomography (CT) and magnetic resonance imaging (MRI) are first-line methods for as-

TABLE 2-1 Examples of Entities Involved in Quality Improvement and Oversight of Clinical and Anatomic Laboratories

Entity	Role in Quality or Oversight
Centers for Disease Control and Prevention (CDC)	The CDC performs research on laboratory testing processes, including quality improvement studies, and develops technical standards and laboratory practice guidelines (CDC, 2014). The CDC also manages the Clinical Laboratory Improvement Advisory Committee (CLIAC), a body that offers guidance to the federal government on quality improvement in the clinical laboratory and revising Clinical Laboratory Improvement Amendments (CLIA) standards.
Centers for Medicare & Medicaid Services (CMS)	CMS regulates laboratories under CLIA (CMS, 2015b). To ensure CLIA compliance, laboratories undergo review of results reporting, laboratory personnel credentialing (i.e., competency assessment), quality control efforts, and procedure documentation. Laboratories are also required to perform proficiency testing (PT), a process in which a laboratory receives an unknown sample to test and report the findings back to the PT program, which evaluates the laboratory's performance.
	CMS grants states or accreditation organizations the authority to deem a laboratory as CLIA-compliant. In most cases the laboratory is deemed compliant by virtue of being accredited by the accreditation organization. Accreditation organizations with deeming authority for CLIA include AABB, the American Association for Laboratory Accreditation, the American Society for Histocompatibility and Immunogenics, COLA, the College of American Pathologists, the Healthcare Facilities Accreditation Program, and The Joint Commission (CMS, 2014).
Food and Drug Administration (FDA)	FDA reviews and assesses the safety, efficacy, and intended use of in vitro diagnostic tests (IVDs) (FDA, 2014a). FDA assesses the analytical validity (i.e., analytical specificity and sensitivity, accuracy, and precision) and clinical validity (i.e., the accuracy with which the test identifies, measures, or predicts the presence or absence of a clinical condition or predisposition), and it develops rules and guidance for CLIA complexity categorization. One subset of IVDs, laboratory developed tests (LDTs), has been granted enforcement discretion from FDA; in 2014 FDA stated its intent to begin regulating LDTs (FDA, 2014b).
American Academy of Family Physicians (AAFP)	The AAFP offers a number of CMS-approved PT programs (AAFP, 2015).

TABLE 2-1 Continued

Entity	Role in Quality or Oversight
American Society for Clinical Pathology (ASCP)	ASCP certifies medical laboratory professionals. ASCP also manages a CMS-approved PT program for gynecologic cytology (ASCP, 2014).
College of American Pathologists (CAP)	CAP accreditation ensures the safety and quality of laboratories and satisfies CLIA requirements. CAP also offers an inter-laboratory peer PT program (CAP, 2013, 2015). This program includes • Q-Tracks: a continuous quality monitoring process • Q-Probes: a short-term study that provides a time slice assessment of performance • Q-Monitors: customized programs that address process-, outcome-, and structure-oriented quality assurance issues
Healthcare Facilities Accreditation Program (HFAP)	HFAP accreditation ensures the safety and quality of laboratories and satisfies CLIA requirements (HFAP, 2015).
The Joint Commission	The Joint Commission accreditation ensures the safety and quality of laboratories and satisfies CLIA requirements (The Joint Commission, 2015).

sessing conditions of the central and peripheral nervous system, while for musculoskeletal and a variety of other conditions, X-ray and ultrasound are often employed first because of their relatively low cost and ready availability, with CT and MRI being reserved as problem-solving modalities. CT procedures are frequently used to assess and diagnose cancer, circulatory system diseases and conditions, inflammatory diseases, and head and internal organ injuries. A majority of MRI procedures are performed on the spine, brain, and musculoskeletal system, although usage for the breast, prostate, abdominal, and pelvic regions is rising (IMV, 2014).

Medical imaging is characterized not just by the increasingly precise anatomic detail it offers but also by an increasing capacity to illuminate biology. For example, magnetic resonance spectroscopic imaging has allowed the assessment of metabolism, and a growing number of other MRI sequences are offering information about functional characteristics, such as blood perfusion or water diffusion. In addition, several new tracers for molecular imaging with PET (typically as PET/CT) have recently been approved for clinical use, and more are undergoing clinical trials, while PET/MRI was recently introduced to the clinical setting. Functional and molecular imaging data may be assessed qualitatively, quantitatively, or both. Although other forms of diagnostic testing can identify a wide array of molecular markers, molecular imaging is unique in its capacity to noninvasively show the locations of molecular processes in patients, and it is expected to play a critical role in advancing precision medicine, particularly for cancers, which often demonstrate both intra- and inter-tumoral biological heterogeneity (Hricak, 2011).

The growing body of medical knowledge, the variety of imaging options available, and the regular increases in the amounts and kinds of data that can be captured with imaging present tremendous challenges for radiologists, as no individual can be expected to achieve competency in all of the imaging modalities. General radiologists continue to be essential in certain clinical settings, but extended training and sub-specialization are often necessary for optimal, clinically relevant image interpretation, as is involvement in multidisciplinary disease management teams. Furthermore, the use of structured reporting templates tailored to specific examinations can help to increase the clarity, thoroughness, and clinical relevance of image interpretation (Schwartz et al., 2011).

Like other forms of diagnostic testing, medical imaging has limitations. Some studies have found that between 20 and 50 percent of all advanced imaging results fail to provide information that improves patient outcome, although these studies do not account for the value of negative imaging results in influencing decisions about patient management (Hendee et al., 2010). Imaging may fail to provide useful information because of modality sensitivity and specificity parameters; for example, the spatial resolution of an MRI may not be high enough to detect very small abnormalities. Inadequate patient education and preparation for an imaging test can also lead to suboptimal imaging quality that results in diagnostic error.

Perceptual or cognitive errors made by radiologists are a source of diagnostic error (Berlin, 2014; Krupinski et al., 2012). In addition, incomplete or incorrect patient information, as well as insufficient sharing of patient information, may lead to the use of an inadequate imaging protocol, an incorrect interpretation of imaging results, or the selection of an inappropriate imaging test by a referring clinician. Referring clinicians often struggle with selecting the appropriate imaging test, in part because of the large number of available imaging options and gaps in the teaching of radiology in medical schools. Although consensus-based guidelines (e.g., the various "appropriateness criteria" published by the American College of Radiology [ACR]) are available to help select imaging tests for many conditions, these guidelines are often not followed. The use of clinical decision support systems at the point of care as well as direct consultations with radiologists have been proposed by the ACR as methods for improving imaging test selection (Allen and Thorwarth, 2014).

There are several mechanisms for ensuring the quality of medical imaging. The Mammography Quality Standards Act (MQSA)—overseen by the Food and Drug Administration—was the first government-mandated accreditation program for any type of medical facility; it was focused on X-ray imaging for breast cancer. MQSA provides a general framework for ensuring national quality standards in facilities that perform screening mammography (IOM, 2005). MQSA requires all personnel at facilities to meet initial qualifications, to demonstrate continued experience, and to complete continuing education. MQSA addresses protocol selection, image acquisition, interpretation and report generation, and the communication of results and recommendations. In addition, it provides facilities with data on diagnostic performance that can be used for benchmarking, self-monitoring, and improvement. MQSA has decreased the variability in mammography performed across the United States and improved the quality of care (Allen and Thorwarth, 2014). However, the ACR noted that MQSA is complex and specified in great detail, which makes it inflexible, leading to administrative burdens and the need for extensive training of staff for implementation (Allen and Thorwarth, 2014). It also focuses on only one medical imaging modality in one disease area; thus, it does not address newer screening technologies (IOM, 2005). In addition, the Medicare Improvements for Patients and Providers Act (MIPPA)[3] requires that private outpatient facilities that perform CT, MRI, breast MRI, nuclear medicine, and PET exams be accredited. The requirements include personnel qualifications, image quality, equipment performance, safety standards, and quality assurance and quality control (ACR, 2015a). There are four CMS-designated accreditation organizations for medical imaging: ACR, the Intersocietal Accreditation Commission, The Joint Commission, and RadSite (CMS, 2015a). MIPPA also mandated that, beginning in 2017, ordering clinicians will be required to consult appropriateness criteria to order advanced medical imaging procedures, and the act called for a demonstration project evaluating clinician compliance with appropriateness criteria (Timbie et al., 2014). In addition to these mandated activities, societies such as ACR and the Radiological Society of North America (RSNA) provide quality improvement programs and resources (ACR, 2015b; RSNA, 2015).

---

[3] Public Law 110-275 (July 15, 2008).

Referral and Consultation

Clinicians may refer to or consult with other clinicians (formally or informally) to seek additional expertise about a patient's health problem. The consult may help to confirm or reject the working diagnosis or may provide information on potential treatment options. If a patient's health problem is outside a clinician's area of expertise, he or she can refer the patient to a clinician who holds more suitable expertise. Clinicians can also recommend that the patient seek a second opinion from another clinician to verify their impressions of an uncertain diagnosis or if they believe that this would be helpful to the patient. Many groups raise awareness that patients can obtain a second opinion on their own (AMA, 1996; CMS, 2015c; PAF, 2012). Diagnostic consultations can also be arranged through the use of integrated practice units or diagnostic management teams (Govern, 2013; Porter, 2010; see Chapter 4).

IMPORTANT CONSIDERATIONS IN THE DIAGNOSTIC PROCESS

The committee elaborated on several aspects of the diagnostic process which are discussed below, including

- diagnostic uncertainty
- time
- population trends
- diverse populations and health disparities
- mental health

Diagnostic Uncertainty

One of the complexities in the diagnostic process is the inherent uncertainty in diagnosis. As noted in the committee's conceptual model of the diagnostic process, an overarching question throughout the process is whether sufficient information has been collected to make a diagnosis. This does not mean that a diagnosis needs to be absolutely certain in order to initiate treatment. Kassirer concluded that:

> Absolute certainty in diagnosis is unattainable, no matter how much information we gather, how many observations we make, or how many tests we perform. A diagnosis is a hypothesis about the nature of a patient's illness, one that is derived from observations by the use of inference. As the inferential process unfolds, our confidence as [clinicians] in a given diagnosis is enhanced by the gathering of data that either favor it or argue against competing hypotheses. Our task is not to attain cer-

tainty, but rather to reduce the level of diagnostic uncertainty enough to make optimal therapeutic decisions. (Kassirer, 1989, p. 1489)

Thus, the probability of disease does not have to be equal to one (diagnostic certainty) in order for treatment to be justified (Pauker and Kassirer, 1980). The decision to begin treatment based on a working diagnosis is informed by: (1) the degree of certainty about the diagnosis; (2) the harms and benefits of treatment; and (3) the harms and benefits of further information-gathering activities, including the impact of delaying treatment.

The risks associated with diagnostic testing are important considerations when conducting information-gathering activities in the diagnostic process. While underuse of diagnostic testing has been a long-standing concern, overly aggressive diagnostic strategies have recently been recognized for their risks (Zhi et al., 2013) (see Chapter 3). Overuse of diagnostic testing has been partially attributed to clinicians' fear of missing something important and intolerance of diagnostic uncertainty: "I am far more concerned about doing too little than doing too much. It's the scan, the test, the operation that I should have done that sticks with me—sometimes for years. . . . By contrast, I can't remember anyone I sent for an unnecessary CT scan or operated on for questionable reasons a decade ago" (Gawande, 2015). However, there is growing recognition that overly aggressive diagnostic pursuits are putting patients at greater risk for harm, and they are not improving diagnostic certainty (Kassirer, 1989; Welch, 2015).

When considering diagnostic testing options, the harm from the procedure itself needs to be weighed against the potential information that could be gained. For some patients, the risk of invasive diagnostic testing may be inappropriate due to the risk of mortality or morbidity from the test itself (such as cardiac catheterization or invasive biopsies). In addition, the risk for harm needs to take into account the cascade of diagnostic testing and treatment decisions that could stem from a diagnostic test result. Included in these assessments are the potential for false positives and ambiguous or slightly abnormal test results that lead to further diagnostic testing or unnecessary treatment.

There are some cases in which treatment is initiated even though there is limited certainty in a working diagnosis. For example, an individual who has been exposed to a tick bite or HIV may be treated with prophylactic antibiotics or antivirals, because the risk of treatment may be felt to be smaller than the risk of harm from tick-borne diseases or HIV infection. Clinicians sometimes employ empiric treatment strategies—or the provision of treatment with a very uncertain diagnosis—and use a patient's response to treatment as an information-gathering activity to help arrive at a working diagnosis. However, it is important to note that response rates to treatment can be highly variable, and the failure to respond to treatment does not necessarily reflect that a diagnosis is incorrect. Nor does improvement in the patient's condition necessarily validate that the treatment conferred this benefit and, therefore, that the empirically tested diagnosis was in fact correct. A treatment that is beneficial for some patients might not be beneficial for others with the same condition (Kent and Hayward, 2007), hence the interest in precision medicine, which is hoped to better tailor therapy to maximize efficacy and minimize toxicity (Jameson and Longo, 2015). In addition, there are isolated cases where the morbidity and the mortality of a diagnostic procedure and the likelihood of disease is sufficiently high that significant therapy has been given empirically. Moroff and Pauker (1983) described a decision analysis in which a 90-year-old practicing lawyer with a new 1.5 centimeter lung nodule was deemed to have a sufficiently high risk for mortality from lung biopsy and high likelihood of malignancy that the radiation oncologists felt comfortable treating the patient empirically for suspected lung cancer.

Time

Of major importance in the diagnostic process is the element of time. Most diseases evolve over time, and there can be a delay between the onset of disease and the onset of a patient's symptoms; time can also elapse before a patient's symptoms are recognized as a specific diagnosis (Zwaan and Singh, 2015). Some diagnoses can be determined in a very short time frame, while months may elapse before other diagnoses can be made. This is partially due to the growing recognition of the variability and complexity of disease presentation. Similar symptoms may be related to a number of different diagnoses, and symptoms may evolve in different ways as a disease progresses; for example, a disease affecting multiple organs may initially involve symptoms or signs from a single organ. The thousands of different diseases and health conditions do not present in thousands of unique ways; there are only a finite number of symptoms with which a patient may present. At the outset, it can be very difficult to determine which particular diagnosis is indicated by a particular combination of symptoms, especially if symptoms are nonspecific, such as fatigue. Diseases may also present atypically, with an unusual and unexpected constellation of symptoms (Emmett, 1998).

Adding to the complexity of the time-dependent nature of the diagnostic process are the numerous settings of care in which diagnosis occurs and the potential involvement of multiple settings of care within a single diagnostic process. Henriksen and Brady noted that this process—for patients, their families, and clinicians alike—can often feel like "a disjointed journey across confusing terrain, aided or impeded by different agents, with no destination in sight and few landmarks along the way" (Henriksen and Brady, 2013, p. ii2).

Some diagnoses may be more important to establish immediately than others. These include diagnoses that can lead to significant patient harm if not recognized, diagnosed, and treated early, such as anthrax, aortic dissection, and pulmonary embolism. Sometimes making a timely diagnosis relies on the fast recognition of symptoms outside of the health care setting (e.g., public awareness of stroke symptoms can help improve the speed of receiving medical help and increase the chances of a better recovery) (National Stroke Association, 2015). In these cases, the benefit of treating the disease promptly can greatly exceed the potential harm from unnecessary treatment. Consequently, the threshold for ordering diagnostic testing or for initiating treatment becomes quite low for such health problems (Pauker and Kassirer, 1975, 1980). In other cases, the potential harm from rapidly and unnecessarily treating a diagnosed condition can lead to a more conservative (or higher-threshold) approach in the diagnostic process.

Population Trends

Population trends, such as the aging of the population, are adding significant complexity to the diagnostic process and require clinicians to consider such complicating factors in diagnosis as comorbidity, polypharmacy and attendant medication side effects, as well as disease and medication interactions (IOM, 2008, 2013b). Diagnosis can be especially challenging in older patients because classic presentations of disease are less common in older adults (Jarrett et al., 1995). For example, infections such as pneumonia or urinary tract infections often do not present in older patients with fever, cough, and pain but rather with symptoms such as lethargy, incontinence, loss of appetite, or disruption of cognitive function (Mouton et al., 2001). Acute myocardial infarction (MI) may present with fatigue and confusion rather than with typical symptoms such as chest pain or radiating arm pain (Bayer et al., 1986; Qureshi et al., 2000; Rich, 2006). Sensory limitations in older adults, such as hearing and vision impairments, can also contribute to challenges in making diagnoses (Campbell et al., 1999). Physical illnesses often present with a change in cognitive status in older individuals without dementia (Mouton et al., 2001). In older adults with mild to moderate dementia, such illnesses can manifest with worsening cognition. Older patients who have multiple comorbidities, medications, or cognitive and functional impairments are more likely to have atypical disease presentations, which may increase the risk of experiencing diagnostic errors (Gray-Miceli, 2008).

Diverse Populations and Health Disparities

Communicating with diverse populations can also contribute to the complexity of the diagnostic process. Language, health literacy, and cultural barriers can affect clinician–patient encounters and increase the potential for challenges in the diagnostic process (Flores, 2006; IOM, 2003; The Joint Commission, 2007). There are indications that biases influence diagnosis; one well-known example is the differential referral of patients for cardiac catheterization by race and gender (Schulman et al., 1999). In addition, women are more likely than men to experience a missed diagnosis of heart attack, a situation that has been partly attributed to real and perceived gender biases, but which may also be the result of physiologic differences, as women have a higher likelihood of presenting with atypical symptoms, including abdominal pain, shortness of breath, and congestive heart failure (Pope et al., 2000).

Mental Health

Mental health diagnoses can be particularly challenging. Mental health diagnoses rely on the *Diagnostic and Statistical Manual of Mental Disorders* (DSM); each diagnosis in the DSM includes a set of diagnostic criteria that indicate the type and length of symptoms that need to be present, as well as the symptoms, disorders, and conditions that cannot be present, in order to be considered for a particular diagnosis (APA, 2015). Compared to physical diagnoses, many mental health diagnoses rely on patient reports and observation; there are few biological tests that are used in such diagnoses (Pincus, 2014). A key challenge can be distinguishing physical diagnoses from mental health diagnoses; sometimes physical conditions manifest as psychiatric ones, and vice versa (Croskerry, 2003a; Hope et al., 2014; Pincus, 2014; Reeves et al., 2010). In addition, there are concerns about missing psychiatric diagnoses, as well as overtreatment concerns (Bor, 2015; Meyer and Meyer, 2009; Pincus, 2014). For example, clinician biases toward older adults can contribute to missed diagnoses of depression, because it may be perceived that older adults are likely to be depressed, lethargic, or have little interest in interactions. Patients with mental health–related symptoms may also be more vulnerable to diagnostic errors, a situation that is attributed partly to clinician biases; for example, clinicians may disregard symptoms in patients with previous diagnoses of mental illness or substance abuse and attribute new physical symptoms to a psychological cause (Croskerry, 2003a). Individuals with health problems that are difficult to diagnose or those who have chronic pain may also be more likely to receive psychiatric diagnoses erroneously.

CLINICAL REASONING AND DIAGNOSIS

Accurate, timely, and patient-centered diagnosis relies on proficiency in clinical reasoning, which is often regarded as the clinician's quintessential competency. Clinical reasoning is "the cognitive process that is necessary to evaluate and manage a patient's medical problems" (Barrows, 1980, p. 19). Understanding the clinical reasoning process and the factors that can impact it are important to improving diagnosis, given that clinical reasoning processes contribute to diagnostic errors (Croskerry, 2003a; Graber, 2005). Health care professionals involved in the diagnostic process have an obligation and ethical responsibility to employ clinical reasoning skills: "As an expanding body of scholarship further elucidates the causes of medical error, including the considerable extent to which medical errors, particularly in diagnostics, may be attributable to cognitive sources, insufficient progress in systematically evaluating and implementing suggested strategies for improving critical thinking skills and medical judgment is of mounting concern" (Stark and Fins, 2014, p. 386). Clinical reasoning occurs within clinicians' minds (facilitated or impeded by the work system) and involves judgment under uncertainty, with a consideration of possible diagnoses that might explain symptoms and signs, the harms and benefits of diagnostic testing and treatment for each of those diagnoses, and patient preferences and values.

The current understanding of clinical reasoning is based on the dual process theory, a widely accepted paradigm of decision making. The dual process theory integrates analytical and non-analytical models of decision making (see Box 2-4). Analytical models (slow system 2) involve a conscious, deliberate process guided by critical thinking (Kahneman, 2011). Nonanalytical models (fast system 1) involve unconscious, intuitive, and automatic pattern recognition (Kahneman, 2011).

Fast system 1 (nonanalytical, intuitive) automatic processes require very little working memory capacity. They are often triggered by stimuli or result from overlearned associations or implicitly learned activities.[4] Examples of system 1 processes include the ability to recognize human faces (Kanwisher and Yovel, 2006), the diagnosis of Lyme disease from a bull's-eye rash, or decisions based on heuristics (mental shortcuts), intuition, or repeated experiences.

In contrast, slow system 2 (reflective, analytical) processing places a heavy load on working memory and involves hypothetical and counterfactual reasoning (Evans and Stanovich, 2013; Stanovich and Toplak, 2012). System 2 processing requires individuals to generate mental models

---

[4] The term "system 1" is an oversimplification because it is unlikely there is a single cognitive or neural system responsible for all system 1 cognitive processes.

BOX 2-4
Models of Clinical Reasoning

Analytical models (slow system 2). Hypothetico-deductivism is an analytical reasoning model that describes clinical reasoning as hypothesis testing (Elstein et al., 1978, 1990). The steps involved in hypothesis testing include

1. Cue acquisition: Clinicians obtain contextual information by taking a history, performing a physical examination, administering diagnostic tests, or consulting with other clinicians.
2. Hypothesis generation (working diagnoses): Clinicians formulate alternative diagnostic possibilities.
3. Cue interpretation (diagnostic modification and refinement): Clinicians interpret the consistency of the information with each of the alternative hypotheses under consideration.
4. Hypothesis evaluation (diagnostic verification): The data are weighed and combined to evaluate whether one of the working diagnoses can be confirmed. If not, further information gathering, hypothesis generation, interpretation, and evaluation is conducted until verification is achieved (Elstein and Bordage, 1988).

Analytical reasoning models have several additional characteristics. First, the generation of a set of hypotheses that occurs after cue acquisition facilitates the construction of a differential diagnosis, with evidence suggesting that the consideration of potential hypotheses prior to gathering information can improve diagnostic accuracy (Kostopoulou et al., 2015). Second, in order to supplement hypotheses retrieved from memory, some clinicians may employ clinical decision support tools. Third, the evolving list of diagnostic hypotheses determines subsequent information-gathering activities (Kassirer et al., 2010). Fourth, the entire process involves, either explicitly or implicitly, clinicians assigning and updating the probability of each potential diagnosis, given the available data (Kassirer et al., 2010).

These models hold that clinical problem-solving tasks, such as diagnosis, require deliberate, logically sound reasoning by clinicians. Thus, clinical reasoning can be improved by developing the critical thinking skills (Papp et al., 2014). They also imply that clinical reasoning uses the presence or absence of specific signs or symptoms to be evidence that either confirms or disproves a diagnosis. Studies

---

of what should or should not happen in particular situations, in order to test possible actions or to explore alternative causes of events (Stanovich, 2009). Hypothetical thinking occurs when one reasons about what should occur if some condition held: For example, if this patient has diabetes, then the blood sugar level should exceed 126 mg/dl after an 8-hour fast, or if prescribed a diabetes medication, the sugar level should improve. Counterfactual reasoning occurs when one thinks about what should occur if the situation differed from how it actually is. The deliberate,

have shown that clinicians do participate in analytical reasoning (Barrows et al., 1982; Elstein et al., 1978; Neufeld et al., 1981). However, studies also suggest that experience is crucial to the development of expertise and that general problem-solving skills, such as hypothesis testing, cannot account for differences in clinical reasoning skills between experts and novices (Elstein and Schwarz, 2002; Groen and Patel, 1985; Neufeld et al., 1981; Norman, 2005). These findings support a role for nonanalytical models of clinical reasoning and the importance of content knowledge and clinical experience.

Nonanalytical models (fast system 1). Broadly construed through a pattern-recognition framework, nonanalytical models attempt to understand clinical reasoning through human categorization and classification practices. These models suggest that clinicians make diagnoses and choose treatments by matching presenting patients to their mental models of diseases (or information about diseases that is stored in memory). Although the nature of these mental models remain under debate, most assume that they are either exemplars (specific patients seen previously and stored in memory as concrete examples) or prototypes (an abstract disease conceptualization that weighs disease features according to their frequency) (Bordage and Zacks, 1984; Norman, 2005; Rosch and Mervis, 1975; Schmidt et al., 1990; Smith and Medin, 1981, 2002).

Expert pattern matching by experienced clinicians may involve illness scripts, in which elaborated disease knowledge includes enabling conditions or risk factors (e.g., physical contact with the Ebola virus); the pathophysiology of the disease (Ebola virus replication, invasion and destruction of endothelial surfaces); and the signs and symptoms of the disease (bleeding from Ebola) (Boshuizen and Schmidt, 2008). After encountering a patient, a clinician may activate a single illness script or multiple scripts. Illness scripts differ from exemplars and prototypes by having more extensive knowledge stored for each disease. As the diagnostic process evolves, the clinician matches the activated scripts against the presenting signs and symptoms, with the best matching script offered as the most likely diagnosis.

While exemplars, prototypes, and illness scripts are assumed to encode different types of information about disease conditions—that is, actual instances versus typical presentation versus multidimensional information—pattern recognition models assume them to play the same role in diagnosis.

conscious, and reflective nature of both hypothetical and counterfactual reasoning illustrates the analytical nature of system 2.

Heuristics—mental shortcuts or cognitive strategies that are automatically and unconsciously employed—are particularly important for decision making (Gigerenzer and Goldstein, 1996). Heuristics can facilitate decision making but can also lead to errors, especially when patients present with atypical symptoms (Cosmides and Tooby, 1996; Gigerenzer, 2000; Kahneman, 2011; Klein, 1998; Lipshitz et al., 2001; McDonald, 1996).

When a heuristic fails, it is referred to as a cognitive bias. Cognitive biases, or predispositions to think in a way that leads to failures in judgment, can also be caused by affect and motivation (Kahneman, 2011). Prolonged learning in a regular and predictable environment increases the success-fulness of heuristics, whereas uncertain and unpredictable environments are a chief cause of heuristic failure (Kahneman, 2011; Kahneman and Klein, 2009). There are many heuristics and biases that affect clinical rea-soning and decision making (see Table 2-2 for medical and nonmedical examples). Additional examples of heuristics and biases that affect deci-sion making and the potential for diagnostic errors are described below (Croskerry, 2003b):

- The representativeness heuristic answers the question, "how likely is it that this patient has a particular disease?" by assessing how typical the patient's symptoms are for that disease. If the symptoms are highly typical (e.g., fever and nausea after contact with an individual from West Africa with Ebola virus), then it is likely the patient will be diagnosed as having that condition (e.g., Ebola virus infection). The representativeness bias refers to the tendency to make decisions based on a typical case, even when this may lead to an incorrect judgment. The representativeness bias helps to explain why an incorrect diagnosis (e.g., a patient diagnosed as not having Ebola virus infection) is made when presenting symptoms are atypical (e.g., no fever or nausea after contact with a person from West Africa).
- Base-rate neglect describes the tendency to ignore the prevalence of a disease in determining a diagnosis. For example, a clinician may think the diagnosis is acid reflux because it is a prevalent condition, even though it is actually an MI, which can present with similar symptoms (e.g., chest pain), but is less likely.
- The overconfidence bias reflects the universal tendency to believe that we know more than we do. This bias encourages individuals to diagnose a disease based on incomplete information; too much faith is placed in one's opinion rather than on carefully gathering evidence. This bias is especially likely to develop if clinicians do not have feedback on their diagnostic performance.
- Psych-out errors describe the increased susceptibility of people with mental illnesses to clinician biases and heuristics due to their mental health conditions. Patients with mental health issues may have new physical symptoms that are not considered seriously because their clinicians attribute them to their mental health issues. Patients with physical symptoms that mimic men-tal illnesses (hypoxia, delirium, metabolic abnormalities, central

TABLE 2-2 Examples of Heuristics and Biases That Influence Decision Making

Heuristic or Bias	Medical Example	Nonmedical Example
Anchoring is the tendency to lock onto salient features in the patient's initial presentation and failing to adjust this initial impression in the light of later information.	A patient is admitted from the emergency department with a diagnosis of heart failure. The hospitalists who are taking care of the patient do not pay adequate attention to new findings that suggest another diagnosis.	We buy a new car based on excellent reviews and tend to ignore or downplay negative features that are noticed.
Affective bias refers to the various ways that our emotions, feelings, and biases affect judgment.	New complaints from patients known to be "frequent flyers" in the emergency department are not taken seriously.	We may have the belief that people who are poorly dressed are not articulate or intelligent.
Availability bias refers to our tendency to more easily recall things that we have seen recently or things that are common or that impressed us.	A clinician who just recently read an article on the pain from aortic aneurysm dissection may tend toward diagnosing it in the next few patients he sees who present with nonspecific abdominal pain, even though aortic dissections are rare.	Because of a recent news story on a tourist kidnapping in Country "A," we change the destination we have chosen for our vacation to Country "B."
Context errors reflect instances where we misinterpret the situation, leading to an erroneous conclusion.	We tend to interpret that a patient presenting with abdominal pain has a problem involving the gastrointestinal tract, when it may be something else entirely: for example, an endocrine, neurologic or vascular problem.	We see a work colleague picking up two kids from an elementary school and assume he or she has children, when they are instead picking up someone else's children.
Search satisficing, also known as **premature closure**, is the tendency to accept the first answer that comes along that explains the facts at hand, without considering whether there might be a different or better solution.	The emergency department clinician seeing a patient with recent onset of low back pain immediately settles on a diagnosis of lumbar disc disease without considering other possibilities in the differential diagnosis.	We want a plane ticket that costs no more than $1,000 and has no more than one connection. We perform an online search and purchase the first ticket that meets these criteria without looking to see if there is a cheaper flight or one with no connections.

nervous infections, and head injuries) may also be susceptible to these errors.

In addition to cognitive biases, research suggests that fallacies in reasoning, ethical violations, and financial and nonfinancial conflicts of interest can influence medical decision making (Seshia et al., 2014a,b). These factors, collectively referred to as "cognitive biases plus," have been identified as potentially undermining the evidence that informs clinical decision making (Seshia et al., 2014a,b).

The interaction between fast system 1 and slow system 2 remains controversial. Some hold that these processes are constantly occurring in parallel and that any conflicts are resolved as they arise. Others have argued that system 1 processes generate an individual's default response and that system 2 processes may or may not intervene and override system 1 processing (Evans and Stanovich, 2013; Kahneman, 2011). When system 2 overrides system 1, this can lead to improved decision making, because engaging in analytical reasoning may correct for inaccuracies. It is important to note that slow system 2 processing does not guarantee correct decision making. For instance, clinicians with an inadequate knowledge base may not have the information necessary to make a correct decision. There are some instances when system 1 processing is correct, and the override from system 2 can contribute to incorrect decision making. However, when system 1 overrides system 2 processing, this can also result in irrational decision making.

Intervention by system 2 is likely to occur in novel situations when the task at hand is difficult; when an individual has minimal knowledge or experience (Evans and Stanovich, 2013; Kahneman, 2011); or when an individual deliberately employs strategies to overcome known biases (Croskerry et al., 2013). Monitoring and intervention by system 2 on system 1 is unlikely to catch every failure because it is inefficient and would require sustained vigilance, given that system 1 processing often leads to correct solutions (Kahneman, 2011). Factors that affect working memory can impede the ability of system 2 to monitor and, when necessary, intervene on system 1 processes (Croskerry, 2009b). For example, if clinicians are tired or distracted by elements in the work system, they may fail to recognize when a decison provided by system 1 processing needs to be reconsidered (Croskerry, 2009b).

System 1 and system 2 perform optimally in different types of clinical practice settings. System 1 performs best in highly reliable and predictable environments but falls short in uncertain and irregular settings (Kahneman and Klein, 2009; Stanovich, 2009). System 2 performs best in relaxed and unhurried environments.

Dual Process Theory and Diagnosis

This section applies the dual process theory of clinical reasoning to the diagnostic process (Croskerry, 2009a,b; Norman and Eva, 2010; Pelaccia et al., 2011). Croskerry and colleagues provide a framework for understanding the cognitive activities that occur in clinicians as they iterate through information gathering, information integration and interpretation, and determining a working diagnosis (Croskerry et al., 2013) (see Figure 2-2).

When patients present, clinicians gather information and compare that information with their knowledge about various diseases. This can

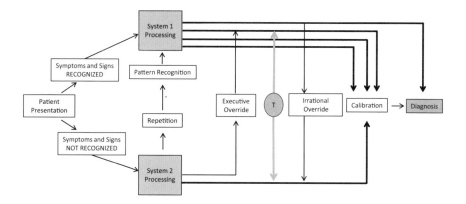

FIGURE 2-2 The dual process model of diagnostic decision making. When a patient presents to a clinician, the initial data include symptoms and signs of disease, which can range from single characteristics of disease to illness scripts. If the symptoms and signs of illness are recognized, system 1 processes are used. If they are not recognized, system 2 processes are used. Repetition of data to system 2 processes may eventually be recognized as a new pattern and subsequently processed through system 1. Multiple arrows stem from system 1 processes to depict intuitive, fast, parallel decision making. Because system 2 processes are slow and serial, only one arrow stems from system 2 processes, depicting analytical decision making. The executive override pathway shows that system 2 surveillance has the potential to overrule system 1 decision making. The irrational override pathway shows the capability for system 1 processes to overrule system 2 analytical decision making. The toggle arrow (T) illustrates how the decision maker may employ both fast system 1 and slow system 2 processes throughout the decision-making process. The manner in which data are processed through system 1 and system 2 determines the calibration of a clinician's diagnostic performance, or a clinician's understanding of his/her diagnostic abilities and limitations.
SOURCE: Adapted by permission from BMJ Publishing Group Limited. Cognitive debiasing 1: Origins of bias and theory of debiasing. P. Croskerry, G. Singhal, and S. Mamede. *BMJ Quality and Safety* 22(Suppl 2):ii58–ii64. 2013.

include comparing a patient's signs and symptoms with clinicians' mental models of diseases (or information about diseases that is stored in memory as exemplars, prototypes, or illness scripts; see Box 2-4). This initial pattern matching is an instance of fast system 1 processing. If a sufficiently unique match occurs, then a diagnosis may be made without involvement of slow system 2.

However, some symptoms or signs may not be recognized or they may trigger mental models for several diseases at once. When this happens, slow system 2 processing may be engaged, and the clinician will continue to gather, integrate, and interpret potentially relevant information until a working diagnosis is generated and communicated to the patient. When this process triggers pattern matches for several mental models of disease, a differential diagnosis is developed. At this point, the diagnostic process shifts to slow system 2 analytical reasoning. Based on their knowledge base, clinicians then use deductive reasoning: If this patient has disease A, what clinical history and physical examination findings might be expected, and does the patient have them? This process is repeated for each condition in the differential diagnosis and may be augmented by additional sources of information, such as diagnostic testing, further history gathering or physical examination, or referral or consultation. The cognitive process of reassessing the probability assigned to each potential diagnosis involves inductive reasoning,[5] or going from observed signs and symptoms to the likelihood of each disease to determine which hypothesis is most likely (Goodman, 1999). This can help refine and narrow the differential diagnosis. Further information gathering activities or treatment could provide greater certainty regarding a working diagnosis or suggest that alternative diagnoses be considered. Throughout this process, clinicians need to communicate with patients about the working diagnosis and the degree of certainty involved.

Task complexity and expertise affect which cognitive system is dominantly employed in the diagnostic process. System 1 processing is more likely to be used when patients present with typical signs and symptoms of disease. However, system 2 processing is likely to intervene in situations marked by novelty and difficulty, when patients present with atypical signs and symptoms, or when clinicians lack expertise (Croskerry, 2009b; Evans and Stanovich, 2013). Novice clinicians and medical students are more likely to rely on analytical reasoning throughout the diagnostic process compared to experienced clinicians (Croskerry, 2009b; Elstein and Schwartz, 2002; Kassirer, 2010; Norman, 2005). Expert clinicians possess better developed mental models of diseases, which support more reliable pattern matching (system 1 processes) (Croskerry, 2009b). As a clinician

---

[5] Inductive reasoning involves probabilistic reasoning (see the following section).

accumulates experience, the repetition of system 2 processing can expand pattern matching possibilities by building and storing in memory mental models for additional diseases that can be triggered by patient signs and symptoms. The ability to create and develop mental models through repetition explains why expert clinicians are more likely to rely on pattern recognition when making diagnoses than are novices—continuous engagement with disease conditions allows the expert to develop more reliable mental models of disease—by retaining more exemplars, creating more nuanced prototypes, or developing more detailed illness scripts.

The way in which information is processed through system 1 and system 2 informs a clinician's subsequent diagnostic performance. Figure 2-3 illustrates the concept of calibration, or the process of a clinician becoming aware of his or her diagnostic abilities and limitations through feedback. Feedback mechanisms—both in educational settings (see Chapter 4) and in learning health care systems (see Chapter 6)—allow

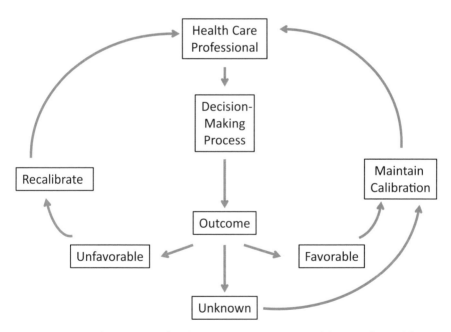

FIGURE 2-3 Calibration in the diagnostic process. Favorable or unfavorable information about a clinician's diagnostic performance provides good feedback and improves clinician calibration. When a patient's diagnostic outcome is unknown, it will be treated as favorable and lead to poor calibration.
SOURCE: Adapted with permission from The feedback sanction. P. Croskerry. *Academic Emergency Medicine* 7(11):1232–1238, 2000.

clinicians to compare their patients' ultimate diagnoses with the diagnoses that they provided to those patients. Calibration enables clinicians to assess their diagnostic accuracy and improve their future performance.

Work system factors influence diagnostic reasoning, including diagnostic team members and tasks, technologies and tools, organizational characteristics, the physical environment, and the external environment. For example, Chapter 6 describes how the physical environment, including lighting, noise, and layout, can influence clinical reasoning. Chapter 5 discusses how health IT can improve or degrade clinical reasoning, depending on the usability of health IT (including clinical decision support), its integration into clinical workflow, and other factors. Box 2-5 describes how certain individual characteristics of diagnostic team members can affect clinical reasoning.

Probabilistic (Bayesian) Reasoning

As described above, the diagnostic process involves initial information gathering that leads to a working diagnosis. The process of ruling in or ruling out a diagnosis involves probabilistic reasoning as findings are integrated and interpreted. Probabilistic (or Bayesian) reasoning provides a formal method to avoid some cognitive biases when integrating and interpreting information. For instance, when patients present with typical symptoms but the disease is rare (e.g., the classic triad of headache, sweating, and rapid heart rate for pheochromocytoma), base rate neglect and the representativeness bias may lead clinicians to overestimate the likelihood of pheochromocytoma among patients presenting with high blood pressure. Using Bayesian reasoning and formally revising probabilities of the various diseases under consideration helps clinicians avoid these errors. Clinicians can then decide whether to pursue additional information gathering or treatment based on an accurate estimate of the likelihood of disease, the harms and benefits of treatment, and patient preferences (Kassirer et al., 2010; Pauker and Kassirer, 1980).

Probabilistic reasoning is most often considered in the context of diagnostic testing, but the presence or absence of specific signs and symptoms can also help to rule in or rule out diseases. The likelihood of a positive finding (the presence of signs or symptoms or a positive test) when disease is present is referred to as sensitivity. The likelihood of a negative finding (the absence of symptoms, signs, or a negative test) when a disease is absent is referred to as specificity. If a sign, symptom, or test is always positive in the presence of a particular disease (100 percent sensitivity), then the absence of that symptom, sign, or test rules out disease (e.g., absence of pain or stiffness means the patient does not have

BOX 2-5
Individual Characteristics That Influence Clinical Reasoning

There are a number of individual characteristics that can affect clinical reasoning, including intelligence and knowledge, age, affect, experience, personality, physical state, and gender.

Intelligence and Knowledge

Intelligence refers to individuals' abilities to engage in high-level cognitive tasks such as reasoning, problem solving, and decision making (Croskerry and Musson, 2009). High scores on intelligence tests indicate that an individual is adept at these cognitive tasks and is more likely to engage system 2 processes to monitor and, when necessary, override system 1 processing (Croskerry and Musson, 2009; Eva, 2002; Evans and Stanovich, 2013). Although intelligence that allows one to monitor and override system 1 processing is important, it rarely suffices by itself for good clinical reasoning. A sufficiently large knowledge base of both biological science and disease conditions is also important. The extent of a clinician's knowledge base depends on memory capacity and training, two factors that can vary among individual clinicians.

Age

It is likely that clinician age has an impact on clinical reasoning abilities (Croskerry and Musson, 2009; Eva, 2002; Singer et al., 2003; Small, 2001). For example, older and more experienced clinicians may be better able to employ system 1 processes in diagnosis, due to well-developed mental models of disease. However, as clinicians age, they tend to have more trouble considering alternatives and switching tasks during the diagnostic process (Croskerry and Musson, 2009; Eva, 2002). Not all individuals experience cognitive or memory decline at the same rate or time though many people start to experience moderate declines in analytical reasoning capacity at some point in their 70s (Croskerry and Musson, 2009).

Affect

Affective factors such as mood and emotional state often play a role (both positive and negative) in clinical reasoning and decision making (Blanchette and Richards, 2009; Croskerry, 2009b; Croskerry et al., 2008; Loewenstein and Lerner, 2003; Slovic and Peters, 2006; Slovic et al., 2002, 2004; Vohs et al., 2007). When an obvious solution to a problem is not present, emotions may help direct people toward an outcome that is better than one that would be produced by random choice (Johnson-Laird and Oatley, 1992; Stanovich, 2009). Decision making guided by one's emotional response to a situation is decision making mediated by the affect heuristic (Slovic et al., 2002).

In cases where precision is important or when an emotional response is unlikely to be a reliable indicator, the affect heuristic can lead to negative consequences. For instance, clinicians may unwittingly allow emotional responses toward their patients to guide their clinical reasoning, even though these feelings are an unreliable indicator of their patients' health problems. In these cases, the

continued

BOX 2-5 Continued

clinicians' reasoning is said to be subject to the affect bias (Croskerry et al., 2008). Affective states such as irritation and stress due to environmental conditions can also affect reasoning, primarily through decreasing the ability of system 2 processes to monitor and override system 1 processes (Croskerry et al., 2008, 2010).

Experience
Novices and experts employ different decision-making practices (Kahneman, 2011). Such differences also occur in the way that expert and novice clinicians reason about their patients' health problems (Eva et al., 2010). Expert nurses, for instance, have been found to collect a wider range of cues than their novice counterparts during clinical decision making (Hoffman et al., 2009). Expert clinicians are more likley to rely on system 1 processing during the diagnostic process, while novice practioners and medical students rely more on conscious, explicit, linear analytical reasoning. Furthermore, expert clinicians are likely to be more accurate than novices when they employ system 1 processes because they have larger stores of developed mental models of disease conditions. While some have argued that experts are more susceptible to premature closure (i.e., accepting a diagnosis before it has been sufficiently verified), there is evidence that experience is more likely to lead to diagnostic flexibility than an explicit metacognitive rule requiring one to "consider alternatives" (Eva and Cunnington, 2006; Eva et al., 2010; McSherry, 1997).

Personality, Physical State, and Gender
Individual personality influences clinical reasoning and decision making (Croskerry and Musson, 2009). Arrogance, for instance, may lead to clinician overconfidence, a personality trait identified as a source of diagnostic error (Berner and Graber, 2008; Croskerry and Norman, 2008). Other personality traits, such as openness to experiences and agreeableness, could improve decision making in some individuals if it increases their openness to divergent views and feedback.
A clinician's physical state can also influence reasoning. Fatigue and sleep deprivation have been found to impede system 2 processing interventions on system 1 processes (Croskerry and Musson, 2009; Zwaan et al., 2009).
Additionally, some research suggests that there are gender-specific effects associated with reasoning, including a male tendency toward risk-taking (Byrnes et al., 1999). Other studies have failed to replicate this proposed gender effect (Croskerry and Musson, 2009).

polymyalgia rheumatica). If a sign, symptom, or test is always negative in the absence of a particular disease (100 percent specificity), then the presence of that symptom, sign, or test rules in disease (e.g., all patients with Kayser–Fleischer rings have Wilson's disease; all patients with Koplik's spots have measles).

However, nearly all signs, symptoms, or test results are neither 100 percent sensitive or specific. For example, studies suggest exceptions for findings such as Kayser–Fleischer rings with other causes of liver disease (Frommer et al., 1977; Lipman and Deutsch, 1990) or Koplik's spots with parvovirus B19 or echovirus (Suringa et al., 1970) and even for Reed-Sternburg cells for Hodgkin's lymphoma (Azar, 1975).

Bayes' theorem provides a framework for clinicians to revise the probability of disease, given disease prevalence, as well as the presence or absence of clinical findings or positive or negative test results (Grimes and Schulz, 2005; Griner et al., 1981; Kassirer et al., 2010; Pauker and Kassirer, 1980). Bayesian calculators are available to facilitate these probability revision analyses (Simel and Rennie, 2008). Box 2-6 works through two examples of probabilistic reasoning. While most clinicians will not formally calculate probabilities, the logical principles behind Bayesian reasoning can help clinicians consider the trade-offs involved in further information gathering, decisions about treatment, or evaluating clinically ambiguous cases (Kassirer et al., 2010). The committee's recommendation on improving diagnostic competencies includes a focus on diagnostic test ordering and subsequent decision making, which relies on the principles of probabilistic reasoning.

BOX 2-6
Examples of Probabilistic (Bayesian) Reasoning

Suppose a clinician considers the possibility of Group A β-hemolytic streptococcus (GABHS) infection in a patient presenting with pharyngitis (sore throat). The absence of nasal congestion occurs in 51 percent of patients with GABHS and in 42 percent of patients without GABHS (Centor et al.,1980). GABHS causes about 10 percent of acute pharyngitis; thus, 90 percent of pharyngitis is not due to GABHS (e.g., viral) (Snow et al., 2001). The likelihood of having GABHS and the absence of nasal congestion is then 5.1 percent (51 percent of 10 percent) and of non-GABHS and the absence of nasal congestion is 37.8 percent (42 percent of 90 percent). Bayesian reasoning then calculates the likelihood of GABHS among those without nasal congestion to be 11.9 percent (5.1 percent divided by [5.1 percent plus 37.8 percent]). The absence of nasal congestion does not help distinguish GABHS from non-GABHS but does illustrate how the absence of a symptom can raise the probability of disease.

However, fever occurs in 24 percent of those with GABHS and 11 percent of those without GABHS (Centor et al., 1980), so 2.9 percent have GABHS without nasal congestion but with fever (11.9 percent with GABHS without nasal congestion times 24 percent), whereas 9.7 percent have non-GABHS without nasal congestion but with fever (88.1 percent with non-GAHBS without nasal conges-

continued

BOX 2-6 Continued

tion times 11 percent). Thus, among patients with an initial 10 percent chance of GABHS, the likelihood of GABHS rises to 23 percent in patients without nasal congestion but with fever (2.9 percent divided by [2.9 percent + 9.7 percent]). Consequently, fever is a distinguishing symptom; if present, it doubles the likelihood of GABHS, and, conversely, its absence would only reduce the likelihood of GABHS to 10.3 percent because it is not a very sensitive symptom (present in only 24 percent of patients with GABHS). The presence of three additional distinguishing symptoms (tonsillar exudates, no cough, and swollen, tender anterior cervical nodes) would raise the likelihood of GABHS to 70 percent, and if those three additional distinguishing symptoms were absent, the likelihood of GABHS would fall to 3 percent (Centor et al., 1980; Snow et al., 2001).

To provide a second example, suppose a woman has a 0.8 percent risk of having breast cancer. Among women with breast cancer, a mammogram will be positive in 90 percent (sensitivity). Among women without breast cancer, a mammogram will be positive in 7 percent (false positive rate or 1 minus a specificity of 93 percent). If the mammogram is positive, what is the likelihood of this woman having breast cancer? Bayes' rule provides the answer. Among 1,000 women, 8 (0.8 percent of 1,000) will have breast cancer and about 7 (90 percent of 8) would have a true positive mammogram. Among the 992 without breast cancer, 69 (7 percent of 992) will have a false positive mammogram. Thus, among the 76 women with a positive mammogram, 7—or 9 percent—will have breast cancer. When a very similar question was presented to practicing physicians with an average of 14 years of experience, their answers ranged from 1 percent to 90 percent, and very few answered correctly (Gigerenzer and Edwards, 2003). Thus, a better understanding of probabilistic reasoning can help clinicians apply signs, symptoms, and test results to subsequent decision making (such as refining or expanding a differential diagnosis, determining the likelihood that a patient has a specific diagnosis on the basis of a positive or negative test result, deciding whether retesting or ordering new tests is appropriate, or beginning treatment) (see Chapter 4).

THE DIAGNOSTIC EVIDENCE BASE AND CLINICAL PRACTICE

Advances in biology and medicine have led to improvements in prevention, diagnosis, and treatment, with a deluge of innovations in diagnostic testing (IOM, 2000, 2013a; Korf and Rehm, 2013; Lee and Levy, 2012). The rising complexity and volume of these advances, coupled with clinician time constraints and cognitive limitations, have outstripped human capacity to apply this new knowledge (IOM, 2011a, 2013a; Marois and Ivanoff, 2005; Miller, 1956; Ostbye et al., 2005; Tombu et al., 2011; Yarnall et al., 2003). The Institute of Medicine report *Best Care Lower Cost: The Path to Continuously Learning Health Care in America* concluded that "diagnostic and treatment options are expanding and changing at an accelerating rate, placing new stresses on clinicians and patients, as well as potentially impacting the effectiveness and efficiency of care delivery" (IOM, 2013a, p. 10). The sheer number of potential diagnoses illustrates this complexity: There are thousands of diseases and related health conditions categorized in the National Library of Medicine's medical subjects headings system and around 13,000 in *International Classification of Diseases, 9th Edition,* with new conditions and diseases added every year (Medicaid.gov, 2015).

With the rapidly increasing number of published scientific articles on health (see Figure 2-4), health care professionals have difficulty keeping up with the breadth and depth of knowledge in their specialties. For example, to remain up to date, primary care clinicians would need to read for an estimated 627.5 hours per month (Alper et al., 2004). McGlynn and colleagues (2003) found that Americans receive only about half of recommended care, including recommended diagnostic processes. Thus, clinicians need approaches to ensure they know the evidence base and are well-equipped to deliver care that reflects the most up-to-date information. One of the ways that this is accomplished is through team-based

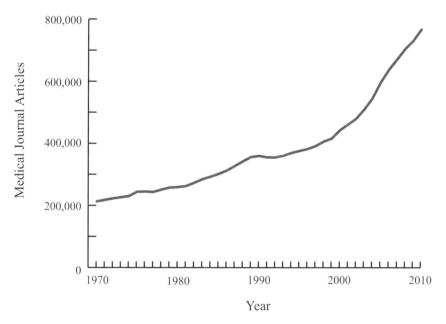

FIGURE 2-4 Number of journal articles published on health care topics per year from 1970 to 2010. Publications have increased steadily over 40 years.
SOURCE: IOM, 2013a.

care; by moving from individuals to teams of health care professionals, patients can benefit from a broader set of resources and expertise to support care (Gittell et al., 2010) (see Chapter 4). In addition, systematic reviews and clinical practice guidelines (CPGs) help synthesize available information in order to inform clinical practice decision making (IOM, 2011a,b).

CPGs came into prominence partly in response to studies that found excessive variation in diagnostic and treatment-related care practices, indicating that inappropriate care was occurring (Chassin et al., 1987; IOM, 1990; Kosecoff et al., 1987; Lin et al., 2008; Song et al., 2010). CPGs are defined as "statements that include recommendations intended to optimize patient care that are informed by a systematic review of the evidence and an assessment of the benefits and harms of alternative care options" (IOM, 2011a, p. 4). CPGs can include diagnostic criteria for specific conditions as well as approaches to information gathering, such as conducting a clinical history and interview, the physical exam, diagnostic testing, and consultations.

CPGs translate knowledge into clinical care decisions, and adherence to evidence-based guideline recommendations can improve health care quality and patient outcomes (Bhatt et al., 2004; IOM, 2011a; Peterson et al., 2006). However, there have been a number of challenges to the development and use of CPGs in clinical practice (IOM, 2011a, 2013a,b; Kahn et al., 2014; Timmermans and Mauck, 2005). Two of the primary challenges are the inadequacy of the evidence base supporting CPGs and determining the applicability of guidelines for individual patients (IOM, 2011a, 2013b). For example, individual patient preferences for possible health outcomes may vary, and with the growing prevalence of chronic disease, patients often have comorbidities or competing causes of mortality that need to be considered. CPGs may not factor in these patient-specific variables (Boyd et al., 2005; Mulley et al., 2012; Tinetti et al., 2004). In addition, the majority of scientific evidence about any diagnostic test typically is focused on test accuracy and not on the impact of the test on patient outcomes (Brozek et al., 2009; Trikalinos et al., 2009). This makes it difficult to develop guidelines that inform clinicians about the role of diagnostic tests within the diagnostic process and about how these tests can influence the path of care and health outcomes for a patient (Gopalakrishna et al., 2014; Hsu et al., 2011). Furthermore, diagnosis is generally not a primary focus of CPGs; diagnostic testing guidelines typically account for a minority of recommendations and often have lower levels of evidence supporting them than treatment-related CPGs (Tricoci et al., 2009). The adoption of available clinical practice guideline recommendations into practice remains suboptimal due to concerns about the trustworthiness of the guidelines as well as the existence of varying and conflicting guidelines (Ferket et al., 2011; Han et al., 2011; IOM, 2011a; Lenzer et al., 2013; Pronovost, 2013).

Health care professional societies have also begun to develop appropriate use or appropriateness criteria as a way of synthesizing the available scientific literature and expert opinion to inform patient-specific decision making (Fitch et al., 2001). With the growth of diagnostic testing and substantial geographic variation in the utilization of these tools (due in part to the limitations in the evidence base supporting their use), health care professional societies have developed appropriate use criteria aimed at better matching patients to specific health care interventions (Allen and Thorwarth, 2014; Patel et al., 2005).

Checklists are another approach that has been implemented to improve the safety of care by, for example, preventing health care–acquired infections or errors in surgical care. Checklists have also been proposed to improve the diagnostic process (Ely et al., 2011; Schiff and Leape, 2012; Sibbald et al., 2013). Developing checklists for the diagnostic process may be a significant undertaking; thus far, checklists have been developed for discrete, observable tasks, but the complexity of the diagnostic process, including the associated cognitive tasks, may represent a fundamentally different type of challenge (Henriksen and Brady, 2013).

REFERENCES

AAFP (American Academy of Family Physicians). 2015. About the AAFP proficiency testing program. www.aafp.org/practice-management/labs/about.html (accessed May 15, 2015).

ACMG (American College of Medical Genetics and Genomics) Board of Directors. 2012. Points to consider in the clinical application in genomic sequencing. *Genetics in Medicine* 14(8):759-761.

ACR (American College of Radiology). 2015a. Accreditation. www.acr.org/quality-safety/accreditation (accessed May 22, 2015).

ACR. 2015b. Quality & safety. www.acr.org/Quality-Safety (accessed May 22, 2015).

Allen, B., and W. T. Thorwarth. 2014. Comments from the American College of Radiology. Input submitted to the Committee on Diagnostic Error in Health Care, November 5 and December 29, 2014, Washington, DC.

Alper, B., J. A. Hand, S. G. Elliott, S. Kinkade, M. J. Hauan, D. K. Onion, and B. M. Sklar. 2004. How much effort is needed to keep up with the literature relevant for primary care? *Journal of the Medical Library Association* 92(4):429–437.

AMA (American Medical Association). 1996. AMA code of ethics. www.ama-assn.org/ama/pub/physician-resources/medical-ethics/code-medical-ethics/opinion8041.page (accessed March 22, 2015).

APA (American Psychiatric Association). 2015. DSM. www.psychiatry.org/practice/dsm (accessed May 13, 2015).

ASCP (American Society for Clinical Pathology). 2014. Patient access to test results. www.ascp.org/Advocacy/Patient-Access-to-Test-Results.html (accessed March 16, 2015).

AvaMedDx. 2013. Introduction to molecular diagnostics: The essentials of diagnostics series. http://advameddx.org/download/files/AdvaMedDx_DxInsights_FINAL(2).pdf (accessed May 22, 2015).

Azar, H. A. 1975. Significance of the Reed-Sternberg cell. *Human Pathology* 6(4):479–484.

Barrows, H. S. 1980. *Problem-based learning: An approach to medical education*: New York: Springer.

Barrows, H. S., G. R. Norman, V. R. Neufeld, and J. W. Feightner. 1982. The clinical reasoning of randomly selected physicians in general medical practice. *Clinical & Investigative Medicine* 5(1):49–55.

Bayer, A. J., J. S. Chadha, R. R. Farag, and M. S. Pathy. 1986. Changing presentation of myocardial infarction with increasing old age. *Journal of the American Geriatrics Society* 34(4):263–266.

Berger, D. 1999. A brief history of medical diagnosis and the birth of the clinical laboratory. Part 4—Fraud and abuse, managed-care, and lab consolidation. *Medical Laboratory Observer* 31(12):38–42.

Berlin, L. 2014. Radiologic errors, past, present and future. *Diagnosis* 1(1):79–84.

Berner, E. S., and M. L. Graber. 2008. Overconfidence as a cause of diagnostic error in medicine. *The American Journal of Medicine* 121(5):S2–S23.

Bhatt, D. L., M. T. Roe, E. D. Peterson, Y. Li, A. Y. Chen, R. A. Harrington, A. B. Greenbaum, P. B. Berger, C. P. Cannon, D. J. Cohen, C. M. Gibson, J. F. Saucedo, N. S. Kleiman, J. S. Hochman, W. E. Boden, R. G. Brindis, W. F. Peacock, S. C. Smith, Jr., C. V. Pollack, Jr., W. B. Gibler, E. M. Ohman, and CRUSADE Investigators. 2004. Utilization of early invasive management strategies for high-risk patients with non-ST-segment elevation acute coronary syndromes: Results from the CRUSADE Quality Improvement Initiative. *JAMA* 292(17):2096–2104.

Blanchette, I., and A. Richards. 2009. The influence of affect on higher level cognition: A review of research on interpretation, judgement, decision making and reasoning. *Cognition and Emotion* 24(4):561–595.

Bluth, E. I., H. Truong, and S. Bansal. 2014. The 2014 ACR Commission on Human Resources Workforce Survey. *Journal of the American College of Radiology* 11(10):948–952.

Bor, J. S. 2015. Among the elderly, many mental illnesses go undiagnosed. *Health Affairs (Millwood)* 34(5):727–731.

Bordage, G., and R. Zacks. 1984. The structure of medical knowledge in the memories of medical students and general practitioners: categories and prototypes. *Medical Education* 18(6):406–416.

Boshuizen, H. P. A., and H. G. Schmidt. 2008. The development of clinical reasoning expertise; Implications for teaching. In J. Higgs, M. Jones, S. Loftus, and N. Christensen (eds.), *Clinical reasoning in the health professions* (pp. 113–121). Oxford: Butterworth Heinemann/Elsevier.

Boyd, C. M., J. Darer, C. Boult, L. P. Fried, L. Boult, and A. W. Wu. 2005. Clinical practice guidelines and quality of care for older patients with multiple comorbid diseases: Implications for pay for performance. *JAMA* 294(6):716–724.

Brozek, J. L., E. A. Akl, R. Jaeschke, D. M. Lang, P. Bossuyt, P. Glasziou, M. Helfand, E. Ueffing, P. Alonso-Coello, J. Meerpohl, B. Phillips, A. R. Horvath, J. Bousquet, G. H. Guyatt, H. J. Schunemann, and G. W. Group. 2009. Grading quality of evidence and strength of recommendations in clinical practice guidelines: Part 2 of 3. The GRADE approach to grading quality of evidence about diagnostic tests and strategies. *Allergy* 64(8):1109–1116.

Byrnes, J. P., D. C. Miller, and W. D. Schafer. 1999. Gender differences in risk taking: A meta-analysis. *Psychological Bulletin* 125(3):367.

Campbell, V.A., J. E. Crews, D. G. Moriarty, M. M. Zack, and D. K. Blackman. 1999. Surveillance for sensory impairment, activity limitation, and health-related quality of life among older adults—United States, 1993–1997. *Morbidity and Mortality Weekly Report* 48(SS08):131–156.

CAP (College of American Pathologists). 2013. Guide to CAP proficiency testing/external quality assurance for international participants. www.cap.org/apps/docs/proficiency_testing/cap_proficiency_testing_guide.pdf (accessed May 15, 2015).

CAP. 2015. Proficiency testing. www.cap.org/web/home/lab/proficiency-testing?_adf.ctrl-state–146u5nip6d_4&_afrLoop=77333689866130 (accessed May 15, 2015).

Carayon, P., A. Schoofs Hundt, B. T. Karsh, A. P. Gurses, C. J. Alvarado, M. Smith, and P. Flatley Brennan. 2006. Work system design for patient safety: The SEIPS model. *Quality & Safety in Health Care* 15(Suppl 1):i50–i58.

Carayon, P., T. B. Wetterneck, A. J. Rivera-Rodriguez, A. S. Hundt, P. Hoonakker, R. Holden, and A. P. Gurses. 2014. Human factors systems approach to healthcare quality and patient safety. *Applied Ergonomics* 45(1):14–25.

CDC (Centers for Disease Control and Prevention). 2008. *Laboratory medicine: A national status report.* Falls Church, VA: The Lewin Group.

CDC. 2010. National hospital ambulatory medical care survey. Hyattsville, MD: Ambulatory and Hospital Care Statistics Branch, National Center for Health Statistics.

CDC. 2014. Clinical Laboratory Improvement Amendments (CLIA). www.cdc.gov/clia (accessed May 15, 2015).

Centor, R. M., J. M. Witherspoon, H. P. Dalton, C. E. Brody, and K. Link. 1980. The diagnosis of strep throat in adults in the emergency room. *Medical decision making: an international journal of the Society for Medical Decision Making* 1(3):239–246.

Chassin, M. R., J. Kosecoff, D. H. Solomon, and R. H. Brook. 1987. How coronary angiography is used: Clinical determinants of appropriateness. *JAMA* 258(18):2543–2547.

CMS (Centers for Medicare & Medicaid Services). 2014. Accreditation organizations/exempt states. www.cms.gov/Regulations-and-Guidance/Legislation/CLIA/Downloads/AOList.pdf (accessed November 3, 2015).

CMS. 2015a. Advanced diagnostic imaging accreditation. www.cms.gov/Medicare/Provider-Enrollment-and-Certification/MedicareProviderSupEnroll/AdvancedDiagnosticImagingAccreditation.html (accessed May 22, 2015).

CMS. 2015b. Clinical Laboratory Improvement Amendments (CLIA). www.cms.gov/Regulations-and-Guidance/Legislation/CLIA/index.html?redirect=/clia (accessed May 15, 2015).

CMS. 2015c. Getting a second opinion before surgery. www.medicare.gov/what-medicare-covers/part-b/second-opinions-before-surgery.html (accessed March 30, 2015).

Cosmides, L., and J. Tooby. 1996. Are humans good intuitive statisticians after all? Rethinking some conclusions from the literature on judgment under uncertainty. *Cognition* 58(1):1–73.

Croskerry, P. 2000. The feedback sanction. *Academic Emergency Medicine* 7(11):1232–1238.

Croskerry, P. 2003a. The Importance of cognitive errors in diagnosis and strategies to minimize them. *Academic Medicine* 78(8):775–780.

Croskerry, P. 2003b. Cognitive forcing strategies in clinical decisionmaking. *Annals of Emergency Medicine* 41(1):110–120.

Croskerry, P. 2009a. Clinical cognition and diagnostic error: Applications of a dual process model of reasoning. *Advances in Health Sciences Education* 14(Suppl 1):27–35.

Croskerry, P. 2009b. A universal model of diagnostic reasoning. *Academic Medicine* 84(8):1022–1028.

Croskerry, P., and D. Musson. 2009. Individual factors in patient safety. In P. Croskerry, K. S. Cosby, S. M. Schenkel, and R. L. Wears (eds.), *Patient Safety in Emergency Medicine* (pp. 269–276). Philadelphia, PA: Lippincott, Williams & Wilkins.

Croskerry, P., and G. Norman. 2008. Overconfidence in clinical decision making. *American Journal of Medicine* 121(5 Suppl):S24–S29.

Croskerry, P., A. A. Abbass, and A. W. Wu. 2008. How doctors feel: affective issues in patients' safety. *Lancet* 372(9645):1205–1206.

Croskerry, P., A. A. Abbass, and A. W. Wu. 2010. Emotional influences in patient safety. *Journal of Patient Safety* 6(4):199–205.

Croskerry, P., G. Singhal, and S. Mamede. 2013. Cognitive debiasing 1: Origins of bias and theory of debiasing. *BMJ Quality and Safety* 22(Suppl 2):ii58–ii64.

Davies, R. H., and B. Rees. 2010. Include "eyeballing" the patient. *BMJ* 340:c291.

Eichbaum, Q., G. S. Booth, and P. S. Young (eds.). 2012. *Transfusion medicine: Quality in laboratory diagnosis*. Edited by M. Laposata. New York: Demos Medical Publishing.

Elstein, A. S., and G. Bordage. 1988. Psychology of clinical reasoning. In J. Dowie and A. Elstein (eds.), *Professional judgment: A reader in clinical decision making* (pp. 109–129). New York: Cambridge University Press.

Elstein, A. S., and A. Schwartz. 2002. Clinical problem solving and diagnostic decision making: Selective review of the cognitive literature. *BMJ* 324(7339):729–732.

Elstein, A. S., L. Shulman, and S. Sprafka. 1978. *Medical problem solving: An analysis of clinical reasoning*. Cambridge, MA: Harvard University Press.

Elstein, A. S., L. S. Shulman, and S. A. Sprafka. 1990. Medical problem solving: A ten-year retrospective. *Evaluation & the Health Professions* 13(1):5–36.

Ely, J. W., M. L. Graber, and P. Croskerry. 2011. Checklists to reduce diagnostic errors. *Academic Medicine* 86(3):307–313.

Emmett, K. R. 1998. Nonspecific and atypical presentation of disease in the older patient. *Geriatrics* 53(2):50–52, 58–60.

Epner, P. L., J. E. Gans, and M. L. Graber. 2013. When diagnostic testing leads to harm: A new outcomes-based approach for laboratory medicine. *BMJ Quality and Safety* 22(Suppl 2):ii6–ii10.

European Society of Radiology. 2010. The future role of radiology in healthcare. *Insights into Imaging* 1(1):2–11.

Eva, K. W. 2002. The aging physician: Changes in cognitive processing and their impact on medical practice. *Academic Medicine* 77(10 Suppl):S1–S6.

Eva, K. W., and J. P. W. Cunnington. 2006. The difficulty with experience: Does practice increase susceptibility to premature closure? *Journal of Continuing Education in the Health Professions* 26(3):192–198.

Eva, K., C. Link, K. Lutfey, and J. McKinlay. 2010. Swapping horses midstream: Factors related to physicians changing their minds about a diagnosis. *Academic Medicine* 85:1112–1117.

Evans, J. P., and M. S. Watson. 2015. Genetic testing and FDA regulation: Overregulation threatens the emergence of genomic medicine. *JAMA* 313(7):669–670.

Evans, J. S. B. T., and K. E. Stanovich. 2013. Dual-process theories of higher cognition: Advancing the debate. *Perspectives on Psychological Science* 8(3):223–241.

FDA (Food and Drug Administration). 2014a. In vitro diagnostics. www.fda.gov/MedicalDevices/ProductsandMedicalProcedures/InVitroDiagnostics/default.htm (accessed May 15, 2015).

FDA. 2014b. Laboratory developed tests. www.fda.gov/MedicalDevices/ProductsandMedicalProcedures/InVitroDiagnostics/ucm407296.htm (accessed May 15, 2015).

Ferket, B. S., T. S. Genders, E. B. Colkesen, J. J. Visser, S. Spronk, E. W. Steyerberg, and M. G. Hunink. 2011. Systematic review of guidelines on imaging of asymptomatic coronary artery disease. *Journal of the American College of Cardiology* 57(15):1591–1600.

Fitch, K., S. J. Bernstein, M. D. Aguilar, B. Burnand, J. R. LaCalle, P. Lazaro, M. v. h. Loo, J. McDonnell, J. Vader, and J. P. Kahan. 2001. The RAND/UCLA appropriateness method user's manual. www.rand.org/pubs/monograph_reports/MR1269 (accessed May 13, 2015).

Flores, G. 2006. Language barriers to health care in the United States. *New England Journal of Medicine* 355(3):229–231.

Frommer, D., J. Morris, S. Sherlock, J. Abrams, and S. Newman. 1977. Kayser-Fleischer-like rings in patients without Wilson's disease. *Gastroenterology* 72(6):1331–1335.

Gandhi, J. S. 2000. Re: William Osler: A life in medicine: Book review. *BMJ* 321:1087.

Gawande, A. 2015. Overkill. *The New Yorker*, May 11. www.newyorker.com/magazine/2015/05/11/overkill-atul-gawande (accessed July 13, 2015).

Gigerenzer, G. 2000. *Adaptive thinking: Rationality in the real world*. New York: Oxford University Press.

Gigerenzer, G. 2013. HIV screening: Helping clinicians make sense of test results to patients. *BMJ* 347:f5151.

Gigerenzer, G., and A. Edwards. 2003. Simple tools for understanding risks: From innumeracy to insight. *BMJ* 327(7417):741–744.

Gigerenzer, G., and D. G. Goldstein. 1996. Reasoning the fast and frugal way: Models of bounded rationality. *Psychology Review* 103:650–669.

Gittell, J. H., R. Seidner, and J. Wimbush. 2010. A relational model of how high-performance work systems work. *Organization Science* 21(2):490–506.

Goodman, S. N. 1999. Toward evidence-based medical statistics. 1: The P value fallacy. *Annals of Internal Medicine* 130(12):995–1004.

Gopalakrishna, G., R. A. Mustafa, C. Davenport, R. J. P. M. Scholten, C. Hyde, J. Brozek, H. J. Schunemann, P. M. M. Bossuyt, M. M. G. Leeflang, and M. W. Langendam. 2014. Applying Grading of Recommendations Assessment, Development and Evaluation (GRADE) to diagnostic tests was challenging but doable. *Journal of Clinical Epidemiology* 67(7):760–768.

Govern, P. 2013. Diagnostic management efforts thrive on teamwork. *Vanderbilt University Medical Center Reporter*, March 7. http://news.vanderbilt.edu/2013/03/diagnostic-management-efforts-thrive-on-teamwork (accessed February 11, 2015).

Graber, M. L. 2005. Diagnostic error in internal medicine. *Archives of Internal Medicine* 165(13):1493–1499.

Gray-Miceli, D. 2008. *Modification of assessment and atypical presentation in older adults with complex illness*. New York: The John A. Hartford Foundation Institute for Geriatric Nursing.

Grimes, D. A., and K. F. Schulz. 2005. Refining clinical diagnosis with likelihood ratios. *Lancet* 365(9469):1500–1505.

Griner, P. F., R. J. Mayewski, A. I. Mushlin, and P. Greenland. 1981. Selection and interpretation of diagnostic tests and procedures: Principles and applications. *Annals of Internal Medicine* 94(4 Pt 2):557–592.

Groen, G. J., and V. L. Patel. 1985. Medical problem-solving: Some questionable assumptions. *Medical Education* 19(2):95–100.

Gunderman, R. B. 2005. The medical community's changing vision of the patient: The importance of radiology. *Radiology* 234(2):339–342.

Han, P. K., C. N. Klabunde, N. Breen, G. Yuan, A. Grauman, W. W. Davis, and S. H. Taplin. 2011. Multiple clinical practice guidelines for breast and cervical cancer screening: perceptions of U.S. primary care physicians. *Medical Care* 49(2):139–148.

Hendee, W. R., G. J. Becker, J. P. Borgstede, J. Bosma, W. J. Casarella, B. A. Erickson, C. D. Maynard, J. H. Thrall, and P. E. Wallner. 2010. Addressing overutilization in medical imaging. *Radiology* 257(1):240–245.

Henriksen, K., and J. Brady. 2013. The pursuit of better diagnostic performance: A human factors perspective. *BMJ Quality and Safety* 22(Suppl 2):ii1–ii5.

HFAP (Healthcare Facilities Accreditation Program). 2015. Notice of HFAP approval by CMS. www.hfap.org/AccreditationPrograms/LabsCMS.aspx (accessed May 15, 2015).

Hickner, J., P. J. Thompson, T. Wilkinson, P. Epner, M. Shaheen, A. M. Pollock, J. Lee, C. C. Duke, B. R. Jackson, and J. R. Taylor. 2014. Primary care physicians' challenges in ordering clinical laboratory tests and interpreting results. *Journal of the American Board of Family Medicine* 27(2):268–274.

Hoffman, K. A., L. M. Aitken, and C. Duffield. 2009. A comparison of novice and expert nurses' cue collection during clinical decision-making: Verbal protocol analysis. *International Journal of Nursing Studies* 46(10):1335–1344.

Hollensead, S. C., W. B. Lockwood, and R. J. Elin. 2004. Errors in pathology and laboratory medicine: Consequences and prevention. *Journal of Surgical Oncology* 88(3):161–181.

Holmboe, E. S., and S. J. Durning. 2014. Assessing clinical reasoning: Moving from in vitro to in vivo. *Diagnosis* 1(1):111–117.

Hope, C., N. Estrada, C. Weir, C. C. Teng, K. Damal, and B. C. Sauer. 2014. Documentation of delirium in the VA electronic health record. *BMC Research Notes* 7:208.

Hricak, H. 2011. Oncologic imaging: A guiding hand of personalized cancer care. *Radiology* 259(3):633–640.

Hsu, J., J. L. Brozek, L. Terracciano, J. Kreis, E. Compalati, A. T. Stein, A. Fiocchi, and H. J. Schunemann. 2011. Application of GRADE: Making evidence-based recommendations about diagnostic tests in clinical practice guidelines. *Implementation Science* 6:62.

IMV. 2014. Ready for replacement? New IMV survey finds aging MRI scanner installed base. www.imvinfo.com/user/documents/content_documents/abt_prs/2014_02_03_16_51_22_809_IMV_MR_Outlook_Press_Release_Jan_2014.pdf (accessed May 3, 2015).

IOM (Institute of Medicine). 1990. *Clinical practice guidelines: Directions for a new program.* Washington, DC: National Academy Press.

IOM. 2000. *Medicare laboratory payment policy: Now and in the future.* Washington, DC: National Academy Press.

IOM. 2003. *Unequal treatment: Confronting racial and ethnic disparties in health care.* Washington, DC: The National Academies Press.

IOM. 2005. *Improving breast imaging quality standards.* Washington, DC: The National Academies Press.

IOM. 2007. *Cancer biomarkers: The promises and challenges of improving detection and treatment.* Washington, DC: The National Academies Press.

IOM. 2008. *Retooling for an aging America: Building the health care workforce.* Washington, DC: The National Academies Press.

IOM. 2010. *Evaluation of biomarkers and surrogate endpoints in chronic disease.* Washington, DC: The National Academies Press.

IOM. 2011a. *Clinical practice guidelines we can trust.* Washington, DC: The National Academies Press.

IOM. 2011b. *Finding what works in health care: Standards for systematic reviews.* Washington, DC: The National Academies Press.

IOM. 2012. *Evolution of translational omics: Lessons learned and the path forward.* Washington, DC: The National Academies Press.

IOM. 2013a. *Best care at lower cost: The path to continuously learning health care in America.* Washington, DC: The National Academies Press.

IOM. 2013b. *Delivering high-quality cancer care: Charting a new course for a system in crisis.* Washington, DC: The National Academies Press.

IOM. 2015a. *Improving genetics education in graduate and continuing health professional education: Workshop summary.* Washington, DC: The National Academies Press.

IOM. 2015b. *Policy issues in the clinical development and use of biomarkers for molecularly targeted therapies.* www.iom.edu/Activities/Research/BiomarkersforMolecularlyTargeted Therapies.aspx (accessed May 22, 2015).

Jameson, J. L., and D. L. Longo. 2015. Precision medicine—Personalized, problematic, and promising. *New England Journal of Medicine* 372(23):2229–2234.

Jarrett, P. G., K. Rockwood, D. Carver, P. Stolee, and S. Cosway. 1995. Illness presentation in elderly patients. *Archives of Internal Medicine* 155(10):1060–1064.

Johansen Taber, K. A., B. D. Dickinson, and M. Wilson. 2014. The promise and challenges of next-generation genome sequencing for clinical care. *JAMA Internal Medicine* 174(2):275–280.

Johnson-Laird, P. N., and K. Oatley. 1992. Basic emotions, rationality, and folk theory. *Cognition & Emotion* 6(3–4):201–223.

The Joint Commission. 2007. "What did the doctor say?" Improving health literacy to protect patient safety. www.jointcommission.org/What_Did_the_Doctor_Say/default. aspx (accessed May 11, 2015).

The Joint Commission. 2015. Eligibility for laboratory accreditation. www.jointcommission. org/eligibility_for_laboratory_accreditation/default.aspx (accessed May 15, 2015).

Jutel, A. 2009. Sociology of diagnosis: A preliminary review. *Sociology of Health and Illness* 31(2):278–299.

Kahn, J. M., M. K. Gould, J. A. Krishnan, K. C. Wilson, D. H. Au, C. R. Cooke, I. S. Douglas, L. C. Feemster, R. A. Mularski, C. G. Slatore, and R. S. Wiener. 2014. An official American thoracic society workshop report: Developing performance measures from clinical practice guidelines. *Annals of the American Thoracic Society* 11(4):S186–S195.

Kahneman, D. 2011. *Thinking, fast and slow.* New York: Farrar, Straus and Giroux.

Kahneman, D., and G. Klein. 2009. Conditions for intuitive expertise: A failure to disagree. *American Psychologist* 64(6):515–526.

Kanwisher, N., and G. Yovel. 2006. The fusiform face area: A cortical region specialized for the perception of faces. *Philosophical Transactions of the Royal Society B: Biological Sciences* 361(1476):2109–2128.

Kassirer, J. P. 1989. Our stubborn quest for diagnostic certainty. A cause of excessive testing. *New England Journal of Medicine* 320(22):1489–1491.

Kassirer, J. P. 2010. Teaching clinical reasoning: Case-based and coached. *Academic Medicine* 85(7):1118–1124.

Kassirer, J. P. 2014. Imperatives, expediency, and the new diagnosis. *Diagnosis* 1(1):11–12.

Kassirer, J. P., J. Wong, and R. Kopelman. 2010. *Learning clinical reasoning.* Baltimore: Williams & Wilkins.

Kent, D. M., and R. A. Hayward. 2007. Limitations of applying summary results of clinical trials to individual patients: The need for risk stratification. *JAMA* 298(10):1209–1212.

Klein, G. 1998. *Sources of power: How people make decisions.* Cambridge, MA: MIT Press.

Kleinman, S., M. P. Busch, L. Hall, R. Thomson, S. Glynn, D. Gallahan, H. E. Ownby, and A. E. Williams. 1998. False-positive HIV-1 test results in a low-risk screening setting of voluntary blood donation: Retrovirus Epidemiology Donor Study. *JAMA* 280(12):1080–1085.

Korf, B. R., and H. L. Rehm. 2013. New approaches to molecular diagnosis. *JAMA* 309(14):1511–1521.

Kosecoff, J., M. R. Chassin, A. Fink, M. F. Flynn, L. McCloskey, B. J. Genovese, C. Oken, D. H. Solomon, and R. H. Brook. 1987. Obtaining clinical data on the appropriateness of medical care in community practice. *JAMA* 258(18):2538–2542.

Kostopoulou, O., A. Rosen, T. Round, E. Wright, A. Douiri, and B. Delaney. 2015. Early diagnostic suggestions improve accuracy of GPs: A randomised controlled trial using computer-simulated patients. *British Journal of General Practice* 65(630):e49–e54.

Krupinski, E. A., K. S. Berbaum, R. T. Caldwell, K. M. Schartz, M. T. Madsen, and D. J. Kramer. 2012. Do long radiology workdays affect nodule detection in dynamic CT interpretation? *Journal of the American College of Radiology* 9(3):191–198.

Kugler, J., and A. Verghese. 2010. The physical exam and other forms of fiction. *Journal of General Internal Medicine* 25(8):756–757.

Laposata, M. 2010. *Coagulation disorders: Quality in laboratory diagnosis.* New York: Demos Medical Publishing.

Laposata, M., and A. Dighe. 2007. "Pre-pre" and "post-post" analytical error: High-incidence patient safety hazards involving the clinical laboratory. *Clinical Chemistry and Laboratory Medicine* 45(6):712–719.

Lee, D. W., and F. Levy. 2012.The sharp slowdown in growth of medical imaging: an early analysis suggests combination of policies was the cause. *Health Affairs (Millwood)* 31(8):1876–1884.

Lenzer, J., J. R. Hoffman, C. D. Furberg, and J. P. Ioannidis, on behalf of the Guideline Panel Review Working Group. 2013. Ensuring the integrity of clinical practice guidelines: A tool for protecting patients. *BMJ* 347:f5535.

Lichstein P. R. 1990. The medical interview. In H. K. Walker, W. D. Hall, and J. W. Hurst (eds.), *Clinical Methods: The History, Physical, and Laboratory Examinations, 3rd edition.* Boston: Butterworths.

Lin, G. A., R. A. Dudley, F. L. Lucas, D. J. Malenka, E. Vittinghoff, and R. F. Redberg. 2008. Frequency of stress testing to document ischemia prior to elective percutaneous coronary intervention. *JAMA* 300(15):1765–1773.

Lipman, R. M., and T. A. Deutsch. 1990. A yellow-green posterior limbal ring in a patient who does not have Wilson's disease. *Archives of Ophthalmology* 108(10):1385.

Lipshitz, R., G. Klein, J. Orasanu, and E. Salas. 2001. Taking stock of naturalistic decision making. *Journal of Behavioral Decision Making* 14(5):331–352.

Loewenstein, G., and J. S. Lerner. 2003. The role of affect in decision making. In R. J. Davidson, K. R. Scherer, and H. H. Goldsmith (eds.), *Handbook of affective sciences* (pp. 619–642). New York: Oxford University Press.

Lundberg, G. D. 1981. Acting on significant laboratory results. *JAMA* 245(17):1762–1763.

Marois, R., and J. Ivanoff. 2005. Capacity limits of information processing in the brain. *Trends in Cognitive Sciences* 9(6):296–305.

McDonald, C. J. 1996. Medical heuristics: the silent adjudicators of clinical practice. *Annals of Internal Medicine* 124(1 Pt 1):56–62.

McGlynn, E. A., S. M. Asch, J. Adams, J. Keesey, J. Hicks, A. DeCristofaro, and E. A. Kerr. 2003. The quality of health care delivered to adults in the United States. *New England Journal of Medicine* 348(26):2635–2645.

McSherry, D. 1997. Avoiding premature closure in sequential diagnosis. *Artificial Intelligence in Medicine* 10(3):269–283.

Medicaid.gov. 2015. ICD-10 Changes from ICD-9. www.medicaid.gov/Medicaid-CHIP-Program-Information/By-Topics/Data-and-Systems/ICD-Coding/ICD-10-Changes-from-ICD-9.html (accessed June 23, 2015).

Meyer, F., and T. D. Meyer. 2009. The misdiagnosis of bipolar disorder as a psychotic disorder: Some of its causes and their influence on therapy. *Journal of Affective Disorders* 112(1–3):174–183.

Miller, G. A. 1956. The magical number seven plus or minus two: Some limits on our capacity for processing information. *Psychological Review* 63(2):81–97.

Moroff, S. V., and S. G. Pauker. 1983. What to do when the patient outlives the literature. *Medical Decision Making.* 3(3):313–338.

Mouton, C. P., O. V. Bazaldua, B. Pierce, and D. V. Espino. 2001. Common infections in older adults. *American Family Physician* 63(2):257–268.

Mulley, A. G., C. Trimble, and G. Elwyn. 2012. Stop the silent misdiagnosis: Patients' preferences matter. *BMJ* 345:e6572.

National Stroke Association. 2015. Act FAST. www.stroke.org/understand-stroke/recognizing-stroke/act-fast (accessed May 14, 2015).

Nelson, C., S. Hojvat, B. Johnson, J. Petersen, M. Schriefer, C. B. Beard, L. Petersen, and P. Mead. 2014. Concerns regarding a new culture method for Borrelia burgdorferi not approved for the diagnosis of Lyme disease. *Morbidity and Mortality Weekly Report* 63(15):333.

Neufeld, V., G. Norman, J. Feightner, and H. Barrows. 1981. Clinical problem-solving by medical students: A cross-sectional and longitudinal analysis. *Medical Education* 15(5):315–322.

NIA (National Institute on Aging). 2008. *A clinician's handbook: Talking with your older patient.* Bethesda, MD: National Institutes of Health.

Nichols, J. H., and C. A. Rauch (eds.). 2013. *Clinical chemistry.* New York: Demos Medical Publishing.

NIH (National Institutes of Health). 2015. Precision Medicine Initiative. www.nih.gov/precisionmedicine (accessed May 22, 2015).

Norman, G. R. 2005. Research in clinical reasoning: Past history and current trends. *Medical Education* 39(4):418–427.

Norman, G. R., and K. W. Eva. 2010. Diagnostic error and clinical reasoning. *Medical Education* 44(1):94–100.

Ostbye, T., K. S. Yarnall, K. M. Krause, K. I. Pollak, M. Gradison, and J. L. Michener. 2005. Is there time for management of patients with chronic diseases in primary care? *Annals of Family Medicine* 3(3):209–214.

PAF (Patient Advocate Foundation). 2012. *Second opinions.* www.patientadvocate.org/help.php/index.php?p=691 (accessed March 30, 2015).

Papp, K. K., G. C. Huang, L. M. Lauzon Clabo, D. Delva, M. Fischer, L. Konopasek, R. M. Schwartzstein, and M. Gusic. 2014. Milestones of critical thinking: A developmental model for medicine and nursing. *Academic Medicine* 89(5):715–720.

Parasuraman, R., T. B. Sheridan, and C. D. Wickens. 2000. A model for types and levels of human interaction with automation. *IEEE Transactions on Systems, Man and Cybernetics—Part A: Systems and Humans* 30(3):286–297.

Patel, M. R., J. A. Spertus, R. G. Brindis, R. C. Hendel, P. S. Douglas, E. D. Peterson, M. J. Wolk, J. M. Allen, and I. E. Raskin. 2005. ACCF proposed method for evaluating the appropriateness of cardiovascular imaging. *Journal of the American College of Cardiology* 46(8):1606–1613.

Pauker, S. G., and J. P. Kassirer. 1975. Therapeutic decision making: A cost-benefit analysis. *New England Journal of Medicine* 293(5):229–234.

Pauker, S. G., and J. P. Kassirer. 1980. The threshold approach to clinical decision making. *New England Journal of Medicine* 302(20):1109–1117.

Pelaccia, T., J. Tardif, E. Triby, and B. Charlin. 2011. An analysis of clinical reasoning through a recent and comprehensive approach: The dual-process theory. *Medical Education Online* March 14:16.

Peterson, E. D., M. T. Roe, J. Mulgund, E. R. DeLong, B. L. Lytle, R. G. Brindis, S. C. Smith, Jr., C. V. Pollack, Jr., L. K. Newby, R. A. Harrington, W. B. Gibler, and E. M. Ohman. 2006. Association between hospital process performance and outcomes among patients with acute coronary syndromes. *JAMA* 295(16):1912–1920.

Pincus, H. 2014. Diagnostic error: Issues in behavioral health. Presentation to the Committee on Diagnostic Error in Health Care, November 6, 2014, Washington, DC.

Plebani, M., and G. Lippi. 2011. Closing the brain-to-brain loop in laboratory testing. *Clinical Chemistry and Laboratory Medicine* 49(7):1131–1133.

Plebani, M., M. Laposata, and G. D. Lundberg. 2011. The brain-to-brain loop concept for laboratory testing 40 years after its introduction. *American Journal of Clinical Pathology* 136(6):829–833.

Pope, J. H., T. P. Aufderheide, R. Ruthazer, R. H. Woolard, J. A. Feldman, J. R. Beshansky, J. L. Griffith, and H. P. Selker. 2000. Missed diagnoses of acute cardiac ischemia in the emergency department. *New England Journal of Medicine* 342(16):1163–1170.

Porter, M. E. 2010. What is value in health care? *New England Journal of Medicine* 363(26):2477–2481.

Pronovost, P. J. 2013. Enhancing physicians' use of clinical guidelines. *JAMA* 310(23):2501–2502.

Qureshi, A. M., L. McDonald, and W. R. Primrose. 2000. Management of myocardial infarction in the very elderly—Impact of clinical effectiveness on practice. *Scottish Medical Journal* 45(6):180–182.

Reeves, R. R., J. D. Parker, R. S. Burke, and R. H. Hart. 2010. Inappropriate psychiatric admission of elderly patients with unrecognized delirium. *Southern Medical Journal* 103(2):111–115.

Rich, M. W. 2006. Epidemiology, clinical features, and prognosis of acute myocardial infarction in the elderly. *American Journal of Geriatric Cardiology* 15(1):7–11; quiz 12.

Rosch, E., and C. B. Mervis. 1975. Family resemblances: Studies in the internal structure of categories. *Cognitive Psychology* 7(4):573–605.

Rosenberg, C. E. 2002. The tyranny of diagnosis: Specific entities and individual experience. *Milbank Quarterly* 80(2):237–260.

RSNA (Radiological Society of North America). 2015. *QI tools*. www.rsna.org/QI_Tools.aspx (accessed May 22, 2015).

SAMHSA (Substance Abuse and Mental Health Services Administration) and HRSA (Health Resources and Services Administration). 2015. Screening tools. www.integration.samhsa.gov/clinical-practice/screening-tools (accessed May 22, 2015).

Sarter, N. 2014. Use(r)-centered design of health IT: Challenges and lessons learned. Presentation to the Committee on Diagnostic Error in Health Care, August, 7, 2014, Washington, DC.

Schiff, G. D., and L. L. Leape. 2012. Commentary: How can we make diagnosis safer? *Academic Medicine* 87(2):135–138.

Schmidt, H. G., G. R. Norman, and H. P. A. Boshuizen. 1990. A cognitive perspective on medical expertise: Theory and implications. *Academic Medicine* 65:611–621.

Schulman, K. A., J. A. Berlin, W. Harless, J. F. Kerner, S. Sistrunk, B. J. Gersh, R. Dube, C. K. Taleghani, J. E. Burke, S. Williams, J. M. Eisenberg, and J. J. Escarce. 1999. The effect of race and sex on physicians' recommendations for cardiac catheterization. *New England Journal of Medicine* 340(8):618–626.

Schwartz, L. H., D. M. Panicek, A. R. Berk, Y. Li, and H. Hricak. 2011. Improving communication of diagnostic radiology findings through structured reporting. *Radiology* 260(1):174–181.

Seshia, S. S., M. Makhinson, D. F. Phillips, and G. B. Young. 2014a. Evidence-informed person-centered healthcare (part I): Do "cognitive biases plus" at organizational levels influence quality of evidence? *Journal of Evaluation in Clinical Practice* 20(6):734–747.

Seshia, S. S., M. Makhinson, and G. B. Young. 2014b. Evidence-informed person-centered health care (part II): Are "cognitive biases plus" underlying the EBM paradigm responsible for undermining the quality of evidence? *Journal of Evaluation in Clinical Practice* 20(6):748–758.

Sharfstein, J. 2015. FDA regulation of laboratory-developed diagnostic tests: Protect the public, advance the science. *JAMA* 313(7):667–668.

Sibbald, M., A. B. de Bruin, and J. J. van Merrienboer. 2013. Checklists improve experts' diagnostic decisions. *Medical Education* 47(3):301–308.

Simel, D., and D. Rennie. 2008. *The rational clinical examination: Evidence-based clinical diagnosis.* McGraw-Hill Professional.

Singer, T., P. Verhaeghen, P. Ghisletta, U. Lindenberger, and P. B. Baltes. 2003. The fate of cognition in very old age: Six-year longitudinal findings in the Berlin Aging Study (BASE). *Psychology and Aging* 18(2):318–331.

Slovic, P., and E. Peters. 2006. Risk perception and affect. *Current Directions in Psychological Science* 15(6):322–325.

Slovic, P., M. L. Finucane, E. Peters, and D. G. MacGregor. 2002. Rational actors or rational fools: Implications of the affect heuristic for behavioral economics. *Journal of Socio-Economics* 31(4):329–342.

Slovic, P., M. L. Finucane, E. Peters, and D. G. MacGregor. 2004. Risk as analysis and risk as feelings: Some thoughts about affect, reason, risk, and rationality. *Risk Analysis* 24(2):311–322.

Small, S. A. 2001. Age-related memory decline: Current concepts and future directions. *Archives of Neurology* 58(3):360–364.

Smith, E. E., and D. L. Medin. 1981. *Categories and concepts.* Cambridge, MA: Harvard University Press.

Smith, E. E., and D. L. Medin. 2002. The exemplar view. In D. J. Levitin (ed.), *Foundations of cognitive psychology: Core readings* (pp. 277–292). Cambridge, MA: Bradford.

Smith, M. B., and P. C. Sainfort. 1989. A balance theory of job design for stress reduction. *International Journal of Industrial Ergonomics* 4(1):67–79.

Snow, V., C. Mottur-Pilson, R. J. Cooper, and J. R. Hoffman. 2001. Principles of appropriate antibiotic use for acute pharyngitis in adults. *Annals of Internal Medicine* 134(6):506–508.

Song, Y., J. Skinner, J. Bynum, J. Sutherland, J. E. Wennberg, and E. S. Fisher. 2010. Regional variations in diagnostic practices. *New England Journal of Medicine* 363(1):45–53.

Sox, H. C., Jr. 1986. Probability theory in the use of diagnostic tests. An introduction to critical study of the literature. *Annals of Internal Medicine* 104(1):60–66.

Stanford Medicine 25 Team. 2015. Stanford medicine 25. http://stanfordmedicine25.stanford.edu/about (accessed July 27, 2015).

Stanovich, K. E. 2009. *Decision making and rationality in the modern world.* New York: Oxford.

Stanovich, K. E., and M. E. Toplak. 2012. Defining features versus incidental correlates of Type 1 and Type 2 processing. *Mind & Society* 11(1):3–13.

Stark, M., and J. J. Fins. 2014. The ethical imperative to think about thinking—Diagnostics, metacognition, and medical professionalism. *Cambridge Quarterly of Healthcare Ethics* 23(4):386–396.

Stratton, C. W. 2011. *Clinical microbiology: Quality in laboratory diagnosis.* New York: Demos Medical Publishing.

Suringa, D. W. R, L. J. Bank, and A. B. Ackerman. 1970. Role of measles virus in skin lesions and Koplik's spots. *New England Journal of Medicine* 283(21):1139–1142.

Timbie, J. W., P. S. Hussey, L. F. Burgette, N. S. Wenger, A. Rastegar, I. Brantely, D. Khodyakov, K. J. Leuschner, B. A. Weidmer, and K. L. Kahn. 2014. *Medicare imaging demonstration final evaluation: Report to Congress*. Santa Monica, CA: RAND.

Timmermans, S., and A. Mauck. 2005. The promises and pitfalls of evidence-based medicine. *Health Affairs (Millwood)* 24(1):18–28.

Tinetti, M. E., S. T. Bogardus, Jr., and J. V. Agostini. 2004. Potential pitfalls of disease-specific guidelines for patients with multiple conditions. *New England Journal of Medicine* 351(27):2870–2874.

Tombu, M. N., C. L. Asplund, P. E. Dux, D. Godwin, J. W. Martin, and R. Marois. 2011. A unified attentional bottleneck in the human brain. *Proceedings of the National Academies of Sciences of the United States of America* 108(33):13426–13431.

Tricoci, P., J. M. Allen, J. M. Kramer, R. M. Califf, and S. C. Smith, Jr. 2009. Scientific evidence underlying the ACC/AHA clinical practice guidelines. *JAMA* 301(8):831–841. [Erratum appears in *JAMA*, 2009, 301(15):1544].

Trikalinos, T. A., U. Siebert, and J. Lau. 2009. Decision-analytic modeling to evaluate benefits and harms of medical tests: Uses and limitations. *Medical Decision Making* 29(5):E22–E29.

Verghese, A. 2011. Treat the patient, not the CT scan. *The New York Times*, February 26. www.nytimes.com/2011/02/27/opinion/27verghese.html (accessed August 5, 2015).

Verghese, A., and R. I. Horwitz. 2009. In praise of the physical examination. *BMJ* 339:b5448.

Verghese, A., E. Brady, C. C. Kapur, and R. I. Horwitz. 2011. The bedside evaluation: ritual and reason. *Annals of Internal Medicine* 155(8):550–553.

Vohs, K. D., R. F. Baumeister, and G. Loewenstein. 2007. *Do emotions help or hurt decision making? A hedgefoxian perspective*. New York: Russell Sage Foundation.

Welch, H. G. 2015. *Less medicine more health: 7 assumptions that drive too much medical care*. Boston, MA: Beacon Press.

WHO (World Health Organization). 2012. *International classification of diseases (ICD)*. Geneva: World Health Organization.

Whiting, P., A. W. S. Rutjes, J. B. Reltsma, A. S. Glas, P. M. M. Bossuyt, and J. Kleljnen. 2004. Sources of variation and bias in studies of diagnostic accuracy. *Annals of Internal Medicine* 140(3):189–202.

Yarnall, K. S., K. I. Pollak, T. Ostbye, K. M. Krause, and J. L. Michener. 2003. Primary care: Is there enough time for prevention? *American Journal of Public Health* 93(4):635–641.

Zhi, M., E. L. Ding, J. Theisen–Toupal, J. Whelan, and R. Arnaout. 2013. The landscape of inappropriate laboratory testing: A 15-year meta-analysis. *PLoS ONE* 8(11):e78962.

Zwaan, L., and H. Singh. 2015. The challenges in defining and measuring diagnostic error. *Diagnosis* 2(2):97–103.

Zwaan, L., A. Thijs, C. Wagner, G. van der Wal, and D. R. Timmermans. 2009. Design of a study on suboptimal cognitive acts in the diagnostic process, the effect on patient outcomes and the influence of workload, fatigue and experience of physician. *BMC Health Services Research* 9:65.

3

Overview of Diagnostic Error in Health Care

This chapter explains the committee's definition of diagnostic error, describes the committee's approach to measurement, and reviews the available information about the epidemiology of diagnostic error. The committee proposes five purposes for measurement: to establish the incidence and nature of the problem of diagnostic error; to determine the causes and risks of diagnostic error; to evaluate interventions; for education and training purposes; and for accountability purposes. Because diagnostic errors have been a very challenging area for measurement, the current focus of measurement efforts has been on understanding the incidence and nature of diagnostic error and determining the causes and risks of diagnostic error. The committee highlighted the way in which various measurement approaches could be applied to develop a more robust understanding of the epidemiology of diagnostic error and the reasons that these errors occur.

DEFINITION OF DIAGNOSTIC ERROR

The Institute of Medicine (IOM) has defined quality of care as "the degree to which health services for individuals and populations increase the likelihood of desired health outcomes and are consistent with current professional knowledge" (IOM, 1990, p. 5). The IOM's report *Crossing the Quality Chasm* further elaborated on high-quality care by identifying six aims of quality: "[H]ealth care should be (1) safe—avoiding injuries to patients from the care that is intended to help them; (2) effective—providing services based on scientific knowledge to all who could benefit and refraining from providing services to those not likely to benefit; (3) patient-centered—providing care that is respectful of and responsive to individual preferences, needs, and values, and ensuring that patient values guide all clinical decisions; (4) timely—reducing waits and sometimes harmful delays for both those who receive and those who give care; (5) efficient—avoiding waste, including waste of equipment, supplies, ideas, and human resources; and (6) equitable—providing care that does not vary in quality because of personal characteristics, such as gender, ethnicity, geography, and socioeconomic status" (IOM, 2001, p. 6). Communicating accurate and timely diagnoses to patients is an important component of providing high-quality care; errors in diagnosis are a major threat to achieving high-quality care.

The IOM defines an error in medicine to be the "failure of a planned action to be completed as intended (i.e., error of execution) and the use of a wrong plan to achieve an aim (i.e., error of planning) [commission]" (IOM, 2004, p. 30). The definition also recognizes the failure of an unplanned action that should have been completed (omission) as an error (IOM, 2004). The IOM report *To Err Is Human: Building a Safer Health System* distinguished among four types of error: diagnostic, treatment, preventive, and other (see Box 3-1). An adverse event is "an event that results in unintended harm to the patient by an act of commission or omission rather than by the underlying disease or condition of the patient" (IOM, 2004, p. 32).

The committee's deliberations were informed by a number of existing definitions and definitional frameworks on diagnostic error (see Appendix C). For instance, Graber and colleagues used a classification of error from the Australian Patient Safety Foundation to define diagnostic error as a "diagnosis that was unintentionally delayed (sufficient information was available earlier), wrong (another diagnosis was made before the correct one), or missed (no diagnosis was ever made), as judged from the eventual appreciation of more definitive information" (Graber et al., 2005, p. 1493). They further divided diagnostic error into three main categories: no-fault errors, system-related errors, and cognitive errors. No-fault errors, originally described by Kassirer and Kopelman (1989), stem from factors outside the control of the clinician or the health care system, including atypical disease presentation or patient-related factors such as providing misleading information. The second category, system-related errors, can include technical or organizational barriers, such as problems with communication and care coordination; inefficient processes; technical failures; and equipment problems. Finally, there are cognitive errors that clinicians may make. The causes of these can include inadequate knowledge, poor critical thinking skills, a lack of competency, problems in data gathering, and failing to synthesize information (Chimowitz et al.,

---

BOX 3-1
Types of Errors Described in
To Err Is Human: Building a Safer Health System

Diagnostic
    Error or delay in diagnosis; failure to employ indicated tests; use of outmoded tests or therapy; failure to act on results of monitoring or testing

Treatment
    Error in the performance of an operation, procedure, or test; error in administering the treatment; error in the dose or method of using a drug; avoidable delay in treatment or in responding to an abnormal test; inappropriate (not indicated) care

Preventive
    Failure to provide prophylactic treatment; inadequate monitoring or follow-up of treatment

Other
    Failure of communication; equipment failure; other system failure

SOURCE: IOM, 2000, p. 36.

1990). Each of these errors can occur in isolation, but they often interact with one another; for instance, system factors can lead to cognitive errors.

Schiff and colleagues (2009, p. 1882) defined diagnostic error as "any mistake or failure in the diagnostic process leading to a misdiagnosis, a missed diagnosis, or a delayed diagnosis." Schiff and colleagues (2005) divide the diagnostic process into seven stages: (1) access and presentation, (2) history taking/collection, (3) the physical exam, (4) testing, (5) assessment, (6) referral, and (7) follow-up. A diagnostic error can occur at any stage in the diagnostic process, and there is a spectrum of patient consequences related to these errors ranging from no harm to severe harm. Schiff and colleagues noted that not all diagnostic process errors will lead to a missed, delayed, or wrong diagnosis, and not all errors (either in the diagnostic process or related to misdiagnosis) will result in patient harm. Relating this model to Donabedian's structure-process-outcome framework, Schiff and colleagues consider diagnosis to be an intermediate outcome of the diagnostic process, and any resulting adverse patient harm would be considered true patient outcomes (Schiff and Leape, 2012; Schiff et al., 2005, 2009).

In describing diagnostic error, Singh focused on defining missed opportunities, where a missed opportunity "implies that something different could have been done to make the correct diagnosis earlier. . . . Evidence of omission (failure to do the right thing) or commission (doing something wrong) exists at the particular point in time at which the 'error' occurred" (Singh, 2014, p. 99). Singh's definition of a missed opportunity takes into account the evolving nature of a diagnosis, making the determination of a missed opportunity dependent on the temporal or sequential context of events. It also assumes that missed opportunities could be caused by individual clinicians, the care team, the system, or patients. Singh also highlighted preventable diagnostic harm—when a missed opportunity results in harm from delayed or wrong treatment or test—as the best opportunity to intervene.

Newman-Toker (2014a,b) developed a conceptual model of diagnostic error that attempted to harmonize the current definitional frameworks. His framing distinguished between diagnostic process failures and diagnostic labeling failures. Diagnostic process failures include problems in the diagnostic workup, and they may include both cognitive and system errors. Diagnosis label failures occur when the diagnosis that a patient receives is incorrect or when there is no attempt to provide a diagnosis label. Newman-Toker identified preventable diagnostic error as the overlap between a diagnostic process failure and a diagnostic label failure, and he noted that this is similar to Singh's conceptualization of a missed opportunity (Singh, 2014). A preventable diagnostic error differs from a near-miss process problem, which is a failure in the diagnostic process without a diagnostic labeling failure. Newman-Toker also identifies unavoidable misdiagnosis, which is a diagnostic labeling failure that may occur in the absence of a diagnostic process failure and corresponds to the no-fault category described earlier. Furthermore, his model illustrates that harm may—or may not—result from diagnostic process failures and diagnostic labeling failures.

In reviewing the diagnostic error literature, the committee concluded that there are varying definitions and terminology currently in use to describe diagnostic error. For example, there is disagreement about exactly what constitutes a diagnostic error as well as about the precise meanings of a delayed diagnosis, a missed diagnosis, and a misdiagnosis (Newman-Toker, 2014b). Some treat the terms "diagnostic error" and "misdiagnosis" as synonyms (Newman-Toker, 2014b; Newman-Toker and Pronovost, 2009). There are some who prefer the term "diagnosis error" rather than "diagnostic error" because they conclude that diagnostic error should refer to the process of arriving at a diagnosis, whereas diagnosis error should refer to the final multifactorial outcome, of which the diagnostic process is only one factor (Berenson et al., 2014). Some use the term "missed diagnosis" solely for situations in which the diagnosis was found upon

autopsy (Graber et al., 2005; Newman-Toker, 2014b). While some definitions of diagnostic error include unavoidable errors, others conceptualize
diagnostic error as something that stems from a failure in the diagnostic
process (Graber et al., 2005; Newman-Toker, 2014b; Schiff et al., 2009). In
part, the various definitions that have arisen reflect the intrinsic dualistic
nature of the term "diagnosis," which has been used to refer both to a
process and to the result of that process. Definitions of diagnostic error
can also vary by stakeholder; for example, a patient's definition of a diagnostic error may be different from a clinician- or research-oriented definition of diagnostic error. Other terms used in the diagnostic error literature
include diagnostic accuracy (Wachter, 2014), misdiagnosis-related harm
(Newman-Toker and Pronovost, 2009), and preventable diagnostic errors
(Newman-Toker, 2014b).

Because of this lack of agreement, the committee decided to formulate
a new definition of diagnostic error. The committee's patient-centered
definition of diagnostic error is:

> *the failure to (a) establish an accurate and timely explanation of the
> patient's health problem(s) or (b) communicate that explanation to
> the patient.*

The definition frames a diagnostic error from the patient's perspective, in recognition that a patient bears the ultimate risk of harm from a
diagnostic error. The committee's definition is two-pronged; if there is a
failure in either part of the definition, a diagnostic error results. It also
conveys that each arm of the definition may be evaluated separately for
measurement purposes (see section on measurement and assessment of
diagnostic error).

The first part of the committee's definition focuses on two major
characteristics of diagnosis: accuracy and timeliness. A diagnosis is not
accurate if it differs from the true condition a patient has (or does not
have) or if it is imprecise and incomplete (lacking in sufficient detail). It is
important to note that a working diagnosis, described in Chapter 2, may
lack precision or completeness but is not necessarily a diagnostic error.
The nature of the diagnostic process is iterative, and as information gathering continues, the goal is to reduce diagnostic uncertainty, narrow down
the diagnostic possibilities, and develop a more precise and complete
diagnosis. The other characteristic the committee highlighted was timeliness. Timeliness means that the diagnosis was not meaningfully delayed.
However, the committee did not specify a time period that would reflect
"timely" because this is likely to depend on the nature of a patient's condition as well as on a realistic expectation of the length of time needed to
make a diagnosis. Thus, the term "timely" will need to be operationalized

for different health problems. Depending on the circumstances, some diagnoses may take days, weeks, or even months to establish, while timely may mean quite quickly (minutes to hours) for other urgent diagnoses.

The second part of the committee's definition focuses on communication. A fundamental conclusion from the committee's deliberations was that communication is a key responsibility in the diagnostic process. From a patient's perspective, an accurate and timely explanation of the health problem is meaningless unless this information reaches the patient so that a patient and health care professionals can act on the explanation. The phrase "explanation of the patient's health problem(s)" was chosen because it was meant to describe the health problem (or problems) involved as well as the manner in which the information is conveyed to a patient. The explanation needs to align with a patient's level of health literacy and to be conveyed in a way that facilitates patient understanding. Because not all patients will be able to participate in the communication process, there will be some situations where the explanation of the health problem may not be feasible to convey or be fully appreciated by the patient (e.g., pediatric patients or patients whose health problems limit or prevent communication). In these circumstances, the communication of the health problem would be between the health care professionals and a patient's family or designated health care proxy. There may also be urgent, life-threatening situations in which a patient's health problem will need to be communicated following treatment. However, even in these urgent situations, patients and their families need to be informed about new developments, so that decision making reflects a patient's values, preferences, and needs. Timely communication is also context-dependent: With some health problems, providing an explanation to a patient can take weeks or months to establish. However, throughout this time clinicians can communicate the working diagnosis, or the current explanation of the patient's health problem, as well as the degree of certainty associated with this explanation.

The phrase "failure to establish" is included in the definition because it recognizes that determining a diagnosis is a process that involves both the passage of time and the collaboration of health care professionals, patients, and their families to reach an explanation. The committee chose the term "health problem" because it is more inclusive than the term "diagnosis" and often reflects a more patient-centered approach to understanding a patient's overall health condition. For example, a health problem could include a predisposition to developing a condition, such as a genetic risk for disease. In addition, there are circumstances when it is important to focus on resolving the symptoms that are interfering with a patient's basic functioning, described as "activities of daily living," rather than focusing exclusively on identifying and following up on all of a patient's potential diagnoses (Gawande, 2007). Individual patient preferences for possible health outcomes can vary substantially, and with the growing prevalence of chronic disease, patients often have comorbidities or competing causes of mortality that need to be taken into consideration when defining a patient's health problem and subsequent plan for care (Gawande, 2014; Liss et al., 2013; Mulley et al., 2012).

There could be situations in which clinicians and health care organizations, practicing conscientiously (e.g., following clinical practice guidelines or established standards of care), may be unable to establish a definitive diagnosis. Sometimes a health care professional will need to acknowledge an inability to establish a diagnosis and will need to refer the patient to other specialists for further assessment to continue the diagnostic process. However, in some cases, this iterative process may still not lead to a firm diagnosis. For example, individuals may have signs and symptoms that have not been recognized universally by the medical community as a specific disease. From the patient's perspective, this could be a diagnostic error, but medicine is not an exact science, and documenting and examining such instances could provide an opportunity to advance medical knowledge and ultimately improve the diagnostic process.

The committee's definition reflects the six aims of high-quality care identified by the IOM (2001). It specifically refers to effectiveness and efficiency (i.e., accuracy), timeliness, and patient-centeredness as important aspects of diagnosis, while assuming safety and equity throughout the diagnostic process. Patients and their families play a key role in the diagnostic process, but a patient's care team is ultimately responsible for facilitating the diagnostic process and the communication of a diagnosis (see Chapter 4).

The committee's definition of diagnostic error differs from previous definitions in that it focuses on the outcome from the diagnostic process (the explanation of the patient's health problem provided to the patient). Other definitions of diagnostic error focus on determining whether or not process-related factors resulted in the diagnostic error. For example, Singh's definition focuses on whether there was a missed opportunity to make a diagnosis earlier (Singh, 2014). Likewise, Schiff and colleagues' (2009) definition of diagnostic error requires a determination that there was a mistake or failure in the diagnostic process. The committee's focus on the outcome from the diagnostic process is important because it reflects what matters most to patients—the communication of an accurate and timely explanation of their health problem. However, identifying failures in the diagnostic process is also critically important, which is reflected in the committee's dual focus on improving the diagnostic process and reducing diagnostic errors. The committee's discussion of measurement includes an emphasis on understanding where failures in the diagnostic process can occur and the work system factors that contribute to these failures (see section on determining the causes and risks of diagnostic error).

Analyzing failures in the diagnostic process provide important information for learning how to improve the work system and the diagnostic process. Some failures in the diagnostic process will lead to diagnostic errors; however, other failures in the diagnostic process will not ultimately lead to a diagnostic error. In this report, the committee describes "failures in the diagnostic process that do not lead to diagnostic errors" as near misses.[1] In other words, a near miss is a diagnosis that was almost erroneous. For example, it would be considered a near miss if a radiologist reported no significant findings from a chest X-ray, but a primary care clinician reviewing the image identified something that required further follow-up (Newman-Toker, 2014b). While there may have been a failure in the diagnostic process, the patient nonetheless received an accurate and timely explanation of the health problem. Examining near misses can help identify vulnerabilities in the diagnostic process as well as strengths in the diagnostic process that compensate for these vulnerabilities (see discussion of error recovery in Chapter 6). Likewise, several of the committee's recommendations focus on identifying both diagnostic errors and near misses because they both serve as learning opportunities to improve diagnosis.

The diagnostic process can lead to a number of outcomes (see Figure 3-1). An accurate and timely diagnosis that is communicated to a patient presents the best opportunity for a positive health outcome because clinical decision making will be tailored to a correct understanding of the patient's health problem. Diagnostic errors and near misses can stem from a wide variety of causes and result in multiple outcomes, and as evidence accrues, a more nuanced picture of diagnostic errors and near misses will develop. For example, further research can be directed at better understanding the causes of diagnostic errors and vulnerabilities in the

---

[1] The term "near miss" is used within many fields—including health care—with varying definitions. For example, an IOM report defined a near miss as "an act of commission or omission that could have harmed the patient but did not cause harm as a result of chance, prevention, or mitigation" (IOM, 2004, p. 227). Because diagnostic errors can have a range of outcomes (including no harm) this definition of near miss is not consistent with the committee's definition of diagnostic error. However, the committee's conceptualization of a near miss is similar to previous uses. For example, the 2004 IOM report states that most definitions of a near miss imply an incident causation model, in which there is a causal chain of events that leads to the ultimate outcome: "Near misses are the immediate precursors to later possible adverse events" (IOM, 2004, p. 227). Rather than focus on adverse events as the outcome of interest, the committee's outcome of interest is diagnostic error. Thus, the committee's definition of a near miss is a failure in the diagnostic process that does not lead to diagnostic error.

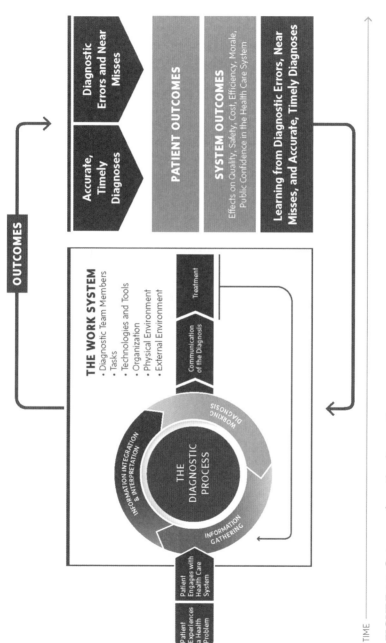

FIGURE 3-1 Outcomes from the diagnostic process.

diagnostic process. Some of the reasons diagnostic errors and near misses occur may be more remediable to interventions than others. In addition, determining which types of diagnostic errors are priorities to address, as well as which interventions could be targeted at preventing or mitigating specific types of diagnostic errors, will be informative in improving the quality of care.

A better understanding of the outcomes resulting from diagnostic errors and near misses will also be helpful. For example, if there is a diagnostic error, a patient may or may not experience harm. The potential harm from diagnostic errors could range from no harm to significant harm, including morbidity or death. Errors can be harmful because they can prevent or delay appropriate treatment, lead to unnecessary or harmful treatment, or result in psychological or financial repercussions. Harm may not result, for example, if a patient's symptoms resolve even with an incorrect diagnosis. Diagnostic errors and near misses may also lead to inefficiency in health care organizations (e.g., the provision of unnecessary treatments) and increase system costs unnecessarily (covering the costs of otherwise unnecessary care or medical liability expenses). Diagnostic errors and near misses influence both the morale of individuals participating in the diagnostic process and public trust in the health care system. Correct diagnoses, diagnostic errors, and near misses can be used as opportunities to learn how to improve the work system and the diagnostic process (Klein, 2011, 2014).

OVERUTILIZATION IN THE DIAGNOSTIC PROCESS AND OVERDIAGNOSIS

There is growing recognition that overdiagnosis is a serious problem in health care today, contributing to increased health care costs, overtreatment, and the associated risks and harms from this treatment (Welch, 2015; Welch and Black, 2010). Overdiagnosis has been described as "when a condition is diagnosed that would otherwise not go on to cause symptoms or death" (Welch and Black, 2010, p. 605). Chiolero and colleagues note that advances in prevention and diagnosis "have changed the diagnostic process, expanding the possibilities of interventions across asymptomatic individuals and blurring the boundaries between health, risk, and disease" (Chiolero et al., 2015, p. w14060). Overdiagnosis has been attributed to the increased sensitivity of diagnostic testing (e.g., improved radiographic resolution); the identification of incidental findings; the widening boundaries or lowered thresholds for defining what is abnormal (e.g., hypertension, diabetes, or cholesterol levels); and clinicians' concerns about missing diagnoses and subsequent medical liability risks (see Chapter 7 for a discussion of defensive medicine concerns) (Chiolero et al., 2015; Gawande, 2015; Moynihan et al., 2012).

Recent discussions in the diagnostic error community have drawn attention to the issue of overdiagnosis and whether overdiagnosis should be defined and classified as an error (Berenson et al., 2014; Newman-Toker, 2014b; Zwaan and Singh, 2015). Although overdiagnosis is a complex and controversial topic, it is distinct from diagnostic error. For example, Chiolero and colleagues (2015, p. w14060) state: "Overdiagnosis is . . . neither a misdiagnosis (diagnostic error), nor a false positive result (positive test in the absence of a real abnormality)." Similarly, Gawande makes the distinction between overdiagnosis and diagnostic error: "Overtesting has also created a new, unanticipated problem: overdiagnosis. This isn't misdiagnosis—the erroneous diagnosis of a disease. This is the correct diagnosis of a disease that is never going to bother you in your lifetime" (Gawande, 2015). Challenges in terminology and the blurry distinctions between diagnosis and treatment add to the confusion between overdiagnosis and diagnostic error. Recent reports in the literature have used the term "overdiagnosis" broadly to incorporate the concept of over-medicalization, including overdetection, overdiagnosis, overtreatment, and overutilization (Carter et al., 2015). For example, widening the criteria used to define a disease may raise important concerns about overmedicalization, but if a diagnosis is consistent with consensus guidelines for medical practice, it would not constitute a diagnostic error as defined by the committee.

A major reason overdiagnosis is not characterized as an error is because it is found primarily with population-based estimates; it is virtually impossible to assess whether overdiagnosis has occurred for an individual patient (Welch and Black, 2010). Our understanding of biology and disease progression is often not advanced enough to determine which individuals are going to be harmed by their health condition, versus the health conditions that are never going to lead to patient harm (e.g., thyroid, breast, and prostate cancers). Thus, clinicians are treating patients based on uncertain prognoses, and many more people are treated compared to those who actually benefit from treatment. Likewise, screening guidelines are intended to identify populations that will most likely benefit from screening, but not all individuals who undergo screening will benefit. For example, screening mammography—like many interventions—is an imperfect test with associated harms and benefits; some breast cancers will be missed, some women will die from breast cancer regardless of being screened, and some cancers that are identified will never lead to harm (Pace and Keating, 2014). Because current diagnostic testing technologies often cannot distinguish the cancers that are likely to progress and lead to patient harm from those that will not, inevitably clinicians treat some patients with breast cancer who will not benefit from the treatment (Esserman et al., 2009). It would be incorrect (and largely impossible) to classify these cases as errors because clinicians are basing screening and treatment decisions on the best available medical knowledge, and the assessment of overdiagnosis is dependent on population-based analysis. For example, once diagnosed and treated for cancer, it is impossible to know whether the patient's outcome would have been different if the tumor (which may have been indolent rather than life-threatening) had never been diagnosed.

However, overdiagnosis represents a true challenge to health care quality, and further efforts are warranted to prevent overdiagnosis and associated overtreatment concerns. Reducing overdiagnosis will likely require improved understanding of disease biology and progression, as well as increased awareness of its occurrence among health care professionals, patients, and their families (Chiolero et al., 2015). In addition, an important strategy that has been suggested for preventing overdiagnosis and associated overtreatment is avoiding unnecessary and untargeted diagnostic testing (Chiolero et al., 2015).

Box 3-2 provides an overview of overutilization of diagnostic testing in health care. Based on the committee's definition of diagnostic error, which focuses on the outcomes for patients, overutilization of diagnostic testing is not necessarily a diagnostic error. Overutilization of diagnostic testing would be considered a failure in the diagnostic process (failure in information gathering—see the measurement section below). Overutilization is a serious concern, and efforts to improve diagnosis need to focus on preventing inappropriate overutilization of diagnostic testing (Newman-Toker, 2014a).

Improving diagnosis should not imply the adoption of overly aggressive diagnostic strategies. Chapter 2 highlights that the goal of diagnostic testing is not to reduce diagnostic uncertainty to zero (an impossible task), but rather to optimize decision making by judicious use of diagnostic testing (Newman-Toker et al., 2013; Kassirer, 1989). This is also why the committee highlighted iterative information gathering and the role of time in the diagnostic process; oftentimes it is not appropriate to test for everything at the outset—further information-gathering activities can be informed by test results, time, and a patient's response to treatment. The committee makes a number of recommendations throughout the report that are targeted at preventing overutilization in the diagnostic process, including improved collaboration and communication among treating clinicians and pathologists, radiologists, and other diagnostic testing health care professionals, as well as increased emphasis on diagnostic testing in health care professional education (see Chapters 4 and 6).

BOX 3-2
Overutilization of Diagnostic Testing

While diagnostic testing has brought many improvements to medical care, advances in diagnostic testing have also led to some challenges, including an under-reliance on more traditional diagnostic tools, such as careful history taking and the physical exam, and the inappropriate utilization of diagnostic testing (Iglehart, 2009; Newman-Toker et al., 2013; Rao and Levin, 2012; Zhi et al., 2013). Inappropriate use has included both overutilization (testing when it is not indicated) and underutilization (not testing when it is indicated).

The use of diagnostic testing to rule out conditions, clinicians' intolerance of uncertainty, an enthusiasm for the early detection of disease in the absence of symptoms, and concerns over medical liability can all contribute to overutilization (Grimes and Schulz, 2002; Newman-Toker et al., 2013; Plebani, 2014). In one survey of physicians in specialties at high risk of litigation (emergency medicine, general surgery, orthopedic surgery, neurosurgery, obstetrics/gynecology, and radiology), 59 percent of respondents reported that they ordered more tests than were medically indicated (Studdert et al., 2005). In an analysis that examined patient understanding of medical interventions, researchers identified a complex array of reasons for overuse, including payment systems that favor more testing over patient interaction, the ease of requesting tests, and patient beliefs that more testing and treatment is equivalent to better care (Croskerry, 2011; Hoffmann and Del Mar, 2015). When a clinician does not have enough time to discuss symptoms and potential diagnoses with a patient, ordering a test is sometimes considered more straightforward and less risky (Newman-Toker et al., 2013). Another contributing factor is an overestimation of the benefits of testing; for example, patients often overestimate the benefits of mammography screening (Gigerenzer, 2014; Hoffmann and Del Mar, 2015).

The overutilization of medical imaging techniques that employ ionizing radiation (such as computed tomography [CT]) is of special concern and has gained considerable attention in the wake of research showing a marked increase in radiation exposure from medical imaging in the U.S. population (Hricak et al., 2011). Epidemiological studies have found reasonable, though not definitive, evidence that exposure to ionizing radiation (organ doses ranging from 5 to 125 millisieverts) result in a very small but statistically significant increase in cancer risk (Hricak et al., 2011). Children are more radiosensitive than adults, and cancer risks increase with cumulative radiation exposure. In addition to age at exposure, genetic considerations, sex, and fractionation and protraction of exposure may influence the level of risk. Medical imaging needs to be justified by weighing its potential benefit against its potential risk. It is important to be sure that imaging is truly indicated and to consider alternatives to the use of ionizing radiation, especially for pediatric patients and those with a history of radiation exposure. In 2010 the Food and Drug Administration launched the Initiative to Reduce Radiation Exposure, aimed at promoting the justification of all imaging examinations and the optimization of imaging protocols so as to minimize radiation doses (FDA, 2015). Studies have shown that the use of clinical decision support and guidelines can minimize unnecessary radiation exposure and that they could prevent as many as 20 to 40 percent of CT scans without compromising patient care (Hricak et al., 2011).

MEASUREMENT AND ASSESSMENT OF DIAGNOSTIC ERROR

For a variety of reasons, diagnostic errors have been more challenging to measure than other quality or safety concepts. Singh and Sittig (2015, p. 103) note that "[c]ompared with other safety concerns, there are also fewer sources of valid and reliable data that could enable measurement" of diagnostic errors. Studies that have evaluated diagnostic errors have employed different definitions, and the use of varying definitions can lead to challenges in drawing comparisons across studies or synthesizing the available information on measurement (Berenson et al., 2014; Schiff and Leape, 2012; Singh, 2014). Even when there is agreement on the definition of diagnostic error, there can be genuine disagreement over whether a diagnostic error actually occurred, and there are often blurry boundaries between different types of errors (e.g., treatment or diagnostic) (Singh and Sittig, 2015; Singh et al., 2012a).

The complexity of the diagnostic process itself, as well as the inherent uncertainty underlying clinical decision making, makes measurement a challenging task (Singh, 2014; Singh and Sittig, 2015). The committee's conceptual model illustrates the complex, time-dependent, and team-based nature of the diagnostic process as well as all of the potential work system factors that can contribute to the occurrence of diagnostic error. The temporal component of the diagnostic process can complicate measurement because the signs and symptoms of a health condition may evolve over time, and there can be disagreement about what an acceptable time frame is in which to make a timely diagnosis (Singh, 2014; Zwaan and Singh, 2015). Clinical reasoning plays a role in diagnostic errors, but clinical reasoning processes are difficult to assess because they occur in clinicians' minds and are not typically documented (Croskerry, 2012; Wachter, 2010). Similarly, some measurement approaches, such as medical record reviews, may not identify diagnostic errors because information related to diagnosis may not be documented (Singh et al., 2012a). Furthermore, many people recover from their health conditions regardless of the treatment or diagnosis they receive, so a diagnostic error may never be recognized (Croskerry, 2012).

The Purposes of Measurement

There are a variety of ways that measurement can be used in the context of the diagnostic process and in assessing the occurrence of diagnostic errors. The committee identified five primary purposes for measuring diagnostic errors: establishing the incidence and nature of the problem of diagnostic error; determining the causes and risks of diagnostic error; evaluating interventions to improve diagnosis and reduce diagnostic

errors; for educational and training purposes; and for accountability purposes (e.g., performance measurement). Each of these purposes is described in greater detail below.

1. *Establish the incidence and nature of the problem of diagnostic error.*
   Today this task is primarily the province of research and is likely
   to remain that way for the foreseeable future. Researchers have
   used a variety of methods to assess diagnostic errors. Attention to
   harmonizing these approaches and recognizing what each method
   contributes to the overall understanding of diagnostic error may
   better characterize the size and dimensionality of the problem and
   may facilitate assessment of diagnostic error rates over time.
2. *Determine the causes and risks of diagnostic error.* This use of measurement and assessment is also primarily undertaken in research
   settings, and this is also likely to continue. Previous research has
   provided numerous insights into causes and risks, but moving
   from these insights to constructing approaches to prevent or detect problems more rapidly will require additional work.
3. *Evaluate interventions.* This report should stimulate the development of programs designed to prevent, detect, and correct diagnostic errors across the spectrum, but these programs will require
   appropriate measurement tools (both quantitative and qualitative) to allow a rigorous assessment of whether the interventions
   worked. This will be particularly challenging for measuring prevention, as is always the case in medical care. Research needs to
   focus on the required attributes of these measurement tools for
   this application.
4. *Education and training.* Given the importance of lifelong learning
   in health care, it will be useful to have measurement tools that
   can assess the initial training of health care professionals, the
   outcomes of ongoing education, and the competency of health
   care professionals. For this application, these tools need to provide an opportunity for feedback and perhaps decision support
   assistance in identifying potential high risk areas. In this instance,
   the measurement tools need to include not only the assessment
   of whether an event occurred or is at risk for occurring but also
   effective methods for feeding back information for learning.
5. *Accountability.* In today's environment, significant pressure exists
   to push toward accountability through public reporting and payment for every area in which a potential problem has been identified in health care. As an aspiration, the committee recognizes that
   transparency and public reporting are worthy goals for helping
   patients identify and receive high-quality care. However, current

pushes for accountability neglect diagnostic performance, and this is a major limitation of these approaches. The committee's assessment suggests that it would be premature either to adopt an accountability framework or to assume that the traditional accountability frameworks for public reporting and payment will be effective in reducing diagnostic error. A primary focus on intrinsic motivation—unleashing the desire on the part of nearly all health care professionals to do the right thing—may be more effective at improving diagnostic performance than programs focused on public reporting and payment. Public awareness may also be a key leverage point, but at this point measurement approaches that reveal weak spots in the diagnostic process and identify errors reliably are lacking. For both health care professionals and patients, it is critical to develop measurement approaches that engage all parties in improving diagnostic performance.

With this in mind, the following discussion elaborates on three of the purposes of measurement: Establishing the incidence and nature of diagnostic error, determining the causes and risks of diagnostic error, and evaluating interventions. This section summarizes the approaches to measurement that are best matched to each purpose. All of the data sources and methods that were identified have some limitations for the committee-defined purposes of measurement.

Issues related to assessing the competency of health care professionals are addressed in Chapter 4; because the committee determined that it is premature to consider diagnostic error from an accountability framework, measurement for the purpose of accountability is not described further in this chapter.

Establishing the Incidence and Nature of the Problem of Diagnostic Error

A number of data sources and methods have been used to understand the incidence and nature of diagnostic error, including postmortem examinations (autopsy), medical record reviews, malpractice claims, health insurance claims, diagnostic testing studies, and patient and clinician surveys, among others (Berner and Graber, 2008; Graber, 2013; Singh and Sittig, 2015).

Before reviewing each of these approaches, the committee sought to identify or construct a summary, population-based estimate of the frequency with which diagnostic errors occur. Such a number can underscore the importance of the problem and, over time, be used to evaluate whether progress is being made. To arrive at such a number, the committee considered the necessary measurement requirements to establish the incidence and nature of diagnostic errors. First, one would need an estimate of the number of opportunities to make a diagnosis each year (denominator) and the number of times the diagnosis (health problem) is not made in an accurate and timely manner or is not communicated to the patient. This formulation takes into consideration the fact that during any given year patients may experience multiple health problems for which a diagnosis is required; each represents an opportunity for the health care system to deliver an accurate and timely explanation of that health problem. About one-third of ambulatory visits are for a new health problem (CDC, 2015). The formulation also reflects the fact that the final product (the explanation of the patient's health problem) needs to be free of defects; that is, it needs to meet all elements of a correct diagnosis (accuracy, timeliness, and communication).

Perhaps not surprisingly, the available research estimates were not adequate to extrapolate a specific estimate or range of the incidence of diagnostic errors in clinical practice today. Even less information is available to assess the severity of harm caused by diagnostic errors. Part of the challenge in gathering such data is the variety of settings in which these errors can occur; these settings include hospitals, emergency departments, a variety of outpatient settings (such as primary and specialty care settings and retail clinics), and long-term-care settings (such as nursing homes and rehabilitation centers). A second part of the challenge is the complexity of the diagnostic process itself. Although there are data available to examine diagnostic errors in some of these settings, there are wide gaps and much variability in the amount and quality of information available. In addition, a number of problems arise when aggregating data across the various research methods (such as postmortem examinations, medical record reviews, and malpractice claims). Each method captures information about different subgroups in the population, different dimensions of the problem, and different insights into the frequency and causes of diagnostic error. Taken together, however, the committee concluded that the evidence suggests that diagnostic errors are a significant and common challenge in health care and that most people will experience at least one diagnostic error in their lifetime. The committee based this observation on its collective assessment of the available evidence describing the epidemiology of diagnostic errors. In each data source that the committee evaluated, diagnostic errors were a consistent quality and safety challenge.

The committee anticipates that its definition of diagnostic error will inform measurement activities. The two components of the definition—(a) accuracy and timeliness and (b) communication—will likely have to be accounted for separately. For example, it is often difficult to determine from a medical record review whether the diagnosis has been communicated to the patient. Other data sources, such as patient surveys, may be helpful in making this determination. Alternatively, medical record charting practices could be improved to emphasize communication because of its importance in improving diagnosis and subsequent care. Measuring each arm of the definition is also consistent with the committee's approach to identifying failures in the diagnostic process; the committee specifies that each step in the diagnostic process can be evaluated for its susceptibility to failures (see section on determining the causes and risks of diagnostic error).

To better understand both the challenges and the opportunities associated with the various measurement methods, the committee examined for each of the data sources (1) the mechanism by which eligible patients were identified for assessment (denominator) and (2) the way that diagnostic errors were identified (numerator). The results are summarized in Table 3-1. In the sections following the table, the committee describes each data source; highlights the features of the data source that enhance or limit its utility for estimating the incidence of diagnostic error; describes the methods that have been used in studies to select cases for review (the denominator); and describes the methods for determining if an error occurred (numerator). Next, a summary of what is known about the incidence of diagnostic errors from studies that use those data sources is offered. Each section ends with a discussion of potential improvements to the methods that use each data source.

TABLE 3-1 Methods for Estimating the Incidence of Diagnostic Errors

Data Source	Key Features of the Data Source	Method(s) for Selecting Cases for Review (Denominator)	Method for Determining if Error Occurred (Numerator)
Postmortem examination (Autopsy)	Deaths only Limited number of reviews Selection bias (typically focused on unexpected deaths) Limited workforce	Consecutive series with criteria Convenience samples Prespecified criteria Requests (from clinicians or families)	Comparison to another data source (medical record, interview, location/circumstance of death) Cause of death determination Effects or indication of disease

TABLE 3-1 Continued

Data Source	Key Features of the Data Source	Method(s) for Selecting Cases for Review (Denominator)	Method for Determining if Error Occurred (Numerator)
Medical records	Rely on documentation (what was recorded, such as clinical history and interview, physical exam, and diagnostic testing)	Prespecified criteria (e.g., trigger tool) Random sample	Implicit review/expert assessment Explicit criteria
Medical malpractice claims	Requires claim to be filed; more likely for negligent care Most studies done on closed claims	Classification criteria (typically based on claim made in suit)	Claims adjudication process (including courts)
Health insurance claims	Requires a billable event Relies on documentation necessary for payment	Criteria-based algorithm (selected) Universe of claims	Criteria-based algorithm
Diagnostic testing	Source data available for review Applies only to diagnoses for which diagnostic testing data are a key factor Focus on interpretation	Random sample Prespecified criteria	Expert assessment compared to original
Medical imaging	Source data available for review Applies only to diagnoses for which medical imaging data are a key factor Focus on interpretation	Random sample Prespecified criteria	Expert assessment compared to original
Surveys of clinicians	Subject to nonresponse bias May be difficult to validate	Sample receiving survey	Descriptive statistics on self-report
Surveys of patients	Subject to nonresponse bias May be difficult to validate	Sample receiving survey	Descriptive statistics on self-report

Postmortem Examinations

Description of the data source Postmortem examinations, often referred to as autopsies, are highly specialized surgical procedures that are conducted to determine the cause of death or extent of disease. Hoyert (2011, p. 1) identifies two primary types of postmortem exams conducted in the United States: (1) "hospital or clinical autopsies, which family or physicians request to clarify cause of death or assess care," and (2) "medicolegal autopsies, which legal officials order to further investigate the circumstances surrounding a death." Postmortem exams may vary from an external-only exam to a full external and internal exam, depending on the request. While this chapter focuses on full-body postmortem exams, Chapter 6 describes the potential future state of postmortem examinations, which may include more minimally invasive approaches, such as medical imaging, laparoscopy, biopsy, histology, and cytology.

Notes about the data source Postmortem exams are considered a very strong method for identifying diagnostic errors because of the extensiveness of the examination that is possible (Graber, 2013; Shojania, 2002). However, there are some limitations to this data source for the purpose of estimating the incidence of diagnostic error. Postmortem exams are conducted on people who have died; thus, the results can only provide information about diagnostic errors that led to the patient's death and about other diseases present that had not been previously identified, whether or not they contributed to the patient's death. A very limited number of postmortem exams are performed annually, and postmortem exam rates can also vary geographically and institutionally. Little information is available for characterizing the relationship between those who receive postmortem exams and the potential number of eligible cases, but those who undergo autopsy are more likely to have experienced a diagnostic error and that error is more likely to have contributed to the patient's (premature) death (an example of selection bias) (Shojania, 2002).

Methods for identifying cases for review (denominator) The decision about whether an individual patient will receive a postmortem exam is based on requests from clinicians or family members as well as on local criteria set by coroners or medical examiners. With the exception of postmortem examinations done for criminal forensic purposes, family members must consent to having the procedure done. There is no systematic information on the frequency with which the request for an autopsy is refused (which would introduce response bias into results). The performance of postmortem exams has declined substantially in the United States in recent decades (Lundberg, 1998). National data on postmortem exams have not been collected since 1994; at that time, fewer than 6 percent of non-forensic deaths underwent a postmortem exam (Shojania et al., 2002).

Research studies that have used postmortem exam results have used consecutive series, prespecified criteria (including randomly selected autopsies), or convenience samples (Shojania, 2002).

Methods for determining if an error occurred (numerator) The results of the postmortem exam typically provide a cause of death and a description of the presence and severity of other diseases. These results are compared to another data source, typically medical records or interviews with treating clinicians or family members. Discrepancies between what was found in the postmortem exam and what was known prior to that are the basis for determining the occurrence of a diagnostic error. Such determinations are subject to the reliability and validity of both the postmortem exam findings and the results from the data collected from the original sources.

What is known Postmortem examinations have been described as an important method for detecting diagnostic errors (Berner and Graber, 2008; Graber, 2013). In their review of postmortem examination data, Shojania and colleagues concluded that "the autopsy continues to detect important errors in clinical diagnosis" (Shojania et al., 2002, p. 51). On average, 10 percent of postmortem exams were associated with diagnostic errors that might have affected patient outcomes (i.e., Class I errors).[2] They estimated that the prevalence of major errors (i.e., Class I and II errors) related to the principal diagnosis or the cause of death was 25 percent. Some incidental findings found during postmortem exams should not be classified as diagnostic errors; of primary importance is identifying diagnostic errors that contributed to a patient's death (Class I errors).[3] Shojania and colleagues noted that some selection bias is reflected in this estimate because the cases in which there was more uncertainty about the diagnosis were more likely to undergo postmortem exam. A systematic review of diagnostic errors in the intensive care unit found that 8 percent of postmortem exams identified a Class I error and that 28 percent identified at least one diagnostic error (Winters et al., 2012). According to Shojania et al. (2003, p. 2849), the rates of autopsy-identified diagnostic errors have

---

[2] A Class I error is a major diagnostic error that likely played a role in the patient's death. A Class II error is a major diagnostic error that did not contribute to the patient's death. A Class III error is a minor diagnostic error that is not related to the patient's cause of death but is related to a terminal disease. A Class IV error is a missed minor discrepancy (Winters et al., 2012).

[3] For example, incidental findings of prostate cancer that are not relevant to the patient's provision of health care, terminal disease, or death may not be appropriate to classify as diagnostic error.

declined over time but remain "sufficiently high that encouraging ongoing use of the autopsy appears warranted." Based on their findings, they
estimated that among the 850,000 individuals who die in U.S. hospitals
each year, approximately 8.4 percent (71,400 deaths) have a major diagnosis that remains undetected (Shojania et al., 2003).

Opportunities for improvement The committee concluded that postmortem exams play a critical role in understanding the epidemiology of
diagnostic errors and that increasing the number of such exams is warranted. In addition, tracking the number of deaths, those eligible and
selected for postmortem exams, and the refusal rate among family members would enable the development of better national estimates of diagnostic error incidence. The committee weighed the relative merits of increasing
the number of postmortem examinations conducted throughout the United
States versus a more targeted approach. The committee concluded that
it would be more efficient to have a limited number of systems who are
highly qualified in conducting postmortem exams participate to produce
research-quality information about the incidence and nature of diagnostic
errors among a representative sample of patient deaths. This approach reflects both financial realities and workforce challenges (i.e., a limited number of pathologists being available and willing to conduct a large number of
such exams) (see also Chapter 6). The systems that are selected to routinely
conduct postmortem exams could also investigate how new, minimally
invasive postmortem approaches compare to full-body postmortem exams.

Medical Records

Description of the data source A medical record is defined as a documented account of a patient's examination and treatment that includes the
patient's clinical history and symptoms, physical findings, the results of
diagnostic testing, medications, and therapeutic procedures. The medical
record can exist in either paper or electronic form.

Notes about the data source Medical records exist only for patients who
have sought care from a clinician, team, or facility. Although there are
some common conventions for structuring medical records (both in paper
and electronic formats), much of the content of the record depends on
what the clinician chooses to include; thus, there may be variations in the
extent to which clinical reasoning is documented (e.g., what alternative
diagnoses were considered, the rationale for ordering [or not ordering]
certain tests, and the way in which the information was collected and
integrated). Both regulatory and local rules affect which members of the
diagnostic team contribute to the documentation in a medical record

and how they contribute. Except in highly integrated systems, patients typically have a separate medical record associated with each clinician or facility from which they have sought care. When patients change their source of care, the information from medical records maintained by the previous clinicians may or may not be incorporated into the new record.

Methods for identifying cases for review (denominator) The most common methods for identifying cases for review are either to draw a random sample of records from a facility (especially hospitals), clinic, or clinician practice or to assemble a criteria-based sample (e.g., a trigger tool). The criteria-based tools typically select events that have been associated with a higher probability of identifying a diagnostic error, such as unplanned readmissions to a hospital, emergency department visits after an outpatient visit, or the failure of a visit to occur after an abnormal test result. Estimates of the incidence of diagnostic errors based on medical records need to account for the probability that an individual is included in the study sample and the likelihood that a visit (or set of visits) requires that a diagnosis be made. Because these factors likely vary by geography and patient populations, arriving at national estimates from studies done in limited geographic areas is difficult.

Methods for determining if an error occurred (numerator) There are two common methods for determining if an error occurred: implicit and explicit. In the implicit method, an expert reviewer, taking into account all of the information that is available in the medical record, determines whether or not an accurate or timely diagnosis was made and, if a defect in the process occurred, the nature of that problem. In the explicit method, specific criteria are developed and data are abstracted from the medical record to determine whether or not an error occurred. The reliability of implicit and explicit methods for assessing quality of care and patient safety has been studied. Generally, implicit methods have been found to be less reliable than explicit methods (Hofer et al., 2004; Kerr et al., 2007). In the Utah and Colorado Medical Practice Study, which was one of the sources for estimating medical errors in the IOM's *To Err Is Human* report, the inter-rater reliability (agreement among reviewers) was $\kappa=0.40$–0.41 (95 percent confidence interval, 0.30–0.51) for identifying adverse events and $\kappa=0.19$–0.24 (95 percent confidence interval, 0.05–0.37) for identifying negligent adverse events (Thomas et al., 2002). These rates are considered moderate to poor (Landis and Koch, 1977). The reliabilities for the Harvard Medical Practice Study were in the same range (Brennan et al., 1991). Zwaan et al. (2010) reported a reliability of $\kappa=0.25$ (95 percent confidence interval, 0.05–0.45) (fair) for identifying adverse events and of $\kappa=0.40$ (95 percent confidence interval, 0.07–0.73) (moderate) for whether the event was preventable. Reliability in turn can affect the event rate that is reported. By contrast, the inter-rater reliability for explicit review of records for quality studies has been reported at approximately 0.80 (McGlynn et al., 2003).

What is known Two studies based on medical record reviews reported in the literature in the 1990s and early 2000s estimated that diagnostic errors account for 7 and 17 percent of adverse events in hospitalized patients, respectively. In the Harvard Medical Practice Study of more than 30,000 patient records, diagnostic errors were identified in 17 percent of the adverse events (Leape et al., 1991). A review of 15,000 records from Colorado and Utah found that diagnostic errors constituted 6.9 percent of adverse events (Thomas et al., 2000).

More recently, Zwaan and colleagues conducted a retrospective patient record review to assess the occurrence of diagnostic adverse events (harm associated with a diagnostic error) within hospitals in the Netherlands (Zwaan et al., 2010). Those researchers found that diagnostic adverse events occurred in 0.4 percent of all hospital admissions and that diagnostic adverse events accounted for 6.4 percent of all adverse events. The researchers had reviewers classify the causes of diagnostic adverse events by human, organizational, technical, patient-related, and other factors (Zwaan et al., 2010). They further divided the "human" category into knowledge-based, rule-based, skill-based, or other (such as violations or failures by deliberate deviations from rules or procedures). They found that human failures were the main cause of diagnostic adverse events—96.3 percent of these events had a human cause.[4] However, organizational and patient-related factors were present in 25.0 percent and 30.0 percent of diagnostic adverse events, respectively. The researchers found that the primary causes of diagnostic adverse events were knowledge-based failures (physicians did not have sufficient knowledge or applied their knowledge incorrectly) and information transfer failures (physicians did not receive the most current updates about a patient).

In another study by Zwaan and colleagues (2012), rather than focusing exclusively on adverse events, the researchers had four internists review 247 patient medical records for patients with dyspnea (shortness of breath) symptoms. The reviewers used a questionnaire to identify failures in diagnostic reasoning, diagnostic errors, and harm. They found that failures in diagnostic reasoning occurred in 66 percent of the cases, that diagnostic errors occurred in 13.8 percent of all cases, and that the patient was harmed in 11.3 percent of cases. Although cases with diag-

---

[4] It is likely that the "human failures" identified in this study actually related to work system factors.

nostic errors and patient harm had more failures in diagnostic reasoning, in 4 percent of the cases diagnostic errors occurred in the absence of diagnostic reasoning failures.

Singh et al. (2014) estimated the frequency of diagnostic error in the outpatient setting using data from three prior studies (Murphy et al., 2014; Singh et al., 2010a, 2012a). Two of the studies used "triggered" electronic queries to identify suspected cases of diagnostic error. In one study these triggers identified medical records in which a patient had a primary care visit followed by an unplanned hospitalization or unscheduled follow-up appointment, while the other study looked for a lack of follow-up for abnormal colorectal cancer findings. The third study examined consecutive cases of lung cancer. Physicians reviewed medical records to determine if there was a diagnostic error (defined as a missed opportunity to make or pursue the correct diagnosis when adequate data were available at the index [i.e., first] visit) (Singh, 2012a). The combined estimate of diagnostic error based on these three datasets was about 5 percent. Extrapolating to the entire U.S. population, Singh et al. (2014) estimated that approximately 12 million adults (or 1 in 20 adults) experience a diagnostic error each year; the researchers suggested that about half of these errors could be potentially harmful. Due to the definition of diagnostic error that Singh and colleagues employed, they asserted—as have other researchers—that this number may be a conservative estimate of the rate of outpatient diagnostic errors (Aleccia, 2014).

Opportunities for improvement Medical records will continue to be an important source of data for assessing diagnostic errors. The advent of electronic forms that make some methods more cost-efficient, combined with mechanisms such as health information exchanges that may make it easier to assemble the entire patient diagnostic episode, may enhance the use of these methods. Developing a standard method that could be applied to a random sample of records (either nationally or in prespecified settings) would enhance opportunities to learn about both the incidence and the variation in the likelihood of patients experiencing a diagnostic error. Greater attention to the reliability with which the method is applied, particularly through the use of explicit rather than implicit methods, would also enhance the scientific strength of these studies.

Medical Malpractice Claims

Description of the data source Medical malpractice claims are defined as the electronic and paper databases maintained by professional liability insurers on claims that have been filed by patients or their families seeking compensation for alleged medical errors, including diagnostic errors;

the information in support of the claims (medical records, depositions, other reports); and the final determination, whether achieved through a settlement or a court ruling. In addition to files maintained by insurers, the Health Resources and Services Administration, an agency within the Department of Health and Human Services (HHS), maintains the National Practitioner Data Bank (NPDB). The NPDB is a repository of clinician names, affiliations, and malpractice payments that have been made. It serves primarily as a system to facilitate comprehensive review of the credentials of clinicians, health care entities, providers, and suppliers, but it has been used for research as well. Many states also require claim reporting for purposes of maintaining a state-level database of paid claim information.

Notes about the data source For a diagnostic error to be included in malpractice claims datasets, a patient must have filed a claim, which is a relatively rare event (Localio et al., 1991), and is more likely if the patient has experienced significant harm or if negligence is a factor. For example, one study using data from the Harvard Medical Practice Study estimated that the probability of negligent injury was 0.43 percent and that the probability of nonnegligent injury was 0.80 percent (Adams and Garber, 2007). Furthermore, the probability that a claim would be filed was 3.6 percent if a negligent injury occurred and 3.2 percent if a nonnegligent injury occurred. The probability that a claim would be paid was 91 percent for negligent injury claims and 21 percent for nonnegligent injury claims. Thus, malpractice claims data provide a small window into the problem of diagnostic errors and are biased toward more serious diagnostic errors. For diagnosis-related claims, an average of 5 years elapses between the incident and the settlement of the claim (Tehrani et al., 2013). The validity of claims is uncertain; some claims will be filed and closed when no error occurred. Many, if not most, errors do not lead to malpractice claims. Cases may also be dismissed even when a true diagnostic error occurred.

Methods for identifying cases for review (denominator) Studies of diagnostic error using malpractice claims data use all malpractice claims (any allegation) as the denominator.

Methods for determining if an error occurred (numerator) In malpractice claims, the allegation in the claim is the basis for a determination; multiple allegations can be associated with a single claim. A number of studies have assessed the validity of malpractice claims (Localio et al., 1991; Studdert et al., 2000, 2006). Generally speaking, studies use only closed claims, that is, those for which the insurer has determined that no further legal action will be taken (claims may be closed due to settlement, verdict, dismissal, abandonment, or other reasons). Data from CRICO's Comparative Benchmarking System indicate that 63 percent of closed diagnosis-related cases were withdrawn, denied, or dismissed with no indemnity payment (CRICO, 2014).

What is known Tehrani et al. (2013) analyzed 25 years of closed medical malpractice claims from the National Practitioner Data Bank in order to characterize the frequency, patient outcomes, and economic consequences of diagnostic errors. The researchers found that diagnostic errors were the leading type of paid malpractice claims (28.6 percent) and were responsible for the highest proportion of total payments (35.2 percent) (Tehrani et al., 2013). Diagnostic errors were almost twice as likely to be associated with patient death as other allegation categories (such as treatment, surgery, medication, or obstetrics claims). Almost 70 percent of diagnostic error claims were from the outpatient setting, but inpatient diagnostic error claims were more likely to be associated with patient death. The researchers estimated that the 2011 inflation-adjusted mean and median per claim payout for diagnostic error were $386,849 and $213,250, respectively.

Schiff and colleagues (2013) reviewed closed primary care malpractice claims in Massachusetts from 2005 to 2009. During that 5-year period, 551 medical malpractice claims were from primary care practices. More than 70 percent of the allegations were related to diagnosis. The diagnoses most often appearing in these claims were cancer, heart diseases, blood vessel diseases, infections, and stroke.

CRICO has conducted comprehensive analyses of its claim files and associated medical records for diagnostic errors (CRICO, 2014; Siegal, 2014). CRICO's database represents about 30 percent of the NPDB and includes around 400 hospitals and health care entities and 165,000 physicians. In CRICO's analysis of data from 2008 to 2012 (including more than 4,500 cases and more than $1 billion total incurred losses), the organization reported that diagnosis-related claims represented 20 percent of cases by volume and 27 percent of indemnity payments. It found that diagnostic errors are more common in the ambulatory care setting than in the inpatient or emergency department setting (56 percent versus 28 percent and 16 percent, respectively). Within the inpatient setting, the top diagnoses represented in closed malpractice claims included myocardial infarction (MI) and cardiac events, complications of care (failure to rescue), and infections/sepsis (Siegal, 2014). In the ambulatory care setting, cancer, cardiac care (including MI), and injury (orthopedic, head, and spine) represented the top diagnoses in paid claims. CRICO found that cancer represented almost one-third of all the diagnosis-related medical malpractice claims.

The Doctors Company, another large national medical liability insurer, compiled information from its 2007–2013 claims database for the committee. In its analysis of diagnosis-related claims, The Doctors Company included information from 10 medical specialties (internal medicine, family medicine, obstetrics, cardiology, gynecology, general surgery, emergency medicine, orthopedics, pediatrics, and hospital medicine). For the 10 specialties, diagnosis-related claims constituted between 9 percent (obstetrics) and 61 percent (pediatrics) of total claims. The analysis included the top five diagnoses associated with each specialty's malpractice claims. That analysis indicated that more than half of the diagnoses appeared within multiple specialties and generally were for commonly encountered diseases (such as acute MI, acute cerebral vascular accident, cancer, and appendicitis) (Troxel, 2014).

Opportunities for improvement For malpractice claims to be useful for estimating the incidence of diagnostic error, it will be necessary to develop a better understanding of the underlying prevalence of diagnostic error as well as of the probability that a claim will be filed if an error has occurred and the likelihood that a filed claim will be settled. This will require significant research activity, and such research would have to explore variations by geography, specialty, type of error, and other factors. Databases from malpractice insurers contain much more clinical detail than the NPDB and are likely to be more useful in describing patterns of diagnostic errors, such as the steps in the diagnostic process that present the highest risk for different diagnoses. CRICO's benchmarking studies demonstrate the utility of these data for understanding where in the diagnostic process errors are most likely to occur and what factors contributed to the error. This can be useful for designing both monitoring and improvement programs.

Health Insurance Claims

Description of the data source The data source consists of electronic databases maintained by health insurance companies that contain the details of bills submitted by health care professionals and organizations for payment of services delivered. Both public (e.g., Medicare, Medicaid) and private (e.g., Aetna, Blue Cross, United Healthcare) entities maintain such databases on the individuals with whom they have a contractual arrangement to provide payment. Typically, health care professionals and organizations bill multiple insurers for services.

Notes about the data source For information to be present in the database, a patient has to have used a service, a claim must have been filed, the service must have been covered, and (usually) payment must have been made. Claims are based on structured coding systems (ICD-9/10, CPT-IV, NDC, DRG) and do not generally include clinical details (e.g., results of history and physical examinations, diagnostic testing results) except as categorical codes. Because data are available electronically and represent the universe of claims filed for any insurer, the probability that a patient or episode of care has been selected for analysis can be calculated. Because health care professionals and organizations bill multiple insurance companies, each of which has different rules, it can be difficult to understand the health care professionals' and organizations' overall practices with data from a single source.

Methods for identifying cases for review (denominator) Although a random sample of claims or groups of claims could be selected, it is more common to focus studies on those with patterns of care consistent with the possibility that a diagnostic error occurred.

Methods for determining if an error occurred (numerator) Frequently, an algorithm is developed to determine when an error likely occurred, such as cases in which there is no evidence that a diagnostic test was done prior to a new diagnosis being made (e.g., breast cancer diagnosis in the absence of a screening mammogram). Health insurance claims data may be linked to other data sources (e.g., National Death Index, diagnostic testing results, medical records) to make a determination that an error occurred.

What is known Within the quality and safety field, improvements in the measurement of both process and outcome measures of quality have been made possible by the expanding use of health information technology (health IT) and health insurance claims databases over the past several decades. For example, health insurance claims databases linked to validated federal death registries have made possible the measurement of 30-day mortality for acute MI, heart failure, and pneumonia, all of which are considered as outcome measures of quality. Similar databases provide the backbone for measuring process quality measures (such as 30-day rehospitalizations, appropriate assessment of left ventricular function in patients with congestive heart failure, and retinopathy screening among patients with diabetes). There are a few examples of the use of these data for investigating diagnostic error. Newman-Toker and colleagues (2014) identified patients who were admitted to the hospital with a diagnosis of stroke who in the previous 30 days had been treated and released from an emergency department for symptoms consistent with a stroke. They found that 12.7 percent of stroke admissions reflected potential missed stroke diagnoses and 1.2 percent reflected probable missed diagnoses.

These rates suggest that 15,000 to 165,000 stroke diagnoses are missed annually in the United States, with a higher risk for missed diagnoses among younger, female, and white patients. The researchers note that their estimates of diagnostic error are inferred rather than confirmed because of the lack of clinical detail in health insurance claims.

Opportunities for improvement Health insurance claims databases maintained by the Centers for Medicare & Medicaid Services (CMS) and by commercial insurers offer the possibility of measuring certain types of diagnostic errors, identifying their downstream clinical consequences and costs, and understanding the system-level, health care professional–level, and patient-level factors that are associated with these errors.

For example, analyses of claims data could be used in "look back" studies to identify the frequency with which acute coronary syndrome is misdiagnosed. Specifically, for those enrollees who are ultimately diagnosed with acute coronary syndrome, analysts could explore how frequently these beneficiaries were seen by health care professionals in the week prior to ultimate diagnosis (either in outpatient, emergency department, or hospital settings), the incorrect diagnoses that were made, and the factors associated with the diagnostic error. For instance, this epidemiologic approach using large administrative databases would make it possible to determine whether the diagnostic error occurs more frequently in specific hospitals, among specific types of clinicians or practice settings, or during particular days of the week when staffing is low or the volume of patients treated is unexpectedly high. The strength of this approach to understanding the epidemiology of diagnostic error is its ability to provide national estimates of diagnostic error rates across a vast array of conditions; to understand how these diagnostic error rates vary across geography and specific settings of care; to study the impact of specific care delivery models on diagnostic error rates (e.g., do accountable care organizations lower diagnostic errors?); and to update measurements as quickly as the administrative data are themselves collected. The main critique of this approach concerns the validity of the findings because of the limited availability of the clinical data necessary to confirm a diagnosis. Thus, this data source may be most useful in combination with other sources.

Diagnostic Testing (Anatomic and Clinical Pathology)

Description of the data source Diagnostic testing includes the examination of secretions, discharges, blood, or tissue using chemical, microscopic, immunologic, or pathologic methods for the purposes of making or ruling out a diagnosis. Analysis of the data may involve automated processes or a visual examination by trained health care professionals (clinical and anatomic pathologists).

Notes about the data source A unique feature of this type of data is that the original source data (the samples) are frequently available for reanalysis or inspection by another health care professional, thus allowing for an independent assessment based on the same data. For the committee's purposes, the focus is on those diagnoses for which diagnostic testing findings are a key information source. A common taxonomy in this field distinguishes among five phases: pre-pre-analytic (i.e., deciding whether or not to order a particular test), pre-analytic (i.e., sample labeling and acquisition, test performance), analytic (i.e., the accuracy of the test or examination of the sample), post-analytic (i.e., the results are reported correctly, interpreted correctly, and communicated back to the ordering clinician in a timely way), and post-post-analytic (i.e., the ordering clinician uses test results to inform patient care) (Plebani et al., 2011). For the purpose of examining the incidence of diagnostic error, the committee focused on those circumstances in which diagnostic testing results are a key information source. One study estimated that at least 10 percent of diagnoses require diagnostic testing results in order to be considered final; this number is likely higher today (Epner et al., 2013; Hallworth, 2011; Peterson et al., 1992). Primary care clinicians order tests in about one-third of patient visits (Hickner et al., 2014). For anatomic pathology specimens, which require visual inspection and clinical judgment, second reviews by another pathologist offer insight into the potential rate of diagnostic error.

Methods for identifying cases for review (denominator) Two methods—random samples and prespecified criteria—are commonly used to identify cases. Both methods allow for the denominator to be characterized (i.e., the probability that a case was reviewed, the characteristics of the cases reviewed as compared to all cases).

Methods for determining if an error occurred (numerator) Because testing involves multiple steps, there are many different methods for identifying errors, including an examination of other data sources such as medical records, malpractice claims, or pharmacy databases (Callen et al., 2011). For second review studies, an error is typically defined as a discrepancy between the findings of the first pathologist and the second pathologist. This review can identify errors in which a finding that leads to a diagnosis was missed and errors in which a finding was inaccurate (i.e., no disease was found by the second reviewer). Second review studies typically assume that the second review is more accurate, but these studies do not typically link to patient outcomes. When second reviews are linked to patient outcomes, Renshaw and Gould (2005) concluded that in many cases, the first reviewer was correct. For other diagnostic tests, errors may be detected in the interpretation or communication of results in a timely manner.

What is known Plebani reported that errors in laboratory medicine studies vary greatly because of the heterogeneity in study designs and the particular step or steps in the process that were examined (Plebani, 2010). A considerable focus on the analytic phase has led to substantial reductions in errors in that step; the pre- and post-analytic phases are seen as more vulnerable to error. A review published in 2002 (that only classified the diagnostic testing process in three phases) found that 32 to 75 percent of errors occurred in the pre-analytic phase, 13 to 32 percent in the analytic phase, and 9 to 31 percent in the post-analytic phase (Bonini et al., 2002). A study of urgent diagnostic testing orders in the hospital, which also classified the diagnostic testing process in three phases, found that 62 percent of errors were in the pre-analytic phase, 15 percent in the analytic phase, and 23 percent in the post-analytic phase (Carraro and Plebani, 2007). One study estimated that 8 percent of errors had the potential to result in serious patient harm (Goldschmidt and Lent, 1995). A systematic review of the literature on follow-up of test results in the hospital found failure rates of 1 to 23 percent in inpatients and 0 to 16.5 percent in emergency department patients (Callen et al., 2011).

As Berner and Graber (2008) note, second reviews in anatomic pathology identify varying discrepancy rates. The College of American Pathologists and the Association of Directors of Anatomic and Surgical Pathology recently published guidelines based on a systematic review of the literature which found a median rate of major discrepancies in 5.9 percent of cases (95 percent confidence interval, 2.1–10.5 percent) (Nakhleh et al., 2015). The study also reported variations in the rate by the service performed (surgical pathology versus cytology), the organ system (single versus multiple), and the type of review (internal versus external). Kronz and Westra (2005) report a diagnostic discrepancy rate for the head and neck found by second review of between 1 and 53 percent for surgical pathology and 17 to 60 percent for cytopathology. A study by Gaudi and colleagues (2013) found that pathologists with dermatopathology fellowship training were more likely to disagree with preliminary diagnoses provided by nonspecialist pathologists.

Opportunities for improvement The contribution of diagnostic testing to diagnosis is substantial, but it has not been systematically quantified recently. The understanding of this critical information source could be improved by developing better methods for identifying and enumerating the diagnoses for which such testing is critical, mechanisms for evaluating the appropriateness of test ordering, and methods for determining the impact on patient outcomes. Additionally, studies that use diagnostic variance as a surrogate for accuracy (second reviews in which the second reviewer is considered more accurate) could benefit from the inclusion of patient outcomes.

Medical Imaging

Description of the data source The data are visual representations of the interior of the body generated using a variety of methods (e.g., X-ray, ultrasound, computed tomography [CT], magnetic resonance imaging, and positron emission tomography) that are collected for the purpose of diagnosis; these visual representations generally require interpretation by a radiologist or, in certain circumstances, physicians in nuclear medicine, emergency medicine, or cardiology. In this context, the medical imaging data are reviewed by at least one other clinician, and the findings of all health care professionals are recorded.

Notes about the data source As with anatomic pathology, a unique feature of this data type is the availability of the original images for review by a second radiologist. The focus is on those diagnoses for which medical imaging results are a key information source. In approximately 15 percent of office visits, an imaging study is ordered or provided (CDC, 2010), whereas one or more medical imaging studies are ordered in approximately 47 percent of emergency department visits (CDC, 2011). In both settings, X-rays are the most common imaging method used.

Methods for identifying cases for review (denominator) Typically a random sample of cases is selected for second review, although some studies have included prespecified criteria (e.g., cases known to have higher potential rates of error in interpretation, or abnormal findings only).

Methods for determining if an error occurred (numerator) An error is assumed to have occurred whenever a discrepancy exists between the two clinicians in interpreting the medical imaging study. Some studies have also involved radiologists conducting a second review of their own previously completed studies.

What is known Berlin noted that medical imaging discrepancy rates as indicated by second review have not changed much over the past 60 years (Berlin, 2014). For instance, a study by Abujudeh and colleagues explored intra- and interobserver variability in medical imaging by having three experienced radiologists review 30 of their own previously interpreted CT exams and 30 CT exams originally interpreted by other radiologists (Abujudeh et al., 2010). They found a major discrepancy rate of 26 percent for interobserver variability and 32 percent for intraobserver variability. Velmahos and colleagues (2001) found an 11 percent discrepancy rate between the preliminary and final readings of CT scans of trauma patients. Discrepancy rates were negatively associated with level of experience: The lower the level of experience of the preliminary reader, the more likely there was to be a discrepancy. In many of the second review studies in imaging, high error rates resulted from using a denominator that consisted only of abnormal cases. Studies that look at real-time errors—that is, devising an error rate using both normal and abnormal exams as the denominator—suggest an error rate in the 3 to 4.4 percent range (Borgstede et al., 2004).

Opportunities for improvement Medical imaging plays a key role in many diagnoses, and errors in the use and interpretation of these studies can contribute to diagnostic error. For the purposes of estimating the incidence of diagnostic error due to errors related to medical imaging, it would be useful to identify the subset of diagnoses for which medical imaging results are central to making the diagnosis and to conduct studies to determine the likelihood of errors, the nature of those errors, and the variation in the circumstances under which errors occur. The role of second reviews in error recovery—identifying and "intercepting" errors before they affect patient outcomes—both for medical imaging and for anatomic pathology is discussed in Chapter 6.

Surveys of Clinicians

Description of the data source The data come from questionnaires (written, telephone, interview, Web-based) that obtain clinicians' self-reports about diagnostic errors they have made or what they know about diagnostic errors made by other clinicians. The information content of such surveys can vary.

Notes about the data source As with all surveys, the results can be affected by a number of biases, including nonresponse bias (nonresponders being systematically different from responders, such as being more or less likely to have committed a diagnostic error) or reporting bias (systematic differences in the information that is revealed or suppressed, such as not reporting more serious errors). Unless the self-report can be compared to an authoritative source, it is difficult to determine the validity of rates based solely on self-report. Surveys usually have the advantage of anonymity, which might make respondents more likely to report their errors accurately than through other methods.

Methods for identifying cases for review (denominator) Surveys are frequently conducted on random samples of clinicians, making the implicit denominator the number of opportunities a clinician had to make a diagnosis in the study period. Convenience samples are also used (e.g., surveys of clinicians participating in a continuing medical education course). Reports of survey findings have used different denominators, but often the denominator is the number of clinicians responding to the survey.

Methods for determining if an error occurred (numerator) An error is judged to have occurred when a clinician self-reports having made one or more diagnostic errors in the study time frame. Some studies have asked about errors known to the clinician that were made by other clinicians or experienced by family members. This approach makes estimating the incidence rate nearly impossible, as the true denominator is unknown.

What is known Schiff et al. (2009) surveyed physicians and asked them to recall instances of diagnostic error. In their analysis of 583 reports of diagnostic error, they found that physicians readily recalled instances of diagnostic error; the most commonly reported diagnostic errors were pulmonary embolism, drug reactions, cancer, acute coronary syndrome, and stroke. Singh and colleagues (2010b, p. 70) surveyed pediatricians about diagnostic errors and found that "more than half of respondents reported that they made a diagnostic error at least once or twice per month." In another survey of physicians, 35 percent reported that they had experienced medical errors either in their own or a family member's care (Blendon et al., 2002).

Opportunities for improvement For the purposes of making national estimates of the incidence of diagnostic errors, it would be useful to have more clearly defined sampling frames, more detailed questions about the nature of the errors and the circumstances surrounding the error, and an opportunity to compare this method to other methods that use different data sources. Surveys have the advantage of being a potentially easy way to get a snapshot of diagnostic error rates, but the quality of the information may make this source less useful for other applications. The biases that are inherent in surveys are difficult to overcome and likely limit the utility of this source.

Surveys of Patients

Description of the data source The data come from questionnaires (written, telephone, interview, Web-based) that obtain patients' self-reports about diagnostic errors they have experienced or their awareness of diagnostic errors experienced by others. The information collected can vary.

Notes about the data source As with all surveys, the results can be affected by nonresponse bias and by reporting bias. Unless there are opportunities to compare answers to other data sources, it may not be possible to confirm the validity of the responses. Patient definitions of diagnostic errors might vary from the definitions of health care professionals. Patient surveys can be very useful in determining whether a new health problem was explained to the patients and whether they understood the explanation.

Methods for identifying cases for review (denominator) Surveys are usually conducted on a sample of patients that is randomly drawn from some population (e.g., geographic area, members of a health plan, and patients who utilize a specific care setting) or selected so that the patients meet certain criteria (similar to the trigger tools discussed above). Convenience samples are also used.

Methods for determining if an error occurred (numerator) The determination of an error is based on self-report by the patient. Some studies inquire about both the patient's own experience and that of others known to the patient. The latter approach makes it impossible to estimate a true incidence rate because of uncertainty around the real size of the denominator.

What is known In one survey of patients, 42 percent reported that they had experienced medical errors either in their own or a family member's care (Blendon et al., 2002). A poll commissioned by the National Patient Safety Foundation found that approximately one in six of those surveyed had experience with diagnostic error, either personally or through a close friend or relative (Golodner, 1997). More recently, 23 percent of people surveyed in Massachusetts indicated that they or someone close to them had experienced a medical error, and approximately half of these errors were diagnostic errors (Betsy Lehman Center for Patient Safety and Medical Error Reduction, 2014). Weissman and colleagues (2008) surveyed patients about adverse events during a hospital stay and compared survey-detected adverse events with medical record review. Twenty-three percent of surveyed patients reported at least one adverse event, compared to 11 percent identified by medical record review.

Opportunities for improvement The particular value of patient surveys is likely to be related to understanding failures at the front end of the diagnostic process (failure to engage) and in the process of delivering an explanation to the patient. Both are critical steps, and patients are uniquely positioned to report on those elements of diagnostic performance. The committee did not have examples of this application, and potential future uses are discussed in Chapter 8.

Other Methods

A variety of other methods have been employed to examine different dimensions of diagnostic error. These methods were not included in the table because they are unlikely to be a major source for estimating the incidence of error.

Patient actors, or "standardized patients," have been used to assess rates of diagnostic error. Patient actors are asked to portray typical presentations of disease, and clinicians are assessed on their diagnostic performance. In one study in internal medicine, physicians made diagnostic errors in 13 percent of interactions with patient actors portraying four common conditions (Peabody et al., 2004). In a more recent multicenter study with unannounced patient actors, Weiner et al. (2010) looked at both biomedical-related errors (such as errors in diagnosis and treatment) and context-related errors (such as the lack of recognition that a patient may be unable to afford a medicine based on certain patient cues) in patient management. They found that physicians provided care that was free from errors in 73 percent of the uncomplicated encounters but made more errors in more complex cases (Weiner et al., 2010).

Many health care organizations in the United States have systems in place for patients and health care professionals to report minor and major adverse events. However, voluntary reporting typically results in underreporting and covers only a limited spectrum of adverse events (AHRQ, 2014b). For example, one study found that over half of voluntary reports concentrated on medication/infusion adverse events (33 percent), falls (13 percent), and administrative events, such as discharge process, documentation, and communication (13 percent) (Milch et al., 2006). In Maine, the use of a physician champion to encourage voluntary diagnostic error reporting was implemented in 2011. During the 6-month pilot, there were 36 diagnostic errors reported. Half of the diagnostic errors were associated with moderate harm, and 22 percent of the diagnostic errors were classified as causing severe harm (Trowbridge, 2014).

Direct observation is another method that has been used to identify medical errors. Andrews and colleagues (1997) conducted observational research within a hospital setting and found that approximately 18 percent of patients in the study experienced a serious adverse event.

There have also been efforts to assess disease-specific diagnostic error rates, using a variety of data sources and methods. Berner and Graber (2008) and Schiff and colleagues (2005) provide examples of diagnostic errors in a variety of disease conditions.

Summary of Approaches to Assess the Incidence of Diagnostic Error

A number of methods have been used to assess the frequency with which diagnostic error occurs. Based on the committee's review, the most promising methods for estimating incidence are postmortem exams, medical record reviews, and medical malpractice claims analysis, but none of these alone will give a valid estimate of the incidence of diagnostic error. This conclusion is consistent with studies in the broader area of medical errors and adverse events. For example, the Office of Inspector General of HHS completed an analysis that compared different measurement methods (nurse reviews, analysis of administrative claims data, patient interviews, analysis of incident reports, and an analysis of patient safety indicators) and found that 46 percent of patient safety events were identified by only one of the methods (Office of Inspector General, 2010). Levtzion-Korach and colleagues (2010) compared information gathered with five different measurement approaches—incident reporting, patient complaints, risk management, medical malpractice claims, and executive WalkRounds—and concluded that each measurement method identified different but complementary patient safety issues. In a related commentary, Shojania concluded that "it appears that a hospital's picture of patient safety will depend on the method used to generate it" (Shojania, 2010, p. 400). This suggests that no one method will perfectly capture the incidence and the nature of medical errors and adverse events in health care: "[A] compelling theme emerged . . . different methods for detecting patient safety problems overlap very little in the safety problems they detect. These methods complement each other and should be used in combination to provide a comprehensive safety picture of the health care organization" (Shekelle et al., 2013, p. 416). This likely applies to the measurement of diagnostic errors; with the complexity of the diagnostic process, multiple approaches will be necessary to provide a more thorough understanding of the occurrence of these errors.

Determining the Causes and Risks of Diagnostic Error

This section describes how measurement can be used to better characterize diagnostic errors by identifying the causes and the risks associated with diagnostic error. Characterization of diagnostic errors requires understanding (1) which aspects in the diagnostic process are susceptible to failures and (2) what the contributing factors to these failures are. The committee used its conceptual model and input from other frameworks to provide a context for the measurement of the causes and the risks of diagnostic error. Measurement can focus on diagnostic process steps, the work system components, or both in order to identify causes and risks of diagnostic error.

The Diagnostic Process and Measurement Approaches to Identifying Potential Failures

Because the diagnostic process is a complex, team-based, iterative process that occurs over varying time spans, there are numerous opportunities for failures. The failures can include (1) the step never occurring, (2) the step being done incompletely or incorrectly (accuracy), and (3) a meaningful delay in taking a step (timeliness). In Figure 3-2, the committee's conceptual model is used to identify where in the diagnostic process these failures can occur, including the failure of engagement in the health care system, failure in the diagnostic process, failure to establish an explanation of the health problem, and failure to communicate the explanation of the health problem.

Table 3-2 is organized around the major steps in the diagnostic process and adapts Schiff and colleagues' (2009) framework to the failures associated with each of these steps. For example, diagnostic testing is part of several diagnostic steps where failures may happen, namely, during information gathering, integration, and interpretation. The last column identifies some of the methods that can be used to identify failures in actual practice settings. Experimental laboratory methods are a complementary approach to the methods in Table 3-2 to understand potential failures related to reasoning (Kostopoulou et al., 2009, 2012; Zwaan et al., 2013). The following discussion includes more information about the measurement approaches that can be used at each of these steps.

Failure of engagement This step primarily involves either patients not recognizing symptoms or health risks rapidly enough to access the health care system or patients experiencing significant barriers to accessing health care. Health care organizations are familiar with routine measures of eligible patients presenting for common screening tests;

120

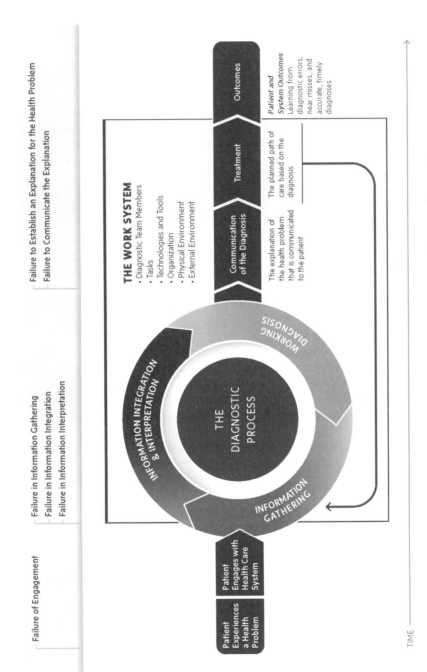

FIGURE 3-2 Places in the diagnostic process where failures can occur that contribute to diagnostic errors.

TABLE 3-2 Methods for Detecting Failures Across the Diagnostic Process

Where in the Diagnostic Process the Failure Occurred	Nature of Failure[a]	Methods for Detecting Failures
Failure to engage in the health care system or in the diagnostic process	• Delay in patient presenting • Patient unable to access care	Analysis of emergency department, urgent care, and other high-risk cohorts Surveys to determine why and what could be done differently
Failure in information gathering	• Failure/delay in eliciting key history, physical exam finding • Failure to order or perform needed tests • Failure to review test results • Wrong tests ordered • Tests ordered in the wrong sequence • Technical errors in the handling, labeling, processing of tests	Random reviews Diagnostic trigger tools (e.g., high-risk cohort algorithms and missed opportunity targets) Comparison to checklists Video recording and debriefing (e.g., "stimulated recall")
Failure in information integration	• Failures in hypothesis generation • Suboptimal weighting and prioritization • Failure to recognize or weight urgency	Debriefing Diagnostic conferences Random exams
Failure in information interpretation	• Inaccurate or failed interpretation of history, physical exam findings, test results	Second review of samples
Failure to establish an explanation (diagnosis)	• Suboptimal weighting and prioritization • Delay in considering diagnosis • Failure to follow up • Scientific knowledge limitations (e.g., signs and symptoms that have not been recognized as a specific disease)	Random reviews Examination of expected follow-up (e.g., Kaiser Permanente's SureNet system) Postmortem examinations
Failure to communicate the explanation to the patient	• Patient not notified • Delay in notification • Incomplete explanation • Patient does not understand explanation	Video recording and debriefing Survey patients Medical record review Shared decision making result

[a] Adapted from Schiff et al., 2009.

these systems can be extended to detect other failures to engage (or reengage) related to routine monitoring for disease progress, follow-up of abnormal test results, and so on (Danforth et al., 2014; Kanter, 2014; Singh et al., 2009). Surveys and interviews with patients can be used to identify approaches that are likely to be successful (and unsuccessful) in reducing delays and increasing engagement. The CRICO benchmarking study found that 1 percent of malpractice claims had an error associated with a failure to engage (CRICO, 2014).

Failure in information gathering The information-gathering step can involve failures to elicit key pieces of information; a failure to order the right diagnostic testing (in the right sequence or with the right specification); or technical errors in the way that samples are handled, labeled, and processed. The CRICO benchmarking study found that 58 percent of cases had one or more errors in the initial diagnostic assessment (CRICO, 2014). Failure to order appropriate diagnostic tests has been found to account for 55 percent of missed or delayed diagnoses in malpractice claims in ambulatory care (Gandhi et al., 2006) and 58 percent of errors in emergency departments (Kachalia et al., 2006). In their examination of physician-reported cases of error, Schiff and colleagues (2009) found that a failure or delay in ordering needed tests was the second most common factor contributing to a diagnostic error. Methods of rapid detection might include random reviews, diagnostic trigger tools, checklists, observation, video or audio recording, and feedback.

Failure in interpretation Inaccurate or failed attempts to interpret information gathered in the diagnostic process can involve such things as diagnostic tests, clinical history and interview, or information received from referral and consultation with other clinicians. CRICO reported that 23 percent of cases in its malpractice benchmarking study had errors in diagnostic test interpretation; 49 percent had errors in medical imaging, 20 percent in medicine, 17 percent in pathology, and 8 percent in surgery (CRICO, 2014). Schiff and colleagues (2009) reported that an erroneous laboratory or radiology reading of a test contributed to 11 percent of the diagnostic errors that they examined. Studies have shown that an incorrect interpretation of diagnostic tests occurs in internal medicine (38 percent reported in Gandhi et al., 2006) and emergency medicine (37 percent reported in Kachalia et al., 2006). Hickner and colleagues (2008) found that 8.3 percent of surveyed primary care physicians reported uncertainty in interpreting diagnostic testing. Failure in interpretations for medical imaging and anatomic pathology can be identified through second reviews conducted by expert clinicians.

Failure in integration Integration failures can be divided into failures in hypothesis generation, the suboptimal weighting and prioritization of information gathered in the diagnostic process, and the failure to recognize or weight urgency of clinical signs or symptoms. In examining major diagnostic errors, Schiff and colleagues (2009) found that 24 percent were the result of a failure to consider or a delay in considering the correct diagnosis. Potential approaches to measuring failure in integration include structured debriefings with the clinicians involved, conferences that review diagnostic errors (such as morbidity and mortality [M&M] conferences and root cause analyses), and random reviews.

Failure to establish an explanation (diagnosis) Failures can also occur when there is a failure to establish the explanation of the patient's health problem. This can include suboptimal weighting and prioritization of clinical signs and symptoms, delays in considering a diagnosis, or failing to follow up with patients (including failing to create and implement an appropriate follow-up plan). CRICO (2014) found that referral errors were common in cancer cases in which there were diagnostic errors (48 percent of cases lacked appropriate referrals or consults). Methods for identifying these failures include random reviews and the analysis of expected follow-up, such as Kaiser Permanente's SureNet system (Danforth et al., 2014; Graber et al., 2014).

Failure to communicate the explanation Failures to communicate the explanation of a patient's health problem can include cases in which no communication was attempted, in which there was a delay in communicating the explanation, or in which the communication occurred but it was not aligned with a patient's health literacy and language needs and was not understood. CRICO (2014) reported that 46 percent of cases in its benchmarking study involved a failure in communication and follow-up, including 18 percent of cases where the clinician did not follow up with the patient and 12 percent of cases where the information was not communicated within the care team. Potential measurement methods for this step include video recording and debriefing, patient surveys, medical record reviews, and shared decision-making results.

Other researchers have employed different classification schemes to illustrate where in the diagnostic process failures occur. For example, some researchers have classified the diagnostic process into three phases: initial diagnostic assessment; diagnostic test performance, interpretation, and results reporting; and diagnostic follow-up and coordination (CRICO, 2014; Lyratzopoulos et al., 2015). Another framework that is useful to depict the steps in the diagnostic testing process where failures can occur is the brain-to-brain loop model described in Chapter 2. The nine-step process was originally developed in the laboratory medicine setting (Lundberg, 1981; Plebani et al., 2011), but it can be applied to anatomic pathology and medical imaging as well. Targeted measurement has shown that the phases of the process that are most prone to errors occur outside of the analytical phase and include test ordering (part of the diagnostic process information-gathering step) and subsequent decision making on the basis of the test results (part of the interpretation step) (Epner et al., 2013; Hickner et al., 2014; Plebani et al., 2011).

*The Work System and Measurement Approaches to
Identifying Potential Vulnerabilities and Risk Factors*

In considering the options for making significant progress on the problem of diagnostic error, it is important to understand the reasons why these failures occur. For this discussion, the committee draws on the general patient safety literature, and applies it specifically to the challenge of diagnostic error. Traditional approaches to evaluating medical errors have focused on identifying individuals at fault. However, the modern patient safety movement has emphasized the importance of a systems approach to understanding medical errors. According to the IOM report *To Err Is Human: Building a Safer Health System*:

> The common initial reaction when an error occurs is to find and blame someone. However, even apparently single events or errors are due most often to the convergence of multiple contributing factors. Blaming an individual does not change these factors and the same error is likely to recur. Preventing errors and improving patient safety for patients require a systems approach in order to modify the conditions that contribute to errors. People working in health care are among the most educated and dedicated workforce in any industry. The problem is not bad people; the problem is that the system needs to be made safer. (IOM, 2000, p. 49)

Often, a diagnostic error has multiple contributing factors. One analogy that has been employed to describe this phenomenon is the Swiss cheese model developed by psychologist James Reason (AHRQ, 2015a; Reason, 1990). In this model, a component of the diagnostic process would represent a slice of cheese in a stack of slices. Each component within the diagnostic process has vulnerabilities to failure (represented by the holes in a slice of Swiss cheese); in a single step of the diagnostic process, this may not affect the outcome. However, if the vulnerabilities (holes in the Swiss cheese) align, a diagnostic error can result.

Another way to think about the causes of diagnostic error is to distinguish between active errors and latent errors. Active errors typically involve frontline clinicians (sometimes referred to as the "sharp end" of patient safety) (IOM, 2000). In contrast, latent errors are more removed from the control of frontline clinicians and can include failures in organizations and design that enable active errors to cause harm (often called the "blunt end" of patient safety) (AHRQ, 2015a; IOM, 2000). In the event of a medical error, too often the focus is on identifying active errors, especially within health care organizations with punitive cultures that focus on individual blame and punishment. But the IOM noted that:

> Latent errors pose the greatest threat to safety in a complex system because they are often unrecognized and have the capacity to result in multiple types of active errors. . . . Latent errors can be difficult for people working in the system to notice since the errors may be hidden in the design of routine processes in computer programs or in the structure or management of an organization. People also become accustomed to design defects and learn to work around them, so they are often not recognized. (IOM, 2000, p. 55)

In line with the IOM's earlier work, the committee took a systems approach to understanding the causes and risks of diagnostic errors. Consistent with the committee's conceptual model, measurement for this purpose examines the different dimensions of the work system to identify the circumstances under which diagnostic errors are more (and less) likely to occur and to identify the risk factors for such errors. Factors contributing to diagnostic errors can be mapped along the components of the work system, including diagnostic team members and their tasks, technologies and tools, organizational characteristics, the physical environment, and the external environment.

Some of the more familiar approaches for assessing the system causes of medical errors are M&M conferences that apply a modern patient safety framework (a focus on understanding contributing factors rather than a focus on individual errors and blame) (Shojania, 2010) and root cause analyses (AHRQ, 2015b). For example, root cause analysis methods were applied to identify the factors that contributed to delays in diagnosis in the Department of Veterans Affairs system (Giardina et al., 2013). Diagnostic errors have also been evaluated in M&M conferences (Cifra et al., 2015).

As the committee's conceptual model shows, the diagnostic process is embedded in a work system. Examining how the various dimensions of the work system contribute to diagnostic errors or how they can be configured to enhance diagnostic performance leads to a deeper understanding of the complexity of the process. Table 3-3 identifies the dimensions of the work system, the contribution each makes to diagnostic errors, and examples of measurement methods that have been used to assess each area. Although diagnostic team members are a critical component of the work system, approaches to ensuring diagnostic competency are addressed in Chapter 4 and they are not included here. The focus here is on the specific measurement tools that are available to help health care organizations better identify aspects of the work system that present vulnerabilities for diagnostic errors. A distinctive feature of some of these methods is

TABLE 3-3 Methods for Assessing the Effect of the Work System on Diagnostic Errors

Work System Dimension	Contribution to Diagnostic Errors	Examples of Methods for Assessing Effects

Tasks and workflow
• Problems with information
  o Amount
  o Accuracy
  o Completeness
  o Appropriateness
• Communication issues
• Task complexity
• Situation awareness
• Poor workflow design
• Interruptions
• Inefficiencies
• Workload
	Information gathering
	Information integration
	Information interpretation
	Information visualization (where, when, and how the information is received in the system)
	Fragmented workflow and lack of support for accurate and timely information flow
	Work-around strategies that increase risk
		Cognitive task and work analysis methods (e.g., decision ladder model)
		
		Observation of care process (e.g., work sampling; task analysis; video recording of care process and debriefing, e.g., stimulated recall)
		
		Situation awareness
		
		Workflow modeling
		
		Proactive risk assessment, including failure mode and effects analysis

Technology
• Inappropriate technology selection
• Poor design
• Poor implementation
• Use error
  o Failure to use technology
  o Failure to respond to signals
• Failure of technology (breakdown)
• Misuse of automation
	Lack of support for stages/steps of diagnostic process: information gathering, information integration, information interpretation
	Data overload
	Information visualization (where, when, and how the information is received in the system)
		Usability evaluation
		Observation of technology in use
		Proactive risk assessment, including failure mode and effect analysis

TABLE 3-3 Continued

Work System Dimension	Contribution to Diagnostic Errors	Examples of Methods for Assessing Effects
Organizational characteristics • Culture • Leadership and management • Staffing • Work organization (distribution of roles, rounding process, etc.) • Scheduling	Not supporting work system design efforts aimed at improving the diagnostic process and preventing/mitigating diagnostic errors Conflicting messages about regulations across the organization Confusion about responsibilities for tasks with unclear roles Reluctance to question people with greater authority	Culture surveys Surveys aimed at assessing leadership and management in quality/safety improvement Interviews or focus groups with clinicians and patients
Physical environment • Noise • Lighting • Poor physical layout	Additional stressors on diagnostic team members that can affect cognitive tasks in diagnostic process: information gathering, information integration, and information interpretation	Physical human factors/ergonomics methods (e.g., direct assessment of noise and lighting [with equipment], survey of diagnostic team members regarding physical environment) Link analysis for assessment of physical layout and team communication

that they can be used proactively to identify risks before an error occurs, versus the measurement methods described above that examine steps leading to an error that has already occurred.

Tasks and workflow The diagnostic process involves a series of tasks and an implicit or explicit workflow that contains and connects those tasks. A variety of challenges can occur with the tasks and workflow that are required to make a diagnosis, including problems with the information (amount, accuracy, completeness, appropriateness), communication issues, the complexity of the task, a lack of situational awareness, poor workflow design, interruptions, and inefficiencies. These issues contribute to diagnostic error at each step in the information gathering, integration, and interpretation process; they can contribute to problems with the timeliness of information availability, and they can lead to problems in cognitive processing.

There are a variety of measurement approaches that can be used to evaluate tasks and workflow. It should be noted that these are best applied in the real-world environment in which the diagnosis is being made. The methods include cognitive task and work analysis (Bisantz and Roth, 2007; Rogers et al., 2012; Roth, 2008); observation of care processes (Carayon et al., 2014); situation awareness (Carayon et al., 2014; Salas et al., 1995); workflow modeling (Kirwan and Ainsworth, 1992); and proactive risk assessment (Carayon et al., 2014). These methods are briefly described below.

Cognitive task and work analysis The purpose of cognitive task and work analysis is to identify and describe the cognitive skills that are required to perform a particular task, such as making a diagnosis. The most common method used for such an analysis is an in-depth interview combined with observations of the specific task of interest (Schraagen et al., 2000). Because cognitive errors are an important contributing factor to diagnostic errors (Croskerry, 2003) these methods are likely to have considerable utility in efforts to reduce errors. Koopman and colleagues (2015) used cognitive task analysis to examine the relationship between the information needs that clinicians had in preparing for an office visit and the information presented in the electronic health record. They found a significant disconnect between clinician needs and the amount of information and the manner in which it was presented. This disconnect can lead to cognitive overload, a known contributor to error (Patel et al., 2008; Singh et al., 2013). The researchers recommended significant reengineering of the clinical progress note so that it matched the workflow and information needs of primary care clinicians.

Observation of care processes Process observation is a means of verifying what exactly occurs during a particular process (CAHPS, 2012). Frequently, these observations are documented in the form of process maps, which are graphical representations of the various steps required to accomplish a task. The approach is able to capture the complex demands imposed on members of the diagnostic team, and it allows for the "documentation of the coordination and communication required between clinicians to complete a task, use their expertise, tools, information and cues to problem solve" (Rogers et al., 2012). For example, Fairbanks and colleagues (2010) used this method to examine workflow and information flow in an emergency department's use of digital imaging by applying both hierarchical task analysis and information process diagrams. The analysis identified gaps in how the information system for imaging supported communication between radiologists and emergency department physicians. In analyzing diagnostic error, this technique can identify the role that contextual or social factors play in assisting or impeding problem resolution (Rogers et al., 2012). Observations of care processes can also provide input for other work system analysis methods, such as cognitive task and work analysis as well as failure mode and effects analysis (FMEA).

Situation awareness Endsley (1995, p. 36) defined situation awareness as "the perception of elements in the environment within a volume of time and space, the comprehension of their meaning, and the projection of their status in the near future." Situation awareness has been applied at the individual, team, and system levels. There are a variety of approaches to measuring situation awareness, including objective and subjective measures, performance and behavioral measures, and process indices. Because of the multidimensional nature of the construct, a combination of approaches is likely most useful. Examples of measurement tools in medicine include the Anesthetists' Non-Technical Skills (ANTS) measure (Fletcher et al., 2003), the Ottawa Global Rating Scales (Kim et al., 2006), and an instrument to measure pediatric residents' self-efficacy skills (which include situation awareness) in crisis resource management (Plant et al., 2011).

Workflow modeling Workflow modeling is a form of prospective analysis used to describe the processes and activities involved in completing clinical tasks. In contrast to observing work processes, modeling techniques allow for quantitative and qualitative estimations of tasks and of the possible paths that can be taken to complete them (Unertl et al., 2009). Challenges to workflow modeling in health care—and diagnosis in particular—include the fact that clinicians must remain flexible because of the need to respond to the nonroutine presentation of symptoms, results, and events as well as the variability in workflow across different health care organizations. Resulting models can be adapted and modified as necessary to reflect observations of care processes. Numerous methods for workflow modeling exist. Carayon et al. (2012) describe 100 methods in 12 categories (e.g., data display/organization methods and process mapping tools) for workflow modeling of the implementation of health IT. Jun et al. (2009) focus on eight workflow or process modeling methods that have been used in quality improvement projects; these include flowcharts and communication diagrams. These methods have great potential for helping to understand the dynamic sequences of tasks performed by various team members in the diagnostic process.

Proactive risk assessment The term "proactive risk assessment" refers to a variety of methods that are used to identify, evaluate, and minimize potential risks or vulnerabilities in a system. An example of such a method is FMEA. Several steps are involved in FMEA, including graphically describing the process, observing the process to ensure that the diagram is an accurate representation, brainstorming about failure modes, conducting a hazard analysis (i.e., different ways in which a particular process can fail to achieve its purpose), and development of a plan to address each failure mode along with outcome measures. DeRosier and colleagues (2002) describe the use of this method by the Department of Veterans Affairs (VA) National Center for Patient Safety and provide concrete examples of its application.

Technology A variety of technologies are used in the diagnostic process, and these can contribute to diagnostic errors for a variety of reasons, including inappropriate technology selection, poor design, poor implementation, use error, technology breakdown or failure, and misuse of automation. Technology failures contribute to problems in information gathering, integration, and interpretation; they may also produce information overload and may interfere with cognitive processes because of problems with the way the information is received and displayed.

Methods for improving the selection, design, implementation, and use of technology involve some of the methods described above, such as workflow modeling, FMEA, and other proactive risk assessment methods. In particular, many health care organizations have been concerned about whether enough attention is being paid to the usability of health IT. For example, in a study of physician job satisfaction, Friedberg and colleagues (2013) found that a number of factors related to electronic health records (EHRs) had a substantial impact on satisfaction, including: poor usability, the time required for data entry, interference in patient interactions, greater inefficiencies in workflow, less fulfilling work content, problems in exchanging information, and a degradation of clinical documentation. This study used a mixed-method design which included semi-structured and structured interviews with physicians. Its findings were consistent with research using other methods to assess the extent to which EHRs are enhancing care delivery (Armijo et al., 2009; Unertl et al., 2009). The American Medical Informatics Association Board of Directors issued recommendations about improving the usability of EHRs that were based in large part on usability studies that had been conducted by Middleton and colleagues (2013). The use of various usability evaluation methods can help in ensuring that usability concerns are addressed as early as possible in the design process. For example, Smith and colleagues incorporated usability testing into the design of a decision-support software tool to catch missed follow-up of abnormal cancer test results in the VA (Smith et al., 2013). These various possible usability evaluation methods include heuristic evaluation methods, scenario-based usability evaluation, user testing, and the observation of technology in use (Gosbee and Gosbee, 2012).

Organizational characteristics Culture, leadership, and management are some of the organizational characteristics that can affect the diagnostic process. Some of the culture-related issues that can contribute to diagnostic error are a lack of organizational support for improvements, conflicting messages about regulations, confusion about task responsibilities, and the perception by people that they should not speak up even when they know a problem is occurring. These issues have been identified in the broader context of patient safety but are likely to affect diagnostic processes as well.

The main mechanisms for assessing these organizational characteristics are surveys (about culture, leadership, management, collaboration, communication) and focus groups. For instance, Shekelle and colleagues (2013) identified a number of survey-based measures in these areas as part of a report on the context-sensitivity of patient safety practices.

Physical environment Various characteristics of the physical environment (e.g., noise, lighting, layout) may affect the diagnostic process (Alvarado, 2012; Parsons, 2000). The physical environment places additional stresses on a diagnostic team that can affect the performance of cognitive tasks and information gathering, integration, and interpretation. For example, the layout and lighting of the radiology reading room may hinder accurate viewing of screens. Emergency departments are another example of a place where it makes sense to examine the effects of the physical environment on diagnostic errors (Campbell et al., 2007).

Human factors/ergonomics methods can be used to evaluate the physical environment. These methods include, for example, making a direct assessment of noise and lighting with specific equipment (e.g., a light meter) and direct observation of care processes to identify challenges related to layout. For instance, observing the physical movements of clinicians can help identify communication among team members and the barriers posed by the physical environment (e.g., lack of available equipment or poorly located equipment; see Potter et al., 2004; Wolf et al., 2006). In addition, surveys can also be used to gather data from a larger population of staff and patients about environmental characteristics, such as the adequacy of lighting and the perception of noise and its impact. In an example of this approach, Mahmood and colleagues (2011) surveyed nurses about the aspects of their physical environment that affected the risk of medication errors. Many of these factors contribute to latent errors—for example, creating conditions under which cognitive functioning is impaired because of the work environment itself.

Summary The committee reviewed a number of methods for assessing the effects of the work system on diagnostic error. This section highlights a number of those methods and illustrates how they have been applied in various health care settings to develop insights into the risks of error and to identify potential areas for improvement. The methods have in common the fact that they combine observation of the actual processes (tasks, communication, interaction with technology) with documentation of those processes. These methods can be relatively labor intensive, and they tend to require application at the individual site level, which implies that this is work that all teams and settings in which diagnoses are made need to become more skilled at undertaking. While standardized tools exist (surveys, methods of observation, and analysis of teams) and might be applied to samples of different types of teams and settings to identify particular vulnerabilities for diagnostic error, the most useful application of these methods is typically for improvement at the local level. The human factors science in this area suggests that a number of likely problems can be readily identified—that is, that deep study may not be necessary—but the complexity of the interactions among these various factors suggests that high levels of vigilance and attention to measurement will likely be necessary throughout the health care system.

Evaluating Interventions

Measurement will be critical to assessing whether changes that are intended to improve diagnosis and reduce diagnostic errors are effective. Changes can be implemented and evaluated as part of a quality improvement program or a research project. For both purposes it would be helpful to develop assessment tools that can be implemented within routine clinical practice to rapidly identify potential failures in the diagnostic process, to alert clinicians and health care organizations to diagnostic errors, and to ascertain trend changes over time. For quality improvement approaches, establishing a baseline (knowing the current rate of failure in a particular step in the diagnostic process using some of the measurement methods in Table 3-2) will provide the main method for understanding whether interventions are having the desired effect. For research studies, the specific aims and change strategy under evaluation will indicate what measurement choice should be made from a broader set or possibilities (e.g., long-term clinical outcomes, diagnostic errors, diagnostic process failures, and contextual variables hypothesized or known to influence diagnostic performance). In some cases the aim of measurement will be to assess whether interventions designed to address specific failures are resulting in lower failure rates. In other cases the aim of measurement will be to assess whether a global intervention reduces multiple causes simultaneously. This purpose relates to the work system focal point for analysis and intervention (Table 3-3 measures). An important contribution to research in this area will be the identification of approaches that can reduce the risk for diagnostic error.

There have been few studies that have evaluated the impact of interventions on improving diagnosis and reducing diagnostic error. McDonald and colleagues (2013) conducted a systematic review to identify interventions targeted at reducing diagnostic error. They found more than 100 evaluations of interventions and grouped them into six categories: "techniques (changes in equipment, procedures, and clinical approaches); personnel changes (the introduction of additional health care professionals or the replacement of certain health care professionals for others); educational interventions (residency training, curricula, and maintenance of certification changes); structured process changes (implementation of feedback mechanisms); technology-based interventions (clinical decision support, text messaging, and pager alerts); and additional review methods (independent reviews of test results)" (McDonald et al., 2013, p. 383). The measures used in these intervention studies included diagnostic accuracy, outcomes related to further diagnostic test use, outcomes related to further therapeutic management, direct patient-related outcomes, time to correct therapeutic management, and time to diagnosis; 26 of the 100 intervention studies examined diagnostic delays. The researchers identified 14 randomized trials (rated as having mostly a low to moderate risk of bias), 11 of which reported interventions that reduced diagnostic errors. The evidence appeared to be strongest for technology-based interventions and specific techniques. The researchers found that very few studies evaluated the impact of the intervention on patient outcomes (e.g., mortality, morbidity), and they suggested that further evaluations of promising interventions should be conducted in large studies across diverse settings of care in order to enhance generalizability (McDonald et al., 2013).

Two previous reviews evaluated the impact of "system-related interventions" and "cognitive interventions" on the reduction of diagnostic errors (Graber et al., 2012; Singh et al., 2012b). For system-related interventions Singh and colleagues concluded, "Despite a number of suggested interventions in the literature, few empirical studies have tested interventions to reduce diagnostic error in the last decade. Advancing the science of diagnostic error prevention will require more robust study designs and rigorous definitions of diagnostic processes and outcomes to measure intervention effects" (Singh et al., 2012b, p. 160). Graber and colleagues identified a variety of possible approaches to reducing cognitive errors in diagnosis. Not all of the suggested approaches had been tested, and of those that had been tested, they generally involved observing trainees in artificial settings, making it difficult to extrapolate the results to actual practice. "Future progress in this area," they concluded, "will require methodological refinements in outcome evaluation and rigorously evaluating interventions already suggested" (Graber et al., 2012, p. 535).

The three systematic reviews of diagnostic interventions draw similar conclusions about the heterogeneity of measures used as well as the dearth of patient-reported outcomes. Synthesizing information from the available interventions is difficult because of the lack of comparable outcomes across studies. As with other areas of quality and patient safety, improved patient outcomes is a common goal, but it may not be practical to assess such patient outcomes during limited-time intervention studies (or quality improvement efforts). Intermediate measures that assess process failures (e.g., the development of algorithms to identify and quantify missed opportunities for making a specific diagnosis among an at-risk population) or cognitive problems (e.g., debriefing to determine what biases are at play and at what frequency) will continue to provide useful information for understanding the influence of an intervention at its point of expected action (as part of the diagnostic process or other component of the work system, or at the sharp or blunt end of care). As with other areas of patient safety research and quality improvement, evidence connecting any intermediate measures to patient outcomes will need proper attention.

Another key area of attention for patient safety intervention research, which applies to diagnostic error measurement, is context-sensitivity. As noted in the section on identifying risks for diagnostic error, work system dimensions have the potential to contribute to diagnostic error. For any diagnostic error reduction intervention, measurement focused on context variables (e.g., dimensions of the work system, as noted in Table 3-3) will allow testing of the hypothesized role of these variables in diagnostic error. Shekelle and colleagues (2013) pointed to the need for evidence about the context in which safety strategies have been adopted and tested in order to help health care organizations understand what works and under what circumstances, so that the intervention strategy can be adapted appropriately to local needs. McDonald summarized domains and measurement options for studying context in relation to quality improvement interventions, which could be extended to new areas such as diagnostic safety interventions. She noted that "efficient and effective means to incorporate the domain of context into research . . . has received relatively minimal attention in health care, even though the salience of this broad topic is well understood by practitioners and policy makers" (McDonald, 2013, p. S51).

In summary, there are a multitude of specific measurement choices when developing and testing interventions for quality improvement or research, but no single repository of options exists. Funders and researchers have developed repositories of measurement tools for various other topics and applications. For example, the Agency for Healthcare Research and Quality's Care Coordination Measures Atlas is a resource that includes a measurement framework, identified measures with acceptable performance characteristics, and maps of these measures to framework domains (AHRQ, 2014a). A similar resource would be useful for those involved in diagnostic error interventions from proof of concept through the spread of successful interventions with widespread applicability (i.e., cases in which an intervention exhibits limited context sensitivity or the cases in which an intervention works well within many contexts). Such a resource could build on the domains and measures shown in Tables 3-2 and 3-3, as well as other sources from quality improvement and patient safety research applicable to diagnostic error.

REFERENCES

Abujudeh, H. H., G. W. Boland, R. Kaewlai, P. Rabiner, E. F. Halpern, G. S. Gazelle, and J. H. Thrall. 2010. Abdominal and pelvic computed tomography (CT) interpretation: Discrepancy rates among experienced radiologists. *European Radiology* 20(8):1952–1957.

Adams, J. L., and S. Garber. 2007. Reducing medical malpractice by targeting physicians making medical malpractice payments. *Journal of Empirical Legal Studies* 4(1):185–222.

AHRQ (Agency for Healthcare Research and Quality). 2014a. Care Coordination Measures Atlas update. www.ahrq.gov/professionals/prevention-chronic-care/improve/coordination/atlas2014/index.html (accessed May 26, 2015.).

AHRQ. 2014b. Patient Safety Network: Voluntary patient safety event reporting (incident reporting). http://psnet.ahrq.gov/primer.aspx?primerID=13 (accessed May 8, 2015).

AHRQ. 2015a. Patient Safety Network: Patient safety primers. Systems approach. http://psnet.ahrq.gov/primer.aspx?primerID=21 (accessed May 8, 2015).

AHRQ. 2015b. Patient Safety Network: Root cause analysis. www.psnet.ahrq.gov/primer.aspx?primerID=10 (accessed May 8, 2015).

Aleccia, J. 2014. Misdiagnosed: Docs' mistakes affect 12 million a year. *NBC News*, April 16. www.nbcnews.com/health/health-news/misdiagnosed-docs-mistakes-affect-12-million-year-n82256 (accessed October 30, 2014).

Alvarado, C. J. 2012. The physical environment in health care. In P. Carayon (ed.), *Handbook of human factors and ergonomics in health care and patient safety* (pp. 215–234). Boca Raton, FL: Taylor & Francis Group.

Andrews, L. B., C. Stocking, T. Krizek, L. Gottlieb, C. Krizek, T. Vargish, and M. Siegler. 1997. An alternative strategy for studying adverse events in medical care. *Lancet* 349(9048):309–313.

Armijo, D., C. McDonnell, and K. Werner. 2009. *Electronic health record usability: Electronic and use case framework.* AHRQ Publication No. 09(10)-0091-1-EF. Rockville, MD: Agency for Healthcare Research and Quality.

Berenson, R. A., D. K. Upadhyay, and D. R. Kaye. 2014. *Placing diagnosis errors on the policy agenda.* Washington, DC: Urban Institute. www.urban.org/research/publication/placing-diagnosis-errors-policy-agenda (accessed May 22, 2015).

Berlin, L. 2014. Radiologic errors, past, present and future. *Diagnosis* 1(1):79–84.

Berner, E. S., and M. L. Graber. 2008. Overconfidence as a cause of diagnostic error in medicine. *American Journal of Medicine* 121(5 Suppl):S2–S23.

Betsy Lehman Center for Patient Safety and Medical Error Reduction. 2014. *The public's views on medical error in Massachusetts.* Cambridge, MA: Harvard School of Public Health.

Bisantz, A., and E. Roth. 2007. Analysis of cognitive work. *Reviews of Human Factors and Ergonomics* 3(1):1–43.

Blendon, R. J., C. M. DesRoches, M. Brodie, J. M. Benson, A. B. Rosen, E. Schneider, D. E. Altman, K. Zapert, M. J. Herrmann, and A. E. Steffenson. 2002. Views of practicing physicians and the public on medical errors. *New England Journal of Medicine* 347(24):1933–1940.

Bonini, P., M. Plebani, F. Ceriotti, and F. Rubboli. 2002. Errors in laboratory medicine. *Clinical Chemistry* 48(5):691–698.

Borgstede, J., R. Lewis, M. Bhargavan, and J. Sunshine. 2004. RADPEER quality assurance program: A multifacility study of interpretive disagreement rates. *Journal of the American College of Radiology* 1(1):59–65.

Brennan, T. A., L. L. Leape, N. M. Laird, L. Hebert, A. R. Localio, A. G. Lawthers, J. P. Newhouse, P. C. Weiler, and H. H. Hiatt. 1991. Incidence of adverse events and negligence in hospitalized patients: Results of the Harvard Medical Practice Study I. *New England Journal of Medicine* 324(6):370–376.

CAHPS (Consumer Assessment of Healthcare Providers and Systems). 2012. The CAHPS improvement guide. www.facs.org/~/media/files/advocacy/cahps/improvement%20guide.ashx (accessed July 12, 2015).

Callen, J., A. Georgiou, J. Li, and J. I. Westbrook. 2011. The safety implications of missed test results for hospitalised patients: A systematic review. *BMJ Quality & Safety in Health Care* 20(2):194–199.

Campbell, S. G., P. Croskerry, and W. F. Bond. 2007. Profiles in patient safety: A "perfect storm" in the emergency department. *Academic Emergency Medicine* 14(8):743–749.

Carayon, P., R. Cartmill, P. Hoonakker, A. S. Hundt, B.-T. Karsh, D. Krueger, M. L. Snellman, T. N. Thuemling, and T. B. Wetterneck. 2012. Human factors analysis of workflow in health information technology implementation. In P. Carayon (ed.), *Handbook of human factors and ergonomics in health care and patient safety* (pp. 507–521). Boca Raton, FL: Taylor & Francis Group.

Carayon, P., Y. Li, M. M. Kelly, L. L. DuBenske, A. Xie, B. McCabe, J. Orne, and E. D. Cox. 2014. Stimulated recall methodology for assessing work system barriers and facilitators in family-centered rounds in a pediatric hospital. *Applied Ergonomics* 45(6):1540–1546.

Carraro, P., and M. Plebani. 2007. Errors in a stat laboratory: Types and frequencies 10 years later. *Clinical Chemistry* 53(7):1338–1342.

Carter, S. M., W. Rogers, I. Heath, C. Degeling, J. Doust, and A. Barratt. 2015. The challenge of overdiagnosis begins with its definition. *BMJ* 350:h869.

CDC (Centers for Disease Control and Prevention). 2010. National Ambulatory Medical Care Survey: 2010 summary tables. www.cdc.gov/nchs/data/ahcd/namcs_summary/2010_namcs_web_tables.pdf (accessed May 26, 2015).

CDC. 2011. National Hospital Ambulatory Medical Care Survey: 2011 emergency department summary tables. www.cdc.gov/nchs/data/ahcd/nhamcs_emergency/2011_ed_web_tables.pdf (accessed May 26, 2015).

CDC. 2015. Ambulatory health care data. www.cdc.gov/nchs/ahcd.htm (accessed May 18, 2015).

Chimowitz, M. I., E. L. Logigian, and L. R. Caplan. 1990. The accuracy of bedside neurological diagnoses. *Annals of Neurology* 28(1):78–85.

Chiolero, A., F. Paccaud, D. Aujesky, V. Santschi, and N. Rodondi. 2015. How to prevent overdiagnosis. *Swiss Medical Weekly* 145:w14060.

Cifra, C. L., K. L. Jones, J. A. Ascenzi, U. S. Bhalala, M. M. Bembea, D. E. Newman-Toker, J. C. Fackler, and M. R. Miller. 2015. Diagnostic errors in a PICU: Insights from the Morbidity and Mortality Conference. *Pediatric Critical Care Medicine* 16(5):468–476.

CRICO. 2014. *Annual benchmarking report: Malpractice risks in the diagnostic process.* Cambridge, MA: CRICO. www.rmfstrategies.com/benchmarking (accessed June 4, 2015).

Croskerry, P. 2003. The importance of cognitive errors in diagnosis and strategies to minimize them. *Academic Medicine* 78(8):775–780.

Croskerry, P. 2011. Commentary: Lowly interns, more is merrier, and the Casablanca Strategy. *Academic Medicine* 86(1):8–10.

Croskerry, P. 2012. Perspectives on diagnostic failure and patient safety. *Healthcare Quarterly* 15(Special issue):50–56.

Danforth, K. N., A. E. Smith, R. K. Loo, S. J. Jacobsen, B. S. Mittman, and M. H. Kanter. 2014. Electronic clinical surveillance to improve outpatient care: Diverse applications within an integrated delivery system. *eGEMS* 2(1):1056.

DeRosier, J., E. Stalhandske, J. P. Bagian, and T. Nudell. 2002. Using health care failure mode and effect analysis™: The VA National Center for Patient Safety's prospective risk analysis system. *Joint Commission Journal on Quality and Patient Safety* 28(5):248–267.

Endsley, M. R. 1995. Toward a theory of situation awareness in dynamic systems. *Human Factors* 37(1):32–64.

Epner, P. L., J. E. Gans, and M. L. Graber. 2013. When diagnostic testing leads to harm: A new outcomes-based approach for laboratory medicine. *BMJ Quality & Safety* 22(Suppl 2):ii6–ii10.

Esserman, L., Y. Shieh, and I. Thompson. 2009. Rethinking screening for breast cancer and prostate cancer. *JAMA* 302(15):1685–1692.

Fairbanks, R., T. Guarrera, A. Bisantz, M. Venturino, and P. Westesson. 2010. Opportunities in IT support of workflow & information flow in the emergency department digital imaging process. *Proceedings of the Human Factors and Ergonomics Society Annual Meeting* 54(4):359–363.

FDA (Food and Drug Administration). 2015. Initiative to reduce unnecessary radiation exposure from medical imaging. www.fda.gov/Radiation-EmittingProducts/Radiation-Safety/RadiationDoseReduction/ucm2007191.htm (accessed May 3, 2015).

Fletcher, G., R. Flin, P. McGeorge, R. Glavin, N. Maran, and R. Patey. 2003. Anaesthetists' Non-Technical Skills (ANTS): Evaluation of a behavioural marker system. *British Journal of Anaesthesia* 90(5):580–588.

Friedberg, M. W., P. G. Chen, K. R. Van Busum, F. Aunon, C. Pham, J. Caloyeras, S. Mattke, E. Pitchforth, D. D. Quigley, and R. H. Brook. 2013. *Factors affecting physician professional satisfaction and their implications for patient care, health systems, and health policy*: Santa Monica, CA: RAND Corporation.

Gandhi, T. K., A. Kachalia, E. J. Thomas, A. L. Puopolo, C. Yoon, T. A. Brennan, and D. M. Studdert. 2006. Missed and delayed diagnoses in the ambulatory setting: A study of closed malpractice claims. *Annals of Internal Medicine* 145(7):488–496.

Gaudi, S., J. M. Zarandona, S. S. Raab, J. C. English, and D. M. Jukic. 2013. Discrepancies in dermatopathology diagnoses: The role of second review policies and dermatopathology fellowship training. *Journal of the American Academy of Dermatology* 68(1):119–128.

Gawande, A. 2007. The way we age now: Medicine has increased the ranks of the elderly. Can it make old age any easier? *The New Yorker*, April 30. www.newyorker.com/magazine/2007/04/30/the-way-we-age-now (accessed May 18, 2015).

Gawande, A. 2014. *Being mortal: Illness, medicine, and what matters in the end*. London, UK: Wellcome Collection.

Gawande, A. 2015. Overkill. *The New Yorker*, May 11. www.newyorker.com/magazine/2015/05/11/overkill-atul-gawande (accessed July 13, 2015).

Giardina, T. D., B. J. King, A. P. Ignaczak, D. E. Paull, L. Hoeksema, P. D. Mills, J. Neily, R. R. Hemphill, and H. Singh. 2013. Root cause analysis reports help identify common factors in delayed diagnosis and treatment of outpatients. *Health Affairs (Millwood)* 32(8):1368–1375.

Gigerenzer, G. 2014. Breast cancer screening pamphlets mislead women. *BMJ* 348:g2636.

Goldschmidt, H. M. J., and R. W. Lent. 1995. From data to information: How to define the context? *Chemometrics and Intelligent Laboratory Systems* 28(1):181–192.

Golodner, L. 1997. How the public perceives patient safety. *Newsletter of the National Patient Safety Foundation* 1(1):1–4.

Gosbee, J., and L. L. Gosbee. 2012. Usability evaluation in health care. In P. Carayon (ed.), *Handbook of human factors and ergonomics in health care and patient safety*, 2nd ed. (pp. 543–555). Boca Raton, FL: Taylor & Francis Group.

Graber, M. L. 2013. The incidence of diagnostic error in medicine. *BMJ Quality and Safety* 22(Suppl 2):ii21–ii27.

Graber, M. L., N. Franklin, and R. Gordon. 2005. Diagnostic error in internal medicine. *Archives of Internal Medicine* 165(13):1493–1499.

Graber, M. L., S. Kissam, V. L. Payne, A. N. Meyer, A. Sorensen, N. Lenfestey, E. Tant, K. Henriksen, K. Labresh, and H. Singh. 2012. Cognitive interventions to reduce diagnostic error: A narrative review. *BMJ Quality and Safety* 21(7):535–557.

Graber, M. L., R. Trowbridge, J. S. Myers, C. A. Umscheid, W. Strull, and M. H. Kanter. 2014. The next organizational challenge: Finding and addressing diagnostic error. *Joint Commission Journal on Quality and Patient Safety* 40(3):102–110.

Grimes, D. A., and K. F. Schulz. 2002. Uses and abuses of screening tests. *Lancet* 359(9309):881–884.

Hallworth, M. J. 2011. The "70% claim": What is the evidence base? *Annals of Clinical Biochemistry* 48(6):487–488.

Hickner, J., D. G. Graham, N. C. Elder, E. Brandt, C. B. Emsermann, S. Dovey, and R. Phillips. 2008. Testing process errors and their harms and consequences reported from family medicine practices: A study of the American Academy of Family Physicians National Research Network. *Quality and Safety in Health Care* 17(3):194–200.

Hickner, J., P. J. Thompson, T. Wilkinson, P. Epner, M. Sheehan, A. M. Pollock, J. Lee, C. C. Duke, B. R. Jackson, and J. R. Taylor. 2014. Primary care physicians' challenges in ordering clinical laboratory tests and interpreting results. *Journal of the American Board of Family Medicine* 27(2):268–274.

Hofer, T., S. Asch, R. Hayward, L. Rubenstein, M. Hogan, J. Adams, and E. Kerr. 2004. Profiling quality of care: Is there a role for peer review? *BMC Health Services Research* 4(1):9.

Hoffmann, T. C., and C. Del Mar. 2015. Patients' expectations of the benefits and harms of treatments, screening, and tests: A systematic review. *JAMA Internal Medicine* 175(2):274–286.

Hoyert, D. L. 2011. The changing profile of autopsied deaths in the United States, 1972–2007. *NCHS Data Brief* 67(August).

Hricak, H., D. J. Brenner, S. J. Adelstein, D. P. Frush, E. J. Hall, R. W. Howell, C. H. McCollough, F. A. Mettler, M. S. Pearce, O. H. Suleiman, J. H. Thrall, and L. K. Wagner. 2011. Managing radiation use in medical imaging: A multifaceted challenge. *Radiology* 258(3):889–905.

Iglehart, J. K. 2009. Health insurers and medical-imaging policy—A work in progress. *New England Journal of Medicine* 360(10):1030–1037.

IOM (Institute of Medicine). 1990. *Medicare: A strategy for quality assurance* (2 vols.). Washington, DC: National Academy Press.

IOM. 2000. *To err is human: Building a safer health system.* Washington, DC: National Academy Press.

IOM. 2001. *Crossing the quality chasm: A new health system for the 21st century.* Washington, DC: National Academy Press.

IOM. 2004. *Patient safety: Achieving a new standard for care.* Washington, DC: The National Academies Press.

Jun, G. T., J. Ward, Z. Morris, and J. Clarkson. 2009. Health care process modelling: Which method when? *International Journal for Quality in Health Care* 21(3):214–224.

Kachalia, A., T. K. Gandhi, A. L. Puopolo, C. Yoon, E. J. Thomas, R. Griffey, T. A. Brennan, and D. M. Studdert. 2006. Missed and delayed diagnoses in the emergency department: A study of closed malpractice claims from 4 liability insurers. *Annals of Emergency Medicine* 49(2):196–205.

Kanter, M. H. 2014. Diagnostic errors—Patient safety. Presentation to the Committee on Diagnostic Error in Health Care, August 7, 2014, Washington, DC.

Kassirer, J. P. 1989. Our stubborn quest for diagnostic certainty. A cause of excessive testing. *New England Journal of Medicine* 320(22)1489–1491.

Kassirer, J. P., and R. I. Kopelman. 1989. Cognitive errors in diagnosis: Instantiation, classification, and consequences. *American Journal of Medicine* 86(4):433–441.

Kerr, E. A., T. P. Hofer, R. A. Hayward, J. L. Adams, M. M. Hogan, E. A. McGlynn, and S. M. Asch. 2007. Quality by any other name? A comparison of three profiling systems for assessing health care quality. *Health Services Research* 42(5):2070–2087.

Kim, J., D. Neilipovitz, P. Cardinal, M. Chiu, and J. Clinch. 2006. A pilot study using high-fidelity simulation to formally evaluate performance in the resuscitation of critically ill patients: The University of Ottawa Critical Care Medicine, High-Fidelity Simulation, and Crisis Resource Management I Study. *Critical Care Medicine* 34(8):2167–2174.

Kirwan, B. E., and L. K. Ainsworth (eds.). 1992. *A guide to task analysis: The Task Analysis Working Group.* Boca Raton, FL: Taylor & Francis Group.

Klein, G. 2011. What physicians can learn from firefighters. Paper presented at the 4th International Diagnostic Error Conference, October 23–26, 2011, Chicago, IL.

Klein, G. 2014. Submitted input. Input submitted to the Committee on Diagnostic Error. December 20, 2014, Washington, DC.

Koopman, R. J., L. M. Steege, J. L. Moore, M. A. Clarke, S. M. Canfield, M. S. Kim, and J. L. Belden. 2015. Physician Information needs and electronic health records (EHRs): Time to reengineer the clinic note. *Journal of the American Board of Family Medicine* 28(3):316–323.

Kostopoulou, O., C. Mousoulis, and B. C. Delaney. 2009. Information search and information distortion in the diagnosis of an ambiguous presentation. *Judgment and Decision Making* 4(5):408–418.

Kostopoulou, O., J. E. Russo, G. Keenan, B. C. Delaney, and A. Douiri. 2012. Information distortion in physicians' diagnostic judgments. *Medical Decision Making* 32(6):831–839.

Kronz, J. D., and W. H. Westra. 2005. The role of second opinion pathology in the management of lesions of the head and neck. *Current Opinion in Otolaryngology and Head and Neck Surgery* 13(2):81–84.

Landis, J. R., and G. G. Koch. 1977. The measurement of observer agreement for categorical data. *Biometrics* 33(1):159–174.

Leape, L. L., T. A. Brennan, N. Laird, A. G. Lawthers, A. R. Localio, B. A. Barnes, L. Hebert, J. P. Newhouse, P. C. Weiler, and H. Hiatt. 1991. The nature of adverse events in hospitalized patients: Results of the Harvard Medical Practice Study II. *New England Journal of Medicine* 324(6):377–384.

Levtzion-Korach, O., A. Frankel, H. Alcalai, C. Keohane, J. Orav, E. Graydon-Baker, J. Barnes, K. Gordon, A. L. Puopulo, E. I. Tomov, L. Sato, and D. W. Bates. 2010. Integrating incident data from five reporting systems to assess patient safety: Making sense of the elephant. *Joint Commission Journal on Quality and Patient Safety* 36(9):402–410.

Liss, M. A., J. Billimek, K. Osann, J. Cho, R. Moskowitz, A. Kaplan, R. J. Szabo, S. H. Kaplan, S. Greenfield, and A. Dash. 2013. Consideration of comorbidity in risk stratification prior to prostate biopsy. *Cancer* 119(13):2413–2418.

Localio, A. R., A. G. Lawthers, T. A. Brennan, N. M. Laird, L. E. Hebert, L. M. Peterson, J. P. Newhouse, P. C. Weiler, and H. H. Hiatt. 1991. Relation between malpractice claims and adverse events due to negligence. Results of the Harvard Medical Practice Study III. *New England Journal of Medicine* 325(4):245–251.

Lundberg, G. D. 1981. Acting on significant laboratory results. *JAMA* 245(17):1762–1763.

Lundberg, G. D. 1998. Low-tech autopsies in the era of high-tech medicine: Continued value for quality assurance and patient safety. *JAMA* 280(14):1273–1274.

Lyratzopoulos, G., P. Vedsted, and H. Singh. 2015. Understanding missed opportunities for more timely diagnosis of cancer in symptomatic patients after presentation. *British Journal of Cancer* 112:S84–S91.

Mahmood, A., H. Chaudhury, and M. Valente. 2011. Nurses' perceptions of how physical environment affects medication errors in acute care settings. *Applied Nursing Research* 24(4):229–237.

McDonald, K. M. 2013. Considering context in quality improvement interventions and implementation: Concepts, frameworks, and application. *Academic Pediatrics* 13(6):S45–S53.

McDonald, K. M., B. Matesic, D. G. Contopoulos-Ioannidis, J. Lonhart, E. Schmidt, N. Pineda, and J. P. Ioannidis. 2013. Patient safety strategies targeted at diagnostic errors: A systematic review. *Annals of Internal Medicine* 158(5 Pt 2):381–389.

McGlynn, E. A., S. M. Asch, J. Adams, J. Keesey, J. Hicks, A. DeCristofaro, and E. A. Kerr. 2003. The quality of health care delivered to adults in the United States. *New England Journal of Medicine* 348(26):2635–2645.

Middleton, B., M. Bloomrosen, M. A. Dente, B. Hashmat, R. Koppel, J. M. Overhage, T. H. Payne, S. T. Rosenbloom, C. Weaver, and J. Zhang. 2013. Enhancing patient safety and quality of care by improving the usability of electronic health record systems: Recommendations from AMIA. *Journal of the American Medical Informatics Association* 20(e1):e2–e8.

Milch, C. E., D. N. Salem, S. G. Pauker, T. G. Lundquist, S. Kumar, and J. Chen. 2006. Voluntary electronic reporting of medical errors and adverse events. *Journal of General Internal Medicine* 21(2):165–170.

Moynihan, R., J. Doust, and D. Henry. 2012. Preventing overdiagnosis: How to stop harming the healthy. *BMJ* 344:e3502.

Mulley, A. G., C. Trimble, and G. Elwyn. 2012. Stop the silent misdiagnosis: Patients' preferences matter. *BMJ* 345(1):e6572.

Murphy, D. R., A. Laxmisan, B. A. Reis, E. J. Thomas, A. Esquivel, S. N. Forjuoh, R. Parikh, M. M. Khan, and H. Singh. 2014. Electronic health record-based triggers to detect potential delays in cancer diagnosis. *BMJ Quality and Safety* 23(1):8–16.

Nakhleh, R. E., V. Nosé, C. Colasacco, L. A. Fatheree, T. J. Lillemoe, D. C. McCrory, F. A. Meier, C. N. Otis, S. R. Owens, S. S. Raab, R. R. Turner, C. B. Ventura, and A. A. Renshaw. 2015. Interpretive diagnostic error reduction in surgical pathology and cytology: Guideline from the College of American Pathologists Pathology and Laboratory Quality Center and the Association of Directors of Anatomic and Surgical Pathology. *Archives of Pathology & Laboratory Medicine.* Epub ahead of print. http://dx.doi.org/10.5858/arpa.2014-0511-SA (accessed December 6, 2015).

Newman-Toker, D. E. 2014a. Prioritization of diagnostic error problems and solutions: Concepts, economic modeling, and action plan. Input submitted to the Committee on Diagnostic Error in Health Care, August 7, 2014, Washington, DC.

Newman-Toker, D. E. 2014b. A unified conceptual model for diagnostic errors: Underdiagnosis, overdiagnosis, and misdiagnosis. *Diagnosis* 1(1):43–48.

Newman-Toker, D. E., and P. J. Pronovost. 2009. Diagnostic errors: The next frontier for patient safety. *JAMA* 301(10):1060–1062.

Newman-Toker, D. E., K. M. McDonald, and D. O. Meltzer. 2013. How much diagnostic safety can we afford, and how should we decide? A health economics perspective. *BMJ Quality and Safety* 22(Suppl 2):ii11–ii20.

Newman-Toker, D. E., E. Moy, E. Valente, R. Coffey, and A. L. Hines. 2014. Missed diagnosis of stroke in the emergency department: A cross-sectional analysis of a large population-based sample. *Diagnosis* 1(2):155–166.

Office of Inspector General. 2010. *Adverse events in hospitals: Methods for identifying events.* Washington, DC: Office of Inspector General. https://oig.hhs.gov/oei/reports/oei-06-08-00221.pdf (accessed June 4, 2015).

Pace, L. E., and N. L. Keating. 2014. A systematic assessment of benefits and risks to guide breast cancer screening decisions. *JAMA* 311(13):1327–1335.

Parsons, K. C. 2000. Environmental ergonomics: A review of principles, methods and models. *Applied Ergonomics* 31:581–594.

Patel, V. L., J. Zhang, N. A. Yoskowitz, R. Green, and O. R. Sayan. 2008. Translational cognition for decision support in critical care environments: A review. *Journal of Biomedical Informatics* 41(3):413–431.

Peabody, J. W., J. Luck, S. Jain, D. Bertenthal, and P. Glassman. 2004. Assessing the accuracy of administrative data in health information systems. *Medical Care* 42(11):1066–1072.

Peterson, M. C., J. H. Holbrook, D. Von Hales, N. L. Smith, and L. V. Staker. 1992. Contributions of the history, physical examination, and laboratory investigation in making medical diagnoses. *Western Journal of Medicine* 156(2):163–165.

Plant, J. L., S. M. van Schaik, D. C. Sliwka, C. K. Boscardin, and P. S. O'Sullivan. 2011. Validation of a self-efficacy instrument and its relationship to performance of crisis resource management skills. *Advances in Health Sciences Education* 16(5):579–590.

Plebani, M. 2010. The detection and prevention of errors in laboratory medicine. *Annals of Clinical Biochemistry* 47(2):101–110.

Plebani, M. 2014. Defensive medicine and diagnostic testing. *Diagnosis* 1(2):151–154.

Plebani, M., M. Laposata, and G. D. Lundberg. 2011. The brain-to-brain loop concept for laboratory testing 40 years after its introduction. *American Journal of Clinical Pathology* 136(6):829–833.

Potter, P., S. Boxerman, L. Wolf, J. Marshall, D. Grayson, J. Sledge, and B. Evanoff. 2004. Mapping the nursing process: A new approach for understanding the work of nursing. *Journal of Nursing Administration.* 34(2):101–109.

Rao, V. M., and D. C. Levin. 2012. The overuse of diagnostic imaging and the Choosing Wisely initiative. *Annals of Internal Medicine* 157(8):574–576.

Reason, J. 1990. *Human error.* New York: Cambridge University Press.

Renshaw, A. A., and E. W. Gould. 2005. Comparison of disagreement and error rates for three types of interdepartmental consultations. *American Journal of Clinical Pathology* 124(6):878–882.

Rogers, M. L., E. S. Patterson, and R. M. L. 2012. Cognitive work analysis in health care. In P. Carayon (ed.), *Handbook of human factors and ergonomics in health care and patient safety,* 2nd ed. (pp. 465–474). Boca Raton, FL: Taylor & Francis Group.

Roth, E. M. 2008. Uncovering the requirements of cognitive work. *Human Factors* 50(3):475–480.

Salas, E., C. Prince, D. P. Baker, and L. Shrestha. 1995. Situation awareness in team performance: Implications for measurement and training. *Human Factors* 37(1):123–136.

Schiff, G. D., and L. L. Leape. 2012. Commentary: How can we make diagnosis safer? *Academic Medicine* 87(2):135–138.

Schiff, G. D., S. Kim, R. Abrams, K. Cosby, A. S. Elstein, S. Hasler, N. Krosnjar, R. Odwanzy, M. F. Wisniewsky, and R. A. McNutt. 2005. *Diagnosing diagnosis errors: Lessons from a multi-institutional collaborative project for the diagnostic error evaluation and research project investigators.* Rockville, MD: Agency for Healthcare Research and Quality.

Schiff, G. D., O. Hasan, S. Kim, R. Abrams, K. Cosby, B. L. Lambert, A. S. Elstein, S. Hasler, M. L. Kabongo, N. Krosnjar, R. Odwazny, M. F. Wisniewski, and R. A. McNutt. 2009. Diagnostic error in medicine: Analysis of 583 physician-reported errors. *Archives of Internal Medicine* 169(20):1881–1887.

Schiff, G. D., A. L. Puopolo, A. Huben-Kearney, W. Yu, C. Keohane, P. McDonough, B. R. Ellis, D. W. Bates, and M. Biondolillo. 2013. Primary care closed claims experience of Massachusetts malpractice insurers. *JAMA Internal Medicine* 173(22):2063–2068.

Schraagen, J. M., S. F. Chipman, and V. L. Shalin. 2000. *Cognitive task analysis.* New York: Psychology Press.

Shekelle, P. G., R. M. Wachter, P. J. Pronovost, K. Schoelles, K. M. McDonald, S. M. Dy, K. Shojania, J. Reston, Z. Berger, B. Johnsen, J. W. Larkin, S. Lucas, K. Martinez, A. Motala, S. J. Newberry, M. Noble, E. Pfoh, S. R. Ranji, S. Rennke, E. Schmidt, R. Shanman, N. Sullivan, F. Sun, K. Tipton, J. R. Treadwell, A. Tsou, M. E. Vaiana, S. J. Weaver, R. Wilson, and B. D. Winters. 2013. *Making health care safer II: An updated critical analysis of the evidence for patient safety practices.* Evidence Reports/Technology Assessments No. 211. Rockville, MD: Agency for Healthcare Research and Quality.

Shojania, K. G. 2010. The elephant of patient safety: What you see depends on how you look. *Joint Commission Journal on Quality and Patient Safety* 36(9):399–401.

Shojania, K. G., E. C. Burton, K. M. McDonald, and L. Goldman. 2002. *The autopsy as an outcome and performance measure.* AHRQ Publication No. 03-E002. Rockville, MD: Agency for Healthcare Research and Quality.

Shojania, K. G., E. C. Burton, K. M. McDonald, and L. Goldman. 2003. Changes in rates of autopsy-detected diagnostic errors over time: A systematic review. *JAMA* 289(21):2849–2856.

Siegal, D. 2014. Analysis of diagnosis-related medical malpractice claims: Input submitted to the Committee on Diagnostic Error in Health Care, August 4, 2014.

Singh, H. 2014. Helping health care organizations to define diagnostic errors as missed opportunities in diagnosis. *Joint Commission Journal on Quality and Patient Safety* 40(3):99–101.

Singh, H., and D. F. Sittig. 2015. Advancing the science of measurement of diagnostic errors in healthcare: The Safer Dx Framework. *BMJ Quality and Safety* 24(2):103–110.

Singh, H., K. Daci, L. A. Petersen, C. Collins, N. J. Petersen, A. Shethia, and H. B. El-Serag. 2009. Missed opportunities to initiate endoscopic evaluation for colorectal cancer diagnosis. *American Journal of Gastroenterology* 104(10):2543–2554.

Singh, H., K. Hirani, H. Kadiyala, O. Rudomiotov, T. Davis, M. M. Khan, and T. L. Wahls. 2010a. Characteristics and predictors of missed opportunities in lung cancer diagnosis: An electronic health record–based study. *Journal of Clinical Oncology* 28(20):3307–3315.

Singh, H., E. J. Thomas, L. Wilson, P. A. Kelly, K. Pietz, D. Elkeeb, and G. Singhal. 2010b. Errors of diagnosis in pediatric practice: A multisite survey. *Pediatrics* 126(1):70–79.

Singh, H., T. D. Giardina, S. N. Forjuoh, M. D. Reis, S. Kosmach, M. M. Khan, and E. J. Thomas. 2012a. Electronic health record-based surveillance of diagnostic errors in primary care. *BMJ Quality and Safety* 21:93–100.

Singh, H., M. L. Graber, S. M. Kissam, A. V. Sorensen, N. F. Lenfestey, E. M. Tant, K. Henriksen, and K. A. LaBresh. 2012b. System-related interventions to reduce diagnostic errors: A narrative review. *BMJ Quality and Safety* 21(2):160–170.

Singh, H., C. Spitzmueller, N. J. Petersen, M. K. Sawhney, and D. F. Sittig. 2013. Information overload and missed test results in electronic health record-based settings. *JAMA Internal Medicine* 173(8):702–704.

Singh, H., A. N. Meyer, and E. J. Thomas. 2014. The frequency of diagnostic errors in outpatient care: Estimations from three large observational studies involving U.S. adult populations. *BMJ Quality and Safety* 23(9):727–731.

Smith, M., D. Murphy, A. Laxmisan, D. Sittig, B. Reis, A. Esquivel, and H. Singh. 2013. Developing software to "track and catch" missed follow-up of abnormal test results in a complex sociotechnical environment. *Applied Clinical Informatics* 4(3):359–375.

Studdert, D. M., E. J. Thomas, H. R. Burstin, B. I. Zbar, E. J. Orav, and T. A. Brennan. 2000. Negligent care and malpractice claiming behavior in Utah and Colorado. *Medical Care* 38(3):250–260.

Studdert, D. M., M. M. Mello, W. M. Sage, C. M. DesRoches, J. Peugh, K. Zapert, and T. A. Brennan. 2005. Defensive medicine among high-risk specialist physicians in a volatile malpractice environment. *JAMA* 293(21):2609–2617.

Studdert, D. M., M. M. Mello, A. A. Gawande, T. K. Gandhi, A. Kachalia, C. Yoon, A. L. Puopolo, and T. A. Brennan. 2006. Claims, errors, and compensation payments in medical malpractice litigation. *New England Journal of Medicine* 354(19):2024–2033.

Tehrani, A., H. Lee, S. Mathews, A. Shore, M. Makary, P. Pronovost, and D. Newman-Toker. 2013. 25-year summary of U.S. malpractice claims for diagnostic errors 1986–2010: An analysis from the National Practitioner Data Bank. *BMJ Quality and Safety* 22:672–680.

Thomas, E. J., D. M. Studdert, H. R. Burstin, E. J. Orav, T. Zeena, E. J. Williams, K. M. Howard, P. C. Weiler, and T. A. Brennan. 2000. Incidence and types of adverse events and negligent care in Utah and Colorado. *Medical Care* 38(3):261–271.

Thomas, E. J., S. R. Lipsitz, D. M. Studdert, and T. A. Brennan. 2002. The reliability of medical record review for estimating adverse event rates. *Annals of Internal Medicine* 136(11):812–816.

Trowbridge, R. 2014. Diagnostic performance: Measurement and feedback. Presentation to the Committee on Diagnostic Error in Health Care. August 7, 2014, Washington, DC.

Troxel, D. 2014. Input submitted to the Committee on Diagnostic Error in Health Care from The Doctors Company Foundation, April 28, 2014.

Unertl, K. M., M. B. Weinger, K. B. Johnson, and N. M. Lorenzi. 2009. Describing and modeling workflow and information flow in chronic disease care. *Journal of the American Medical Informatics Association* 16(6):826–836.

Velmahos, G. C., C. Fili, P. Vassiliu, N. Nicolaou, R. Radin, and A. Wilcox. 2001. Around-the-clock attending radiology coverage is essential to avoid mistakes in the care of trauma patients. *American Surgeon* 67(12):1175–1177.

Wachter, R. M. 2010. Why diagnostic errors don't get any respect—and what can be done about them. *Health Affairs (Millwood)* 29(9):1605–1610.

Wachter, R. M. 2014. Diagnostic errors: Central to patient safety, yet still in the periphery of safety's radar screen. *Diagnosis* 1(1):19–21.

Weiner, S. J., A. Schwartz, F. Weaver, J. Goldberg, R. Yudkowsky, G. Sharma, A. Binns-Calvey, B. Preyss, M. M. Schapira, S. D. Persell, E. Jacobs, and R. I. Abrams. 2010. Contextual errors and failures in individualizing patient care: A multicenter study. *Annals of Internal Medicine* 153(2):69–75.

Weissman, J. S., E. C. Schneider, S. N. Weingart, A. M. Epstein, J. David-Kasdan, S. Feibelmann, C. L. Annas, N. Ridley, L. Kirle, C. Gatsonis. 2008. Comparing patient-reported hospital advere events with medical record review: Do patients know something that hospitals do not? *Annals of Internal Medicine* 149(2):100–108.

Welch, H. G. 2015. *Less medicine more health: 7 assumptions that drive too much medical care*. Boston, MA: Beacon Press.

Welch, H. G., and W. C. Black. 2010. Overdiagnosis in cancer. *Journal of the National Cancer Institute* 102(9):605–613.

Winters, B., J. Custer, S. M. Galvagno, E. Colantuoni, S. G. Kapoor, H. Lee, V. Goode, K. Robinson, A. Nakhasi, and P. Pronovost. 2012. Diagnostic errors in the intensive care unit: A systematic review of autopsy studies. *BMJ Quality and Safety* 21(11):894–902.

Wolf, L., P. Potter, J. A. Sledge, S. B. Boxerman, D. Grayson, and B. Evanoff. 2006. Describing nurses' work: Combining quantitative and qualitative analysis. *Human Factors* 48(1):5–14.

Zhi, M., E. L. Ding, J. Theisen-Toupal, J. Whelan, and R. Arnaout. 2013. The landscape of inappropriate laboratory testing: A 15-year meta-analysis. *PLoS ONE* 8(11):e78962.

Zwaan, L., and H. Singh. 2015. The challenges in defining and measuring diagnostic error. *Diagnosis* 2(2):97–103.

Zwaan, L., M. de Bruijne, C. Wagner, A. Thijs, M. Smits, G. van der Wal, and D. R. Timmermans. 2010. Patient record review of the incidence, consequences, and causes of diagnostic adverse events. *Archives of Internal Medicine* 170(12):1015–1021.

Zwaan, L., A. Thijs, C. Wagner, G. van der Wal, and D. R. Timmermans. 2012. Relating faults in diagnostic reasoning with diagnostic errors and patient harm. *Academic Medicine* 87(2):149–156.

Zwaan, L., G. D. Schiff, and H. Singh. 2013. Advancing the research agenda for diagnostic error reduction. *BMJ Quality and Safety* 22:(Suppl 2):ii52-ii57.

4

Diagnostic Team Members and Tasks: Improving Patient Engagement and Health Care Professional Education and Training in Diagnosis

This chapter describes the team-based nature of the diagnostic process, the importance of clinicians partnering with patients and their families throughout the process, and the education and training that health care professionals need to participate effectively in the diagnostic process. Making accurate and timely diagnoses requires teamwork among health care professionals, patients, and their family members. In terms of the committee's conceptual model of the diagnostic process, the focus of this chapter is on two of the elements of the work system: diagnostic team members (health care professionals, patients, and their families) and the tasks they perform in the diagnostic process (see Figure 4-1). The committee makes two recommendations targeted at improving teamwork and patient engagement in the diagnostic process and preparing health care professionals to effectively participate in the diagnostic process.

THE DIAGNOSTIC PROCESS AS A TEAM ENDEAVOR

This study was originally titled "Diagnostic Error in Medicine," but based on discussions at its first meeting, the committee concluded that "Diagnostic Error in Health Care" was a more accurate description because it better reflected the patient-centered and teamwork-oriented aspects of the diagnostic process. This conceptualization of diagnosis grew out of the recognition that too often the diagnostic process is characterized as a solitary activity, taking place exclusively within an individual physician's mind. While the task of integrating relevant information and communicating a diagnosis to a patient is often the responsibility of an

The Work System

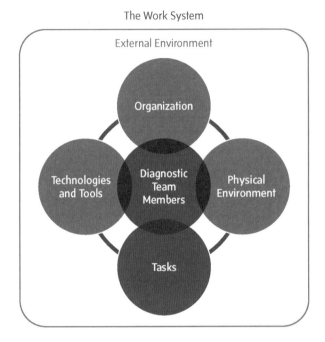

FIGURE 4-1 Diagnostic team members and the tasks they perform are two elements of the work system in which the diagnostic process occurs.

individual clinician, the diagnostic process ideally involves collaboration among multiple health care professionals, the patient, and the patient's family. Patients and their families play a pivotal role in the diagnostic process. Thus, arriving at accurate and timely diagnoses—even those made by an individual clinician working with a single patient—involves teamwork. The number of health care professionals involved in the diagnostic process can vary substantially depending on the nature of the patient's health problem: For example, McDonald (2014) noted that a diagnostic process could involve a single clinician if the suspected diagnosis is considered something straightforward, such as a common cold. However, at the other end of the spectrum, the diagnostic process could be quite complex and involve a broad array of health care professionals, such as primary care clinicians, diagnostic testing health care professionals, multiple specialists if different organ systems are suspected to be involved, nurses, pharmacists, and others.

Even though some diagnoses continue to be made by individual clinicians working independently, this solitary approach to the diagnostic process is likely to be insufficient given the changing nature of health care (see Chapter 2). The mounting complexity of health care, including ever-increasing options for diagnostic testing and treatment and the movement toward precision medicine; the rapidly rising levels of biomedical and clinical evidence to inform clinical practice; and the frequent comorbidities among patients due to the aging of the population will require greater reliance on team-based diagnosis (IOM, 2008, 2013b). To manage the increasing complexity in health care and medicine, clinicians will need to collaborate effectively and draw on the knowledge and expertise of other health care professionals, as well as patients and families, throughout the diagnostic process. The committee recognizes that reframing the diagnostic process as a team-based activity may require changing norms of health care professional roles and responsibilities and that these changes may take some time and may meet some resistance. Nevertheless, the committee concluded that improving diagnosis will require a team-based approach to the diagnostic process, in which all individuals collaborate toward the goal of accurate and timely diagnoses. Consistent with the committee's conclusion, recent reports in the literature make the case that the diagnostic process is a team-based endeavor (Graedon and Graedon, 2014; Haskell, 2014; Henriksen and Brady, 2013; McDonald, 2014). For example, Schiff noted that the new paradigm for diagnosis is that it is carried out by a well-coordinated team of people working together through reliable processes; in this view, diagnosis is the collective work of the team of health care professionals and the patient and his or her family (Schiff, 2014b).

In health care, teamwork has been described as a "dynamic process involving two or more health [care] professionals with complementary backgrounds and skills, sharing common health goals and exercising concerted physical and mental effort in assessing, planning, or evaluating patient care. This is accomplished through interdependent collaboration, open communication and shared decision-making" (Xyrichis and Ream, 2008, p. 238). Five principles of team-based care have been identified by the Institute of Medicine (IOM): shared goals, clear roles, mutual trust, effective communication, and measurable processes and outcomes (see Box 4-1). Research by a number of organizations, including the IOM, has highlighted the important role that teamwork plays in health care (Borrill et al., 2000; Boult et al., 2009; IOM, 2001, 2013a,b; Josiah Macy Jr. Foundation and Carnegie Foundation for the Advancement of Teaching, 2010; Naylor et al., 2010; WHO, 2010). A report commissioned by the Robert Wood Johnson Foundation identified several factors that are important to fostering and sustaining interprofessional collaboration: patient-centeredness, leadership commitment, effective communication, awareness of roles and responsibilities, and an organizational structure

---

BOX 4-1
Principles of Team-Based Health Care

Shared goals: The team—including the patient and, where appropriate, family members or other support persons—works to establish shared goals that reflect patient and family priorities and that can be clearly articulated, understood, and supported by all team members.

Clear roles: There are clear expectations for each team member's functions, responsibilities, and accountabilities, which optimizes the team's efficiency and often makes it possible for the team to take advantage of a division of labor, thereby accomplishing more than the sum of its parts.

Mutual trust: Team members earn each others' trust, creating strong norms of reciprocity and greater opportunities for shared achievement.

Effective communication: The team prioritizes and continuously refines its communication skills. It has consistent channels for candid and complete communication, which are accessed and used by all team members across all settings.

Measurable processes and outcomes: The team agrees on and implements reliable and timely feedback on successes and failures in both the functioning of the team and achievement of the team's goals. These are used to track and improve performance immediately and over time.

SOURCE: Adapted from IOM, 2012c.

---

that integrates interprofessional practice (CFAR et al., 2015). A review by the United Kingdom's National Health Service found that teamwork has "been reported to reduce hospitalization time and costs, improve service provision, [and] enhance patient satisfaction, staff motivation and team innovation" (Borrill et al., 2000, p. 14). One study found that a "culture of collaboration" is a key feature shared by academic medical centers considered to be top performers in quality and safety (Keroack et al., 2007), and a literature review found moderate evidence for an association between teamwork and positive patient outcomes, with the most consistent evidence from the intensive care unit setting (Sorbero et al., 2008). Another study found that surgical teams that did not engage in teamwork had worse patient outcomes, including a higher likelihood of death or serious complications (Mazzocco et al., 2009). These findings are consistent with those from other sectors. For example, in the aviation and nuclear power industries, teamwork and training in team-based skills have been found to improve performance and reduce errors related to communication and coordination problems (Leonard et al., 2004; Salas et al., 2008; Weaver et al., 2014).

Compared to teamwork in other areas of health care, teamwork in the diagnostic process has not received nearly as much attention. Teamwork in diagnosis is likely to be somewhat distinct from the teamwork that occurs after a diagnosis is made, in part due to the fluid, or unstable, collection of health care professionals involved in the diagnostic process. Fluid team membership has been recognized as a strategy to deal with fast-paced, complex tasks such as diagnosis where preplanned coordination may not be possible and where communication and coordination are a necessity (Bushe and Chu, 2011; Edmondson, 2012; Vashdi et al., 2013). Fluid team membership can introduce new challenges, such as a reduced sense of belonging to the team and a decrease in team efficacy (Bushe and Chu, 2011; Dineen and Noe, 2003; Shumate et al., 2010). A number of strategies have been identified as ways to lessen the negative impacts of fluid teams, including standardizing roles and skills, reducing task interdependence, and increasing health care professionals' understanding of others' roles (Bushe and Chu, 2011). Although teams focused on patient treatment may also exhibit fluidity, the uncertainty and complexity of the diagnostic process make unstable team membership more likely in the diagnostic process.

The committee concluded that literature on the role of teams in diagnosis is limited and that lessons from teamwork in other settings, including the treatment setting, are applicable to the diagnostic process. In testimony to the committee, Eduardo Salas of the University of Central Florida said that teamwork was likely to improve diagnosis and reduce diagnostic errors because teamwork has been found to mitigate communication and coordination challenges in other areas of health care. These same challenges have been found to have an impact on diagnostic performance (Gandhi, 2014; IOM, 2013b; The Joint Commission, 2014; Schiff, 2014a; Singh, 2014; Sutcliffe et al., 2004). Emerging research also suggests that teamwork will improve the diagnostic process; one study found that medical students working in teams made fewer diagnostic errors than those working individually, and other research has found that collaboration among treating clinicians and clinical pathology teams resulted in better diagnostic test selection (Hautz et al., 2015; Seegmiller et al., 2013).

Diagnosis depends on health care professionals with differing educational and training backgrounds working together and practicing to the full extent of their education and training (IOM, 2001, 2012c). Having clear roles and responsibilities leaves "those with greater training or responsibility free to perform tasks or to solve problems for which they are uniquely equipped" (Baldwin and Tsukuda, 1984, p. 427), while other tasks in the diagnostic process can be distributed to health care professionals within their own scope of practice (Baldwin and Tsukuda, 1984; IOM, 2011a). Improving diagnostic performance requires participating individuals to recognize the importance of teamwork as well as the contributions of other health care professionals to the diagnostic process.

In recognition that the diagnostic process is a dynamic team-based activity, health care organizations should ensure that health care professionals have the appropriate knowledge, skills, resources, and support to engage in teamwork in the diagnostic process. Ensuring that individuals participating in the diagnostic process have the appropriate resources and support extends beyond the purview of this chapter and requires a systems approach to diagnosis, including consideration of health information technology (health IT) resources (see Chapter 5), an organizational culture and work system that supports teamwork (see Chapter 6), and payment and care delivery models that promote teamwork (see Chapter 7). This chapter focuses on describing the individuals involved in the diagnostic process, identifying opportunities to facilitate patient engagement and intra- and interprofessional collaboration in the diagnostic process, and ensuring that team members have and maintain appropriate competencies in the diagnostic process.

Participants in the Diagnostic Process

The committee described diagnostic teamwork as the collaboration of interrelated individuals working toward the goal of establishing and communicating an accurate and timely explanation of a patient's health problem (Salas et al., 2008). Teamwork in the diagnostic process involves the collaboration of patients and their families; diagnosticians, such as physicians, physician assistants (PAs), and advanced practice nurses (APNs); and health care professionals who support the diagnostic process, such as nurses, pharmacists, laboratory scientists, radiology technologists, medical assistants, and patient navigators.

Figure 4-2 illustrates the relationship among individuals participating in the diagnostic process. Patients and their family members are located at the center because the ultimate goal of the diagnostic process is to explain a patient's health problem and to inform subsequent decision making about a patient's care. Surrounding patients and their families are diagnosticians, health care professionals whose tasks include making diagnoses. Encircling the diagnosticians are health care professionals who support the diagnostic process. Although Figure 4-2 distinguishes between diagnosticians and health care professionals who support the diagnostic process, this distinction may be less clear in practice. For example, triage—a complex cognitive nursing task designed to identify patients

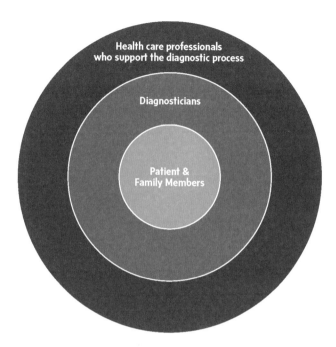

FIGURE 4-2 Teamwork in the diagnostic process includes the collaboration of a patient and his or her family members, diagnosticians, and health care professionals who support the diagnostic process.

needing immediate medical care—has not typically been included as a component in the diagnostic process, but it can often play a de facto role because a nurse may identify a suspected diagnosis during this process (Soni and Dhaliwal, 2012). Similarly, incorrect triage decisions can also introduce cognitive biases (such as framing or anchoring effects) that can contribute to diagnostic errors (see Chapter 2). The overlapping nature of the diagnostic team members in Figure 4-2 reflects the importance of effective communication and collaboration among all individuals in the diagnostic process.

Teamwork in the diagnostic process rarely involves static, fixed diagnostic teams; instead, participation in diagnosis is often dynamic and fluctuates over time, depending on what areas of expertise are needed to diagnose a specific patient and where the patient engages in the diagnostic process. The teamwork involved in the diagnostic process is illustrated in Figure 4-3. If there is good care coordination, a partnership is formed between a patient and his or her primary care team. If a patient develops

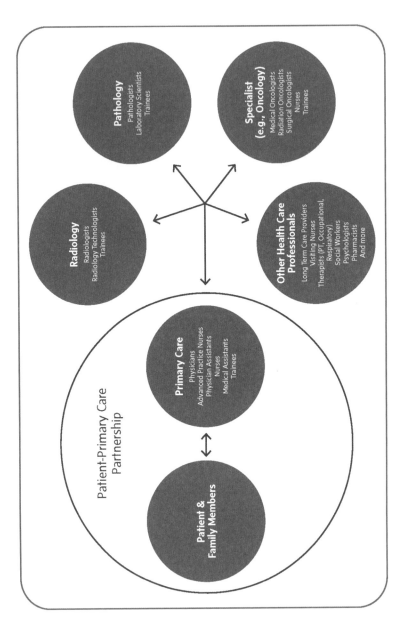

FIGURE 4-3 An example of diagnostic teamwork and the potential participants in the diagnostic process. The arrows in the figure illustrate the importance of communication among team members.
NOTE: PT = physical therapist.

symptoms that require further evaluation, the primary care team can collaborate with other health care professionals (such as pathologists, radiologists, and specialty care clinicians) in the diagnostic process and coordinate subsequent care. The depiction in Figure 4-3 of the various ways that patients and health care professionals interact during the diagnostic process is likely an idealization of clinical practice. For example, patients and their families will often take on a significant burden of care coordination because of the fragmentation of the health care system, a lack of interoperability of patients' electronic health records (EHRs), and payment incentives that do not promote care coordination (Bodenheimer, 2008; Press, 2014). In addition, patients may lack a usual source of primary care, which can hinder care coordination efforts (CDC, 2014; HHS, 2013).

Patients and Their Family Members

The goal of patient engagement in diagnosis is to improve patient care and outcomes by enabling patients and their families to contribute valuable input that will facilitate an accurate and timely diagnosis and improve shared decision making about the path of care. Because patients are a heterogeneous population with varying needs, values, and preferences, their roles in diagnosis need to be individually tailored. Patients hold critical knowledge that informs the diagnostic process, such as knowledge of their health history, their symptoms, their exposure to individuals or environmental factors, the course of their condition, the medications they are taking, as well as knowledge gained from information searches that they conducted in advance of their appointment. In addition, patients and their families may also maintain a more complete version of their own medical records, and they can help ensure that test results are received and facilitate communication among their clinicians (Gruman, 2013).

Diagnosticians

Diagnosticians are health care professionals (physicians, PAs, APNs, and others) who are educated and licensed to provide patients with diagnoses. Although a diagnostician is defined as any health care professional with diagnosis in his or her scope of work, in general, physicians are expected to deal with a greater complexity of diagnostic tasks than other diagnosticians. In addition to diagnosing patients' health problems, diagnosticians often participate in a variety of other health care tasks, such as the provision of preventive care and the management of patients' chronic and acute health conditions. Diagnosticians work in all health care settings and include both general and specialist practitioners. Their clinical reasoning skills come into play as they collect and integrate information from a patient's clinical history, interview, physical exam, diagnostic testing, and consultations with or referrals to other health care professionals (see Chapter 2).

Pathologists and radiologists are diagnosticians who provide information and consultations that are critical to diagnosing patients' health problems, such as advising on the appropriate diagnostic testing for a particular patient and conveying the implications of the test results to treating health care professionals.[1] Despite the important roles that laboratory medicine, anatomic pathology, and medical imaging play in a diagnosis, pathologists and radiologists have sometimes been treated as ancillary or support services. Expert testimony to the committee found that many pathologists and radiologists have not been adequately engaged in the diagnostic process and that better collaboration among all diagnostic team members is necessary (Allen and Thorwarth, 2014; Kroft, 2014). The committee concluded that a culture that perpetuates the notion of anatomic pathology, laboratory medicine, and medical imaging as ancillary health care services will inhibit efforts to improve diagnosis. **Thus, the committee recommends that health care organizations should facilitate and support collaboration among pathologists, radiologists, other diagnosticians, and treating health care professionals to improve diagnostic testing processes.** This includes collaboration throughout the testing process, including the ordering of appropriate tests or images, analysis and interpretation, the reporting and communication of results, and subsequent decision making. Depending on a patient's health problem, treating clinicians may also need to work collaboratively with other diagnosticians, such as sleep specialists, cardiologists, and others. Education and training of health care professionals also needs to ensure that they are prepared to work in this manner.

Health Care Professionals Who Support the Diagnostic Process

In addition to diagnosticians, the diagnostic process may involve an array of health care professionals, including nurses, medical assistants, radiology technologists, laboratory scientists, pharmacists, patient navigators, social workers, therapists, nutritionists, and many others. These health care professionals play a crucial role by facilitating the diagnostic process through the performance of their tasks.

Nurses in particular play a key role in the diagnostic process (see Box 4-2). Nurses may ensure communication and care coordination among diagnostic team members, monitor a patient over time to see if the patient's course is consistent with a working diagnosis, and identify

---

[1] Treating health care professionals are clinicians who directly interact with patients.

BOX 4-2
Suggested Actions for Nurses to Improve
Diagnosis and Reduce Diagnostic Error

1. Know the major diagnoses of your patients.
2. Be the voice of your patients and their advocate in navigating their health care.
3. Be the eyes of the diagnostic team in detecting, reporting, and documenting changes in your patients' symptoms, signs, complaints, or conditions.
4. Be the monitor of the diagnostic team. Is your patient responding to treatment as expected?
5. Help optimize communication between your patient and the care team:
   a. Help patients tell their story and relate all of their symptoms.
   b. Check patients' understanding of their diagnoses and what they've been told.
6. Be the watchdog for appropriate care coordination.
7. Educate patients about the diagnostic process.
8. Learn about how diagnostic errors arise and how they can be avoided.
9. Educate patients about diagnostic tests and explain why they are needed, what the patient will experience, and what the results will reveal.
10. Help patients with the emotional and psychological difficulties that arise when a diagnosis is not yet known or is known to be bad.

SOURCE: Adapted from SIDM and NPSF, 2014. Reprinted, with permission, from the Society to Improve Diagnosis in Medicine and the National Patient Safety Foundation.

---

potential diagnostic errors. Nurses facilitate patient engagement in the diagnostic process by communicating with patients about their history, actively listening to patients' descriptions of their reasons for a visit, documenting patients' symptoms, assessing vital signs, and conveying this information to other clinicians. Nurses need to be full and active members of the diagnostic team, with opportunities to present their observations and conclusions to other team members. The committee's understanding of nurses as crucial contributors to the diagnostic process builds on the recommendations of the IOM report *The Future of Nursing: Leading Change, Advancing Health* (IOM, 2011a). This report provided a road map for transforming nursing practice in the United States. To achieve the necessary changes, the report offered four key recommendations (IOM, 2011a):

- Nurses should practice to the full extent of their education and training.
- Nurses should achieve higher levels of education and training through an improved education system that promotes seamless academic progression.

- Nurses should be full partners, with physicians and other health professionals, in redesigning health care in the United States.
- Effective workforce planning and policy making require better data collection and an improved information infrastructure.

In the 5 years since the report's release, there has been increased awareness of and growing support for these recommendations in nursing schools, health care professional societies, and health care organizations. For example, AARP and the Robert Wood Johnson Foundation recently launched the "Future of Nursing: Campaign for Action," an initiative designed to drive implementation of the report's recommendations.[2] Despite these efforts, progress in the implementation of these recommendations has been uneven. Reenvisioning the roles that nurses play in the diagnostic process is one component of these larger efforts to transform the practice of nursing in the United States.

Radiology technologists and laboratory scientists also play important roles in the diagnostic process. In some cases, radiology technologists take images and make decisions, such as how many and what type of images to take. For example, ultrasound technologists will capture images of normal structures and take additional images of any abnormalities they find. If the radiology technologist does not notice an abnormality, important information may not be conveyed to the radiologist, which may negatively impact the diagnostic process. Laboratory scientists are tasked with procuring samples, preparing samples for analysis, performing analyses, and ensuring that the testing tools are functioning properly. In some cases, these scientists may detect a specimen abnormality during the analysis process that suggests an unsuspected diagnosis or necessitates further investigation.

Pharmacists can make important contributions to the diagnostic process, especially in identifying and averting health problems that stem from drug side effects and interactions (Hines and Murphy, 2011; Malone et al., 2005). Pharmacists and treating clinicians can collaborate to identify whether a patient's symptoms may be due to the side effects of a particular drug or the interaction of multiple medications. Because clinicians may not be aware of all possible drug side effects or interactions, pharmacists may also provide input in the selection of medications for a patient's health problem.

---

[2] See www.campaignforaction.org.

Facilitating Teamwork in Clinical Practice

Health care organizations play a critical role in ensuring effective teamwork. **Thus, the committee recommends that health care organizations should facilitate and support intra- and interprofessional teamwork in the diagnostic process.** There are a number of strategies that health care organizations can employ to improve teamwork in the diagnostic process. Creating a culture that encourages intra- and interprofessional collaboration is critical, as is designing a work system that is supportive of effective teamwork, including the use of results reporting tools that convey important information to the diagnostic team members (see Chapter 6). For example, the use of health IT and telemedicine may help facilitate communication and collaboration among team members, especially when geographically distant health care professionals are involved in the diagnostic process (see Chapter 5). The following section describes several opportunities for improving collaboration, such as care delivery reforms, treatment planning conferences, diagnostic management teams, integrated practice units, morbidity and mortality conferences, and multidisciplinary rounds.

Care Delivery Reforms

Two care delivery reforms—patient-centered medical homes (PCMHs) and accountable care organizations (ACOs)—have recently been implemented across the country as a means to improve patient care coordination and increase communication among health care professionals (see Chapter 7). PCMHs are designed to improve the quality of primary care by fostering a sense of partnership among patients and clinicians and by designating a particular health care practice as being accountable for a patient's care (*Health Affairs*, 2010; Schoen et al., 2007). PCMHs can improve team-based care by acting as the nexus of coordination and communication for a patient and his or her health care professionals; recent evidence suggests that attempts to improve primary care by enhancing its role in coordination have shown some success in improving patient and staff experiences and reducing hospitalization (AHRQ, 2010a). Some PCMH demonstrations are still under evaluation, and other PCMHs are trying new formats; for example, Maryland Blue Cross Blue Shield is offering incentives for physicians to form virtual panels that serve as de facto PCMHs (CMS, 2013; Dentzer, 2012). Barriers to PCMHs include the high up-front costs associated with implementing the health IT infrastructure necessary for improved communication and collaboration and also difficulties in incentivizing outside clinicians to work with those in the PCMH (Crabtree et al., 2010; Rittenhouse et al., 2009).

ACOs are organized groups of health care professionals, practices, or hospitals that work together to assume responsibility for and provide cost-effective care to a defined population of beneficiaries. The Affordable Care Act created ACOs to address delivery system fragmentation and to align incentives to improve communication and collaboration among health care professionals (Berwick, 2011). Although the evidence needed to evaluate the impact of ACOs on improved communication and care coordination is still being collected, there are early indications that ACOs can improve patient care. For example, the Medicare Physician Group Practice, the predecessor to ACOs, demonstrated achievement of 29 of 32 quality measures (Iglehart, 2011), and an early study shows that some Pioneer ACOs were able to reduce overall costs (CMS, 2013). As with PCMHs, high initial costs associated with health IT implementation are a barrier to implementation (Kern, 2014).

Treatment Planning Conferences

Treatment planning conferences (also referred to as tumor boards) are a form of case review in which a multidisciplinary team of health care professionals "review and discuss the medical condition and treatment options of a patient" (NCI, 2015). Treatment planning conferences are often held for specific types of cancers, and their participants may include surgeons, medical oncologists, radiologists, radiation oncologists, pathologists, nurses, and other collaborating health care professionals. These conferences generally serve two purposes: to help diagnose complex cases involving cancer and to consider treatment options for patients with a cancer diagnosis. An advantage of this approach is that it provides a collaborative environment where an intra- and interprofessional team of clinicians can share information and opinions. The evidence on whether treatment planning conferences improve patient outcomes is inconclusive; although a number of studies have found that a small percentage of initial cancer diagnoses changed after review in a treatment planning conference (Chang et al., 2001; Cohen et al., 2009; Newman et al., 2006; Pawlik et al., 2008; Santoso et al., 2004), a multisite study found that treatment planning conferences did not significantly improve the quality of care of patients (Keating et al., 2012). Despite the mixed evidence, treatment planning conferences may help to identify and avoid potential diagnostic errors by bringing multiple perspectives to challenging diagnoses. This approach could also be applied to diagnoses other than cancer, especially ones with serious health consequences or complex symptom presentations.

Diagnostic Management Teams

Health care organizations can support teamwork among pathologists, radiologists, other diagnosticians, and treating health care professionals by forming diagnostic management teams (DMTs).[3] For example, Vanderbilt University's DMT is designed to improve diagnosis through improved communication and access to diagnostic specialists; it offers participating health care professionals assistance in selecting appropriate diagnostic tests and interpreting diagnostic test results (Govern, 2013). DMT consultations consider a patient's clinical information to provide a context for the test result, and they ensure that a clinically valuable interpretation is included in the test result report. Clinicians who participate in this process report a favorable view of DMTs, and although perceived high initial costs are a potential barrier, there is some evidence that DMTs can lower overall costs (Seegmiller et al., 2013).

Integrated Practice Units

Integrated practice units (IPUs) have been proposed as a way to improve the value of health care and to address the communication problems that result from system fragmentation (Porter, 2010; Porter and Lee, 2013). An IPU is a group of clinicians and non-clinicians who are responsible for the comprehensive care of a specific medical condition and the associated complications or for a set of closely related conditions (Porter and Lee, 2013). The members of an IPU have expertise in the relevant condition and work together as a team to provide total care for patients, including inpatient care, outpatient care, and health care education. The IPU model, which has been applied to such conditions as breast cancer and joint replacement, has been shown to improve patient outcomes. For example, patients treated by a spinal care IPU were found to miss fewer days of work, require fewer physical therapy visits, and fewer magnetic resonance images to evaluate their back problems (Porter and Lee, 2013).

Morbidity and Mortality Conferences

Morbidity and mortality (M&M) conferences are forums that bring clinicians together to review cases involving medical errors and adverse events that have occurred. M&M conferences have been used to better understand how errors occur and to help health care organizations identify work system failures and develop interventions to address these failures

---

[3] Personal communication, M. Laposata, August 8, 2014.

(AHRQ, 2008). These conferences have been used to elucidate the causes of diagnostic error and to help improve diagnostic performance (Cifra et al., 2014, 2015).

Multidisciplinary Rounds

Multidisciplinary rounds (also referred to as interdisciplinary rounds) bring health care professionals from different disciplines together to consider the diagnosis and treatment of specific patients. These rounds may involve interacting with patients, or may be part of a lecture with a patient-actor. They provide an opportunity for health care professionals to learn how other health care professionals approach medical issues and to interact with health care professionals from different disciplines. Multidisciplinary rounds have been associated with improvements in care quality, shortened length of stays, and enhancements in resident education (O'Mahony et al., 2007).

PATIENT ENGAGEMENT IN DIAGNOSIS

The IOM report *Crossing the Quality Chasm: A New Health System for the 21st Century* highlighted patient-centeredness as a core aim of the health care system and defined it as "providing care that is respectful of and responsive to individual patient preferences, needs, and values and ensuring that patient values guide all clinical decisions" (IOM, 2001, p. 6). A critical feature of patient-centeredness is the active engagement and shared decision making of patients and their families in the patients' health care. Patient engagement has been defined as "actions [people] take to support their health and benefit from health care" (CFAH, 2015) and has been shown to increase patient satisfaction with care and to improve health outcomes (Boulding et al., 2011; Etchegaray et al., 2014; Glickman et al., 2010; Lucian Leape Institute, 2014; Safran et al., 1998; Sequist et al., 2008; Weingart, 2013). The goal of patient engagement in diagnosis is to improve patient care and outcomes by enabling patients and their families to contribute valuable input that will facilitate an accurate and timely diagnosis and improve shared decision making about the path of care. There are a variety of factors that present challenges to patient engagement in diagnosis, and the committee makes one recommendation to improve patient and family engagement in the diagnostic process.

Challenges to Patient Engagement in Diagnosis

Patients and their families may not be effectively engaged in the diagnostic process for a variety of reasons, including both patient-related factors and health care professional and system factors (see Box 4-3).

Patient-Related Factors

The patient-related factors that prevent active engagement in the diagnostic process can include unfamiliarity with and poor access to the health care system; difficulty with communication due to language, health literacy, and cultural barriers; and a patient's lack of comfort in taking

---

BOX 4-3
Challenges to Effective Patient and Family
Engagement in the Diagnostic Process

Patients and families may:
- Fear complaining and being seen as difficult
- Feel a lack of control or vulnerability for many reasons (sick, scared, social status)
- Not always take their own problems seriously enough
- Lack understanding of the health care system or opportunities to become involved
- Encounter inexperienced health care professionals
- Have language and health literacy barriers
- Be unsure how to seek resolution to a problem when issues are not resolved at the point of care

Health care professionals may:
- Dismiss patients' complaints and knowledge
- Act on implicit or explicit biases and stereotypes
- Incorrectly assume that a patient does not want to be involved in his or her care

Health care systems may exhibit:
- Disjointed care through a lack of coordination and teamwork
- Breakdowns in communication among health care professionals
- Failure to transmit information to patients
- Failure to adequately review or follow up on diagnostic testing results
- Lack of disclosure or apology after diagnostic errors

SOURCE: McDonald et al., 2013. Adapted by permission from BMJ Publishing Group Limited. The patient is in: Patient involvement strategies for diagnostic error mitigation. McDonald, K. M., C. L. Bryce, and M. L. Graber. *BMJ Quality and Safety* 22(2):30–36. 2013.

an active role in diagnosis. Patients are a heterogeneous population, and their needs, values, preferences, and ability to engage in the diagnostic process vary considerably.

Some patients may fear asserting themselves in the diagnostic process because they do not want to appear to be difficult and risk alienating their clinician, which could affect the quality of their care (Frosch et al., 2012). In one study involving cancer patients who thought there had been a serious breakdown in their care, 87 percent did not formally report their concern to the health care organization (Mazor et al., 2012). A patient may also feel uncomfortable asking for a referral to seek a second opinion or asking to see a more experienced clinician (Entwistle et al., 2010). The stress that patients feel related to their health, to navigating the health care system, to missing work, or to dealing with insurance issues can make them less likely to participate in their own care (Evans, 2013). A patient's symptoms and severity of illness can also prevent active engagement in the diagnostic process.

Access to the health care system varies across patients, depending on factors such as health insurance coverage, socioeconomic status and the affordability of health care, and health care delivery system attributes, which in turn can affect the patient's care. For example, the location of health care facilities and the hours of availability for patient care can affect a patient's access to health care. Poor access to, and unfamiliarity with, the health care system may contribute to delays in seeking care for symptoms, which can result in a disease being more advanced when it is diagnosed, leading to a worse prognosis or a more invasive treatment which could have been avoided. Certain populations are more likely to have difficulty obtaining care, including racial and ethnic minorities and individuals of low socioeconomic status (AHRQ, 2013a,b).

Cultural and language barriers can be significant challenges that prevent patients from fully engaging in the diagnostic process. Approximately 22 percent of the 60 million people living in the United States who speak a language other than English at home report not being able to speak English well or at all (Ryan, 2013). The IOM report *Unequal Treatment: Confronting Racial and Ethnic Disparities in Health Care* noted that "Language barriers may affect the delivery of adequate care through poor exchange of information, loss of important cultural information, misunderstanding of physician instruction, poor shared decision making, or ethical compromises (e.g., difficulty obtaining informed consent)" (IOM, 2003b, p. 17). In addition, The Joint Commission has found that miscommunications and misunderstandings increase the risk for adverse events in health care (The Joint Commission, 2007). These barriers have also been associated with diagnostic errors (Flores, 2006; Marcus, 2003; Price-Wise, 2008). To meet the needs of patients with limited English proficiency, some health care organizations have instituted policies to ensure that language services, such as those provided by interpreters, are available and that educational literature is provided in languages other than English (HHS, 2015). Despite these steps, a study found that even when hospitals have a policy regarding language services, they often do not provide staff with the training necessary to access language services, they do not assess the competency of interpreters, and there is little oversight of the quality of the translated literature (Wilson-Stronks, 2007).

Even if a patient speaks the same language as his or her clinicians, there can be communication challenges if the patient has limited health literacy or if clinicians use unfamiliar medical terminology (IOM, 2004). In the United States more than 80 million adults have a poor level of health literacy, which has been defined as "the degree to which individuals have the capacity to obtain, process, and understand basic health information and services needed to make appropriate health decisions" (AHRQ, 2011, p. ES-1). Health literacy requires applying a complex set of skills involving reading, listening, analysis, and decision making to health settings (NNLM, 2013). Patients lacking health literacy skills may be limited in their ability to participate in the diagnostic process and in decision making about the planned path of care (Peters et al., 2007). A recent study indicated that a group of medical trainees, including PA and MD students, lacked confidence in their ability to communicate effectively with patients with low health literacy (Ali et al., 2014).

There is a tremendous amount of information and resources available on the Internet and mobile applications to help patients identify potential diagnoses and to plan for health care appointments. A 2013 Pew Research Center study found that 35 percent of American adults have used online resources to diagnose a condition in themselves or someone else (Fox and Duggan, 2013). These resources have varying levels of accuracy, and patients may have difficulty assessing the quality of the information available to them (NLM, 2012b; Semigran et al., 2015). Clinicians may also react negatively to patients' use of this information in clinical visits (Julavits, 2014).

Patients' level of comfort with actively engaging in care decisions, such as asking questions, stating preferences, or seeking alternative opinions, may differ considerably from one patient to another. Some patients may prefer to be actively involved in all aspects of the decision-making process, while others would rather defer to their clinicians' judgment (Fowler, 2011). In a national survey, the majority of respondents reported that they would like clinicians to effectively engage them in health care decision making by talking about their diagnosis and explaining the options available, including the risks and their impact on quality of life and the costs associated with them (IOM, 2012b). Another survey found that 96 percent of respondents desired to be asked questions and to be given choices regarding their care, and approximately half preferred to have their clinicians make the final decisions (Levinson et al., 2005). Clinicians may not be aware of—or they may misjudge—the role that a patient desires to play in decision making, and as a result they may make decisions that are misaligned with patient preferences, a phenomenon that has been referred to as a preference misdiagnosis (Mulley et al., 2012). Factors such as age, gender, medical history, familiarity with the health care system, socioeconomic status, and cultural issues can factor in to patients' preferences regarding engagement and shared decision making (Boyer et al., 2001; Cox et al., 2012; Lipson et al., 2003; Longtin et al., 2010). Several studies have found that female patients who are younger and have more education tend to prefer a more active role in decisions regarding their health (Arora and McHorney, 2000; Deber et al., 2007; Say et al., 2006). A survey of low-income patients faced with major medical decisions found that 75 percent wanted to be very involved in the decision-making process (BSCF, 2014).

Health Care Professional and System Factors

A major concern cited by health care professionals is a lack of time to truly engage patients in the diagnostic process (Anderson and Funnell, 2005; Sarkar et al., 2012, 2014; Stevenson, 2003). Compared to more procedure-oriented tasks, fee-for-service payment does not incentivize the time spent on evaluation and management services that reflect the cognitive expertise and skills that clinicians employ in the diagnostic process (National Commission on Physician Payment Reform, 2013). This creates an environment in which communication, such as the clinical history and interview, may be rushed and patients may not have time to thoroughly discuss their symptoms and health concerns, although new models of payment and care delivery may make this a higher priority (AHRQ, 2014c; Cosgrove et al., 2013; Roades, 2013) (see Chapter 7). Time pressures may also lead to an overreliance on diagnostic testing in place of patient engagement, even when these may be inappropriate (Newman-Toker et al., 2013; Rao and Levin, 2012; Zhi et al., 2013) (see Chapter 3). The use of EHRs may also lead to problems with patient engagement, as health care professionals may be distracted from communicating with patients as they enter information in the EHR (O'Malley et al., 2010; Spain, 2014) (see Chapter 5).

Although many clinicians are positive about engaging with their patients (Stevenson, 2003), there are indications that some may be resistant to active patient involvement (Graedon and Graedon, 2014; Haskell, 2014; IOM, 2013a; Julavits, 2014). In interactions with patients, certain clinician behaviors can discourage open communication and patient engagement, including being dismissive of a patient's complaints and their knowledge of their symptoms, not listening, or interrupting frequently (Dyche and Swiderski, 2005; Marvel et al., 1999; McDonald et al., 2013). For example, one study found that after a clinician entered the room, patients spoke without being interrupted for an average of only 12 seconds; the clinicians frequently interrupted the patients before they had finished speaking (Rhoades et al., 2001). Clinicians' vulnerability to cognitive and affective biases may also contribute to behaviors that hinder patient engagement and contribute to diagnostic errors (Croskerry, 2013; Klein, 2005). Clinicians may exhibit biases in regard to gender, race, ethnicity, sexual orientation, age, obesity, a patient's health problem (e.g., chronic pain, mental health), or other factors (IOM, 2003b, 2011b,c, 2012e; Puhl and Brownell, 2001; Schwartz et al., 2003). For example, clinicians may be judgmental or blame patients for their illnesses, and this could affect a patient's willingness to participate in the diagnostic process (Croskerry, 2003). Patients may fear disclosing sensitive information to their clinicians, such as their sexual orientation, due to a fear that such disclosure could negatively affect their care (Durso and Meyer, 2013; Foglia and Fredriksen-Goldsen, 2014; IOM, 2011b). If this information is not disclosed, Foglia and Fredriksen-Goldsen (2014) note that it could result in diagnostic error, such as a delay in diagnosing a serious health problem. The *Unequal Treatment* report found that "bias, stereotyping, prejudice, and clinical uncertainty on the part of health care providers may contribute to racial and ethnic disparities in healthcare" (IOM, 2003b, p. 12). For example, one study found that a patient's race and gender independently influenced how physicians managed chest pain; physicians were significantly more likely to refer white men exhibiting signs of coronary artery disease for cardiac catheterization than to refer black women with the same symptoms (Schulman et al., 1999). Clinicians may also disregard symptoms in patients with previous diagnoses of mental illness or substance abuse and may attribute new physical symptoms to a psychological cause without a proper evaluation. Alternatively, clinicians may incorrectly diagnose or assume psychiatric, alcohol, or drug abuse diagnoses for serious medical conditions, such as hypoxia, delirium, metabolic abnormalities, or head injuries; a mistake known as a "psychout error" (Croskerry, 2003).

Fragmentation of health care and poor coordination of care hinder patient engagement and can contribute to errors in diagnosis (CFAH, 2014c; Gandhi and Lee, 2010; Gandhi et al., 2006; IOM, 2013a; Schiff, 2008; Starfield, 2000). In cases where there is poor care coordination and communication among clinicians, patients and their families may need to convey their information among their health care professionals. For example, one survey found that approximately 25 percent of patients reported that their doctors did not share information about their medical history or test results with other health care professionals involved in a patient's care (Stremikis et al., 2011). Limited interoperability among EHRs and laboratory and medical informatics systems may also prevent the flow of information among clinicians and health care settings (see Chapter 5).

Improving Patient Engagement in the Diagnostic Process

Patients and their families play a crucial role in the diagnostic process but the ultimate responsibility for supporting and enabling patient and family engagement in the diagnostic process rests with health care professionals and organizations. Health care professionals need to embrace patients and their families as essential partners in the diagnostic process, with valuable contributions that can improve diagnosis and avert diagnostic errors. **Thus, the committee recommends that health care professionals and organizations should partner with patients and their families as diagnostic team members and facilitate patient and family engagement in the diagnostic process, aligned with their needs, values, and preferences.**

Learning About the Diagnostic Process

To facilitate patient and family engagement, the committee recommends that health care professionals and organizations provide patients with opportunities to learn about the diagnostic process. One of the challenges that patients and their families face with diagnosis is their unfamiliarity with the process; thus, informing patients and their families about it has the potential to improve engagement and reduce diagnostic errors. Patients may be unfamiliar with the terminology related to the diagnostic process, such as a "differential diagnosis" or a "working diagnosis,"[4] and also with the role of time in the process. For example, a health care professional may propose a working diagnosis if there is some uncertainty in the diagnosis, and this may change with new information. For some health problems, watchful waiting is appropriate, and patients need to be informed that time can give clinicians a better understanding of their health problem. It is also important that patients understand when and who to contact if their symptoms do not resolve or if they experience new symptoms that do not seem to fit with a working diagnosis. Providing information explaining the roles and tasks of the various individuals

---

[4] A differential diagnosis is a list of possible diagnoses ranked from most probable to least probable based on the available information. A working diagnosis is a preliminary or provisional diagnosis, and it may be in the form of a differential diagnosis.

involved in diagnosis could also facilitate more active engagement in the diagnostic process.

A number of groups have developed information and resources to help patients become more actively involved in their health care, including the diagnostic process (CFAH, 2014c; The Joint Commission, 2015; Josiah Macy Jr. Foundation, 2014; Lucian Leape Institute, 2014). The Center for Advancing Health has developed a variety of resources to help patients gain maximum benefit from their health care, including information about communicating with clinicians, organizing health care, seeking knowledge about health, and other topics (CFAH, 2014a,b). The Speak Up™ Program offers materials to help patients become more actively involved in their care and avoid errors (The Joint Commission, 2015). The National Patient Safety Foundation, the Society to Improve Diagnosis in Medicine, and Kaiser Permanente have developed resources to help patients get the right diagnosis (see Boxes 4-4 and 4-5) (Kaiser Permanente, 2012; NPSF and SIDM, 2014). The actions suggested in the resources include having a thorough knowledge of medical history, formulating notes about symptoms and questions to bring to appointments, and maintaining a list of medications (such as prescriptions, over-the-counter medications, dietary supplements, and complementary and alternative medicines). Health care professionals and organizations can also inform patients and families about the reliability and accuracy of online resources and direct them to reputable sources (FamilyDoctor.org, 2014; Mayo Clinic, 2015; NLM, 2012a,b; Semigran et al., 2015).

Health Care Environments That Are Supportive of Patient and Family Engagement

Health care professionals and the organizations in which they practice can facilitate patient engagement in the diagnostic process by improving communication and shared decision making and by addressing health literacy barriers. **Thus, the committee recommends that health care professionals and organizations should create environments in which patients and their families are comfortable engaging in the diagnostic process and sharing feedback and concerns about diagnostic errors and near misses.** Health care organizations will need to carefully consider whether their care delivery systems and processes fully support patient engagement and work to improve systems and processes that are oriented primarily toward meeting the needs of health care professionals rather than patients and their families. One of the most important actions that health care professionals can take to implement this recommendation is to improve their communication skills because effective patient–clinician communication is critical to making accurate diagnoses and to averting diagnostic errors. Several organizations offer communication training

BOX 4-4
Checklist for Getting the Right Diagnosis

1. Tell Your Story Well: Be clear, complete, and accurate when you tell your clinician about your illness.
   - Be Clear – Take some time to think about when your symptoms started, what made your symptoms better or worse, or if your symptoms were related to taking medications, eating a meal, exercising, or a certain time of day.
   - Be Complete – Try to remember all of the important information about your illness. Write down some notes and bring them with you. A family member may be able to help you with this.
   - Be Accurate – Sometimes you may see multiple clinicians during a medical appointment. Make sure your clinicians hear the same story regarding your illness.

2. Be a Good Historian:
   - Remember what treatments you have tried in the past, if they helped, and what, if any, side effects you experienced.
   - Think about how your illness has progressed over time.
   - Think about your family's medical history and if you may be at risk for similar illnesses.

3. Keep Good Records:
   - Keep your own records of test results, referrals, and hospital admissions.
   - Keep an accurate list of your medications.
   - Bring your medication list with you when you see your clinician or pharmacist.

4. Be an Informed Consumer:
   - Learn about your illness by looking at reliable sources on the Internet or visit a local library.
   - Learn about the tests or procedures you are having done.
   - Learn about your medications:
     o Know the names of your medications (both brand names and generic). For example: Tylenol (brand name) and acetaminophen (generic name)
     o Know what the medication is for.
     o Know the amount (dose) you need to take.
     o Know the time(s) you need to take it during the day.
     o Know the side effects to watch for and report to your clinician.
     o Know if the medication interacts with any food or drugs.

5. Take Charge of Managing Your Health:
   - When meeting with your clinician, use the Ask Me 3 brochure, *Good Questions for Getting the Right Diagnosis*:
     1. What could be causing my problem?
     2. What else could it be?
     3. When will I get my test results, and what should I do to follow up?
   - If you have more than one clinician, make sure each clinician knows what the other person is thinking and planning.
   - Make sure each clinician knows all of your test results, medications, or other treatments.
   - Be informed and involved in decisions about your health.

6. Know Your Test Results:
   - Make sure both you and your clinician get the results from any tests that are done.
   - Don't assume that no news is good news; call and check on your test results.
   - Ask what the test results mean and what needs to be done next.

7. Follow Up:
   - Ask when you need to make another appointment (follow up) with your clinician once you start treatment.
   - Ask what to expect from the treatment or what it will do for you.
   - Ask what you need to do if you get new symptoms or start to feel worse.

8. Make Sure It Is the Right Diagnosis:
   - Sometimes your diagnosis is the most "likely" thing that is wrong, but it may not be the "right" diagnosis.
   - Don't be afraid to ask "What else could this be?"
   - Encourage your clinicians to think about other possible reasons for your illness.

9. Record Your Health Information and Monitor Your Progress:
   - Track your health information and share it with your health care team in a structured format.[a]

---

[a] One available resource is SIDM's patient toolkit (SIDM, 2015).

SOURCES: Adapted from NPSF, 2015a; NPSF and SIDM, 2014. Reprinted, with permission, from the National Patient Safety Foundation and Society to Improve Diagnosis in Medicine. Ask Me 3 is a registered trademark of Pfizer Inc. and is licensed to the National Patient Safety Foundation.

BOX 4-5
Smart Partners About Your Health

SMART CHECKLIST
- **Symptoms**
  Tell your clinician what's currently wrong . . . why you are here. Is this a new symptom, when did it start, what home remedies have you tried?
- **Medical/medication history**
  Provide medical information about your past. Be prepared to discuss your current medications and over-the-counter medicines or supplements that you take (Ibuprofen, vitamins, etc.) with your clinician.
- **Assessment**
  Describe what you think is going on. Express your feelings and your concerns.
- **Review**
  After your clinician diagnoses your condition, ask if it could be something else. Make sure you understand what is causing your symptoms. In your own words describe the diagnosis back to your clinician. Talk about things that might keep you from following your treatment plan.
- **To do**
  Make sure you understand what you need to do next. Repeat your treatment plan and the information you received from your clinician. Be sure to ask for your after-visit summary and follow all your clinician's instructions or let him or her know if you can't.

SMART SCRIPT
- **Symptoms**
  "I'm concerned about . . ."
  "Symptoms I've been having . . ."
- **Medical/medication history**
  "Some of my medical history that might be important includes (a close family member had cancer)."
  "To help me remember I have a list of my current medications and supplements."
- **Assessment**
  "I'm worried I might have ___ and I have tried . . ."
  After your clinician diagnoses your condition, ask questions and verify next steps.
- **Review**
  "Could you tell me what else it could be or if more than one thing is going on?"
- **To do**
  "Just to make sure I haven't missed anything, I need to . . ."

BEFORE YOUR VISIT THINK ABOUT . . .
- **What you want to talk about during your visit**
  What symptoms are you having?
  How long have you had them?
  Do they go away?
  Have you tried any home treatments? If so, what?
- **Inviting someone to go with you**
  Bringing someone to your appointment can help you to answer questions and give your clinician information.
- **Write down your questions or some words that will help remind you**
  What concerns do you have about your symptoms?
  What concerns are most important to you?
- **Be prepared**
  Be prepared to go over your medications, vitamins, and supplements.
  Make sure you mention any changes that you have made.

DURING YOUR VISIT . . .
- **Confirm with your clinician why you are there**
- **Your symptoms**
  When did your symptoms start?
  Do they go away?
  Where are they located?
  How do they affect your daily activities?
- **Share what home treatments you have tried**
  Did they help or make your symptoms worse?
- **Share your worries about your symptoms**
- **Share what you think might be going on**

YOUR DIAGNOSIS: CONSIDER ASKING THE CLINICIAN:
- **What else could it be?**
- **Do all my symptoms match your diagnosis?**
- **Could there be more than one thing going on?**

AT THE END OF YOUR VISIT . . .
- **Make sure you understand what you need to do next**
  Repeat your treatment plan and the information you received from your clinician.
  If you don't understand ask your clinician to explain any words or ideas that are confusing.
  Talk about things that you feel might keep you from following the treatment plan.
  Talk about other treatment plans or options.
- **Be sure to ask for your after-visit summary**
- **Follow all your clinician's instructions or let them know if you can't**

courses for clinicians, including the Institute for Healthcare Communication and the American Academy on Communication in Healthcare (AACH, 2015; IHC, 2015).

There are several techniques and strategies that clinicians can use to improve communication and patient engagement. One of the most well-known methods is teach-back, which involves a clinician explaining a concept and then asking the patient to repeat in his or her own words what was said (Nouri and Rudd, 2015; Schillinger et al., 2003). The clinician can then evaluate whether the patient has a good understanding and, if the patient does not, can explain the concept further using a different approach in order to improve the patient's comprehension. Patient–clinician communication can also be improved by using clear and simple language, encouraging questions, listening actively, allowing the patient to speak without interruption, and responding to the patient's emotions. Such techniques may also help some patients overcome their fear of discussing their concerns and become more likely to share sensitive information that could provide valuable input to the diagnostic process. If patients are upset or anxious, they may be less likely to give a thorough and accurate account of their symptoms and health concerns. Inclusion of a patient's family in a patient's care may also facilitate engagement and comprehension.

Supportive health care environments are places where patients and families feel comfortable sharing their concerns about diagnostic errors and near misses and providing feedback on their experiences with diagnosis. As discussed in the education section of this chapter, providing feedback to health care professionals about the accuracy of their diagnoses can help improve their diagnostic performance. However, health care professionals often do not have opportunities to hear from patients about their diagnostic performance (Berner and Graber, 2008; Schiff, 2008). For example, a patient discharged from the emergency department may then see a primary care clinician, and the emergency department clinician may never hear whether the diagnosis on discharge was correct. To improve diagnostic performance, health care professionals and organizations should encourage patients and their families to follow up with their health care professionals to let them know about their experiences. Health care organizations can facilitate feedback from patients and their families by, for example, implementing procedures to follow up with patients after their visits. This feedback could also be used as a routine part of assessing patient satisfaction with clinicians and health care organizations.

In order to establish environments where patients and families can share their concerns, clinicians need to be ready to communicate with patients about the occurrence of diagnostic errors. A study involving 13 focus groups found that patients who have experienced a medical error wanted clinicians to disclose all harmful errors (Gallagher et al., 2003).

These patients sought information about what happened, why the error happened, how to mitigate the consequences of the error, and how clinicians would prevent recurrences (Gallagher et al., 2003). Clinicians have been reluctant to disclose medical errors to patients and their families because of the fear of litigation as well as anxiety over communicating these errors; however, disclosing errors has been broadly recognized as the right thing to do (AHRQ, 2014a). There is evidence that disclosure improves patient outcomes and may reduce malpractice claims and costs (AHRQ, 2014a; Hendrich et al., 2014; Kachalia et al., 2003; Mello et al., 2014) (see Chapter 7).

Fostering shared decision making, which is defined as "a collaborative process that allows patients and their providers to make health care decisions together, taking into account the best scientific evidence available, as well as the patient's values and preferences" (IMDF, 2014), can also improve patient and family engagement in the diagnostic process. Tools to promote shared decision making are decision aids, which provide objective, evidence-based information on options that patients may have so that they can make informed decisions (IMDF, 2014; MedPAC, 2010). Although many decision aids are focused on treatment and screening decisions, some have been developed for diagnostic situations, such as an evaluation for low back pain or whether to do imaging studies for chest discomfort (Ronda et al., 2014; SCAI, 2014).

Addressing health literacy barriers may also improve patient and family engagement in the diagnostic process. Acknowledging that the health care system can place unreasonably high health literacy demands on patients and families, an IOM discussion paper identified 10 attributes of health-literate health care organizations, summarized in Box 4-6 (IOM, 2012a). For example, health care organizations can encourage the use of tools—such as Ask Me 3, Getting the Right Diagnosis, Smart Partners About Your Health, and Speak Up—in order to improve communication among patients and their clinicians. If health care organizations make it easier for patients and families to navigate, understand, and use health care services, then patients and their families can become more engaged in the diagnostic process. In addition, health care professionals and organizations can ensure that health care environments reflect cultural and language competencies (AHRQ, 2012). Some health care organizations have instituted policies to ensure that language services, such as those provided by interpreters, are available and that educational literature is provided in languages other than English. The IOM recommended the broader use of interpretation services where community need exists (IOM, 2003b), and the Department of Health and Human Services (HHS) has established national standards for culturally and linguistically appropriate care (HHS, 2015). Many health care professional schools offer cultural

---

BOX 4-6
Attributes of Health Literate Health Care Organizations

A health literate organization:

1. Has leadership that makes health literacy integral to its mission, structure, and operations
2. Integrates health literacy into planning, evaluation measures, patient safety, and quality improvement
3. Prepares the workforce to be health literate and monitors progress
4. Includes populations served in the design, implementation, and evaluation of health information and services
5. Meets the needs of populations with a range of health literacy skills while avoiding stigmatization
6. Uses health literacy strategies in interpersonal communications and confirms understanding at all points of contact
7. Provides easy access to health information and services and navigation assistance
8. Designs and distributes print, audiovisual, and social media content that is easy to understand and act on
9. Addresses health literacy in high-risk situations, including care transition and communications about medicines
10. Communicates clearly what health plans will cover and what individuals will have to pay for services

SOURCE: IOM, 2012a.

---

competency courses, and there are continuing education programs designed to increase cultural competency and sensitivity. Though there is evidence that improving cultural competency can improve patient satisfaction with care (Castro and Ruiz, 2009; Paez et al., 2009), the evidence connecting cultural competency with improvements in patient outcomes is limited (Beach et al., 2005; Lie et al., 2011).

Health care organizations can also facilitate patients' reengagement with the health care system for unresolved symptoms or in other instances (such as a missed follow-up appointment). For example, Kaiser Permanente's SureNet Program identifies people who have inadvertent lapses in care and uses electronic surveillance and staff to follow up with these patients (Danforth et al., 2014; Kanter, 2014). Closed-loop communication systems that require all information from referrals and consultations to be relayed to the treating clinician may also help ensure that patients reengage the health care system when necessary (Gandhi, 2014; Schiff, 2014a) (see Chapter 6).

Patient Access to Their Electronic Health Information

Another opportunity to encourage patient engagement in the diagnostic process is to make a patient's health information more accessible and transparent. One way to accomplish this is through open medical records, or records that "patients, and others authorized by them, are allowed to read. . . . When used properly, they let patients see themselves through the eyes of their caregivers and give them insight into diagnoses and treatment options. Having access to such information permits patients to take a more active role in decisions about their care" (Frampton et al., 2009, p. 59). **Thus, the committee recommends that health care professionals and organizations should ensure patient access to EHRs, including clinical notes and diagnostic testing results, to facilitate patient engagement in the diagnostic process and patient review of health records for accuracy.** The Office of the National Coordinator for Health Information Technology's Meaningful Use 2 requirements include patient access to their electronic health information (such as medication lists, diagnostic test results, allergies, and clinical problem lists), and organizations have begun to employ patient portals in order to enable patient access to this information (Adler-Milstein et al., 2014; Bruno et al., 2014; Furukawa et al., 2014; HealthIT.gov, 2015). Unfortunately, many organizations are having trouble meeting the Meaningful Use 2 requirement that 5 percent of patients "view, download, or transmit their health information" (Adler-Milstein, 2015).

The OpenNotes initiative, available to almost five million patients, has promoted even greater transparency of patients' health information by inviting patients to view the notes recorded by health care professionals during a clinical visit (OpenNotes, 2015). In an analysis of patients who were invited to read their notes over the course of 1 year, approximately 70 to 80 percent surveyed said that they read their notes, understood their care plan better, and were better prepared for visits (Bell et al., 2014; Delbanco et al., 2012). Clinicians report that implementing OpenNotes results in few, if any, disruptions to their practice (Bell et al., 2014; Walker et al., 2014).

In input that was provided to the committee, the OpenNotes developers suggested that initiatives like OpenNotes have the potential to reduce diagnostic errors by enabling patients and families to catch errors within clinician notes, by encouraging patients to speak up, and by preventing diagnostic delay by helping patients better remember recommendations for tests and procedures. In addition, the developers cited transparency as a means to help patients better understand their clinicians' thought processes, to enhance trust, and to engage family caregivers. In a pilot study, the developers found that patients with access to their medical information were more likely than those without such access to have questions, to identify inaccuracies, and to offer additional information regarding the data in their health records (NORC, 2014).

Direct patient access to diagnostic testing results is also important to patient engagement because diagnostic errors commonly occur within the testing steps of the diagnostic process (Gandhi et al., 2006; Schiff et al., 2009). In 2014, HHS strengthened patients' rights to directly access their laboratory test results (HHS, 2014). Prior to the implementation of this regulation, an analysis found that only 3 in 10 laboratories allowed patients or their legal representatives access to their clinical test results (Swain and Patel, 2014). Similarly, the Mammography Quality Standards Act mandated the direct reporting of mammography results to patients with a summary of the report written in easily understood terms. A study found that direct reporting improved patient satisfaction with mammography and the timeliness of the results reporting, although it did not significantly reduce patient anxiety or improve patient adherence to the recommendations (Priyanath et al., 2002). Although there is some concern that providing patients direct access to diagnostic testing results before they consult with their clinician may not be appropriate in all cases (e.g., for worrisome test results or for test results that patients may have difficulty in interpreting), there are a number of advantages to direct patient access, including reducing the likelihood that patients do not receive a test result and improving subsequent decision making and treatment (ASCP, 2014). Some organizations have implemented time delays to enable clinicians to communicate directly with patients before the patients access their diagnostic testing results electronically (Butcher, 2014).

Involvement of Patients and Families in Efforts to Improve Diagnosis

Patients and their families have unique insights into the diagnostic process, their health outcomes, and the occurrence of diagnostic errors (Etchegaray et al., 2014; Gertler et al., 2014; Schiff et al., 2014). Their perspectives are critical to identifying errors and near misses, especially ones that health care professionals may not be aware of, and they can also inform efforts to improve the diagnostic process (Gertler et al., 2014; Weingart et al., 2005). **Thus, the committee recommends that health care professionals and organizations should identify opportunities to include patients and their families in efforts to improve the diagnostic process by learning from diagnostic errors and near misses.** Some of the opportunities for learning include participation in root cause analyses and M&M conferences (Gertler et al., 2014; NPSF, 2015b; Schiff et al., 2014;

Zimmerman and Amori, 2007).[5] For example, patients and family members may have information that is unavailable to health care professionals that can be used during a root cause analysis to identify contributors to a diagnostic error (Etchegaray et al., 2014). Participation in these events may also be satisfying to patients and their families because they have an opportunity to help improve safety and reduce the chance of future errors (Zimmerman and Amori, 2007). However, it is important for health care organizations to tailor patient and family involvement according to individual needs and preferences and to be aware of the legal constraints to involving patients and families in these efforts.

Health care organizations can also create patient and family advisory councils and use their input to design more patient-centered diagnostic processes. Patient and family advisory councils may be involved in the development, implementation, or evaluation of new programs; the design of materials or tools to improve patient–clinician relationships; and other activities (AHRQ, 2014b). These councils can involve patients and families in the design of care and can leverage their experiences in order to implement patient-centered changes, including changes that may reduce diagnostic errors (Coulter et al., 2008; IOM, 2013a). For example, a patient and family advisory council at Inova Health System played a role in designing a shift-change procedure for nursing staff that could reduce the potential for errors related to care transitions (Friesen et al., 2013).

HEALTH CARE PROFESSIONAL EDUCATION AND TRAINING

There are indications that health care professionals may not receive adequate preparation to function optimally in the diagnostic process (Brush, 2014; Dhaliwal, 2014; Durning, 2014; Richardson, 2007; ten Cate, 2014; Trowbridge et al., 2013). Education and training-related challenges include methods that have not kept pace with advances in the learning sciences[6] and an insufficient focus on areas critical to the diagnostic process, such as clinical reasoning, teamwork, communication, and the use of diagnostic testing and health IT. Because there is limited research on how education and training can affect diagnosis, the committee drew from a broader literature that included research on the impact of education and training in other areas of health care, in other industries, as well as submitted expert input to the committee. Education and training across the career trajectory plays an important role in improving the diagnostic

---

[5] Root cause analysis is a problem-solving method that attempts to identify the factors that contributed to an error. M&M conferences are forums that allow clinicians to discuss and learn from errors that have occurred within an organization.

[6] The learning sciences study how people learn in order to optimize education and training.

process and reducing diagnostic errors and near misses. This section describes the challenges to health care professional education and training and presents the committee's recommendation. Though the focus is on leveraging changes in education and training to improve diagnosis, recommended actions could also have broader impact on clinical practice. For example, ensuring that clinicians have clinical reasoning skills may also improve clinicians' abilities to treat and manage patients' health problems. Although this section's emphasis is on diagnosticians, the challenges and solutions are relevant to many health care professionals who participate in the diagnostic process.

Educational Approaches

The learning sciences are an interdisciplinary field that studies learning methods and principles in an effort to understand how to optimize learning (Torre et al., 2006). The findings from this field—including the importance of developing deep conceptual understandings, participative learning, building on prior knowledge, the use of reflection, and appropriate learning environments—are relevant to health care professional education and training (see Box 4-7) (Sawyer, 2006). For example, students often gain deeper knowledge when their learning involves activities that mimic those of professionals engaged in the relevant discipline, a learning style that has been described as "authentic practice" (Sawyer, 2008). The learning sciences have also found that some learning styles are better suited for some individuals than others (Dunn et al., 2002; Lujan and DiCarlo, 2006).

Health care professional education programs may not be adequately informed by advances in the learning sciences (Cooke et al., 2010; Rolfe and Sanson-Fisher, 2002). For example, programs may continue to emphasize memorization without helping students develop the deeper conceptual understandings that are needed to apply knowledge in novel, practice-based situations (Myers, 2013). This may result in them having difficulty diagnosing conditions in nonstandard contexts, such as cases involving atypical presentations or comorbidities. Educational experts have asserted that there is a tendency to focus learning on prototypical and representational cases of disease rather than on real-life presentations (AHRQ, 2010b; Papa, 2014a). While this may be appropriate for the early stages of learning, students need exposure to actual patient cases, including atypical cases, in order to be prepared to diagnose disease in practice (Dhaliwal, 2014). Programs that delay student interaction with patients until the later stages of education also miss opportunities to provide students with authentic practice (ten Cate, 2014). Given the mismatch of training and practice environments, it may be challenging to provide stu-

---

BOX 4-7
The Learning Sciences

The following are important aspects of learning, identified by the learning sciences, for individuals engaged in knowledge work—i.e., professions that rely on using, manipulating, and generating knowledge.

1. **Developing deeper conceptual understanding**
   Students can apply learned material more broadly and across contexts if they have developed a deep conceptual understanding of the material. A deeper understanding requires learners to: (1) relate novel ideas to previous knowledge, (2) integrate knowledge into conceptual systems, (3) seek out patterns and connecting principles, (4) consider new ideas critically, (5) understand the structure of arguments and the process through which knowledge is generated, and (6) reflect on how they learn and what they understand.

2. **Focusing on learning**
   Students learn in different ways and these differences need to be considered as educational programs are designed and implemented. Programs that include participatory learning may benefit students and should be considered.

3. **Creating learning environments**
   Specifically designed learning environments can positively impact the learning process.

4. **Building on prior knowledge**
   Learning processes that move from concrete to abstract facts facilitate the knowledge integration and retention necessary to develop deep conceptual understandings.

5. **Reflecting on one's knowledge**
   Taking time to reflect on one's state of knowledge enhances the learning process.

SOURCE: Sawyer, 2006.

---

dents with authentic practice; for example, a majority of graduate medical education (GME) training occurs in inpatient settings, even though many physicians will work in outpatient settings (ACGME, 2015; Cooke et al., 2010; IOM, 2014; Josiah Macy Jr. Foundation, 2011).

Some health care professional education programs may not be providing learners adequate opportunities to achieve expertise in diagnosis. For example, educators may attempt to teach students to think like experienced clinicians even though they lack the experience and knowledge base necessary to function in this manner (ten Cate, 2014). Programs may also place insufficient emphasis on developing the skills and methods required to pursue self-motivated, lifelong learning. Individuals who lack these skills may find it more difficult to develop diagnostic skills beyond the formal education setting, leading to challenges in remaining abreast of findings throughout a clinician's career (IOM, 2010, 2011a).

The evaluation of students may need to be better aligned with best practices from the learning sciences. Some health care professional schools rely on training time as a means of evaluating student performance, but it has been suggested that competency-based evaluation (CBE), which evaluates students based on their competency in certain areas, may be a better method because it is a better predictor of future performance (Holmboe et al., 2010). CBE is still in development, however, and there is some disagreement about using it exclusively to assess learners' abilities. There is limited evidence connecting CBE to improvements in student learning, and it is difficult to assess certain characteristics, such as professionalism, through a competency-based approach (Jarvis-Selinger et al., 2012; Lurie, 2012; Morcke et al., 2013).

A number of methods to assess competency have been proposed, including written and computerized testing, performance appraisals, medical record reviews, and simulations; some methods may be better suited for assessing specific competencies than others (Kak et al., 2001). Psychometric testing methods such as multiple choice and vignette-based exams have been used to evaluate clinicians' medical knowledge, though they often do not capture key aspects of clinical reasoning that contribute to diagnostic expertise (Holmboe and Durning, 2014) (see Chapter 2). Given the importance of clinical reasoning to practice, there is now a growing movement to develop assessment methods that are better able to evaluate clinical reasoning competencies (ABIM, 2014; Holmboe and Durning, 2014). For example, the American Board of Internal Medicine's Assessment 2020 Initiative is focused on improving cognitive assessment in internal medicine. It is evaluating the role of computer-based clinical simulations, in which a simulated patient's condition changes as clinicians make decisions in the diagnostic and treatment processes (ABIM, 2015). Oral exams, such as chart stimulated recall and case-based discussions, as well as audio and video reviews of actual clinical encounters have also been suggested as assessment methods for clinical reasoning (Holmboe and Durning, 2014). Simulation exercises have been used to assess teamwork skills and communication competencies (Scalese et al., 2008).

Experts who provided input to the committee focused on the use of feedback to improve diagnostic performance and promote self-reflection (Schiff, 2014a; Singh, 2014; Trowbridge, 2014). Feedback is an integral part of continuous learning and can help health care professionals understand how well they are performing (Croskerry, 2000b). However, there are indications that current educational settings are not providing sufficient opportunities for learners to receive timely feedback, and students often perceive that they receive inadequate feedback (Hekelman et al., 1993; Milan et al., 2011; Nutter and Whitcomb, 2001). Insufficient time for feedback, teacher reluctance to provide feedback, a lack of continuity in the learner–teacher relationship, and a lack of observation time necessary for feedback may all contribute to an inadequate focus on providing feedback (Bernard et al., 2011; Schiff, 2008).

A recent IOM report concluded that continuing education is also disconnected from theories of how adults learn and from the delivery of patient care (IOM, 2010). Many continuing education requirements and evaluations focus on achieving credit hours instead of on educational outcomes and competencies (IOM, 2010). The result is a continuing education system that does not meet the needs of health care professionals in practice; for example, didactic activities such as lectures are large components of continuing education, even though participatory learning opportunities may be more appropriate (Hager et al., 2008).

In light of these findings, the committee concluded that health care professional education and training needs to better reflect findings from the learning sciences. **Thus, the committee recommends that educators should ensure that curricula and training programs across the career trajectory employ educational approaches that are aligned with evidence from the learning sciences.** Given the heterogeneity of learners and the variety of educational objectives, it is important that educational programs consider the spectrum of learning sciences approaches when developing curricula and training opportunities. Although it is beyond the committee's charge to recommend specific changes that should be made in health care professional education, the committee identified a number of opportunities for educators to consider. For example, programs may need to accommodate different learning styles, to include mechanisms to provide immediate feedback to learners (both positive and negative), to use CBE to assess performance, to increase the time allotted for clinical experience and patient interaction, and to place a larger emphasis on self-directed learning (Cooke et al., 2010; Hirsh et al., 2014; McLaughlin et al., 2014; Trowbridge, 2014). It may also be necessary to develop more effective forms of instruction and instructional media (Mayer, 2010), including the use of simulation-based exercises (McGaghie et al., 2011; Patel et al., 2009a). Employing deliberate practice approaches that focus on "frequent practice, rapid feedback to understand and correct errors, and raising bars with new attempts" may also be helpful (Durning, 2014; ten Cate, 2014). Changes to GME could include replacing traditional discipline-specific block rotations with longitudinal integrated clerkships in order to improve relationship building skills, both interprofessionally and among patients and clinicians (Teherani et al., 2013; ten Cate, 2014; Thibault,

2013). In addition, the IOM report *The Future of Nursing: Leading Change, Advancing Health* recommended the development and implementation of nursing residency programs to facilitate nursing graduates' transition to practice and to ensure that nurses develop the knowledge and skills to deliver safe, high-quality care (IOM, 2011a). This report also emphasized the importance of developing an expectation for lifelong learning.

A number of academic institutions have implemented changes in their health professional programs, including a major shift toward incorporating more authentic practice. For example, most medical schools have introduced clinical practice experience much earlier in their curriculum rather than delaying this experience until after students have completed the basic sciences training. Programs are also experimenting with innovative ways to help students develop a deeper conceptual understanding of human biology and disease, including an increased emphasis on individualized learning, self-teaching and assessment, and an exposure to more and varied cases of disease (OHSU, 2014). Northwestern University's Feinberg School of Medicine is adopting CBE, removing time requirements for degree completion, and moving from lecture-based instruction to small group and practice-based learning (Feinberg School of Medicine, 2015).

There is a growing recognition of the need to better align training and practice environments. For example, the Health Resources and Services Administration's Teaching Health Center Graduate Medical Education program is providing more opportunities for authentic practice by funding community-based primary care residency programs (HRSA, 2015). The IOM report *Graduate Medical Education That Meets the Nation's Health Needs* concluded that the Medicare GME payment system discourages physician training outside of the hospital setting and may not provide graduates the skills necessary for office-based practice, even though most are likely to practice in community settings (IOM, 2014). In addition, *The Future of Nursing* report highlighted the need to develop nursing expertise outside of hospital-based care settings. Because of the aging of the population and the shift from hospital-based to community-based care settings, there is a greater "need for nursing expertise in chronic illness management, care of older adults in home settings, and transitional services" (IOM, 2011a, p. 121).

Though many programs are beginning to initiate changes that better align with current knowledge about health care professional education, a larger focus on aligning education with the learning sciences is warranted across the career trajectory. This includes a focus on continuing education to ensure that individuals maintain and continue to develop the competencies necessary for the diagnostic process. Models of continuing education that are competency based or that focus on quality improvement have been proposed and may improve the effectiveness of continuing education (Campbell et al., 2010; Shojania et al., 2012).

The Diagnostic Process

Improving the content of health care professional education can improve diagnostic performance and reduce the potential for diagnostic errors and near misses. **Thus, the committee recommends that educators should ensure that curricula and training programs across the career trajectory address performance in the diagnostic process. The committee identified a number of areas of performance that could be improved. These are**

- **Clinical reasoning**
- **Teamwork**
- **Communication with patients, their families, and other health care professionals**
- **Appropriate use of diagnostic tests and the application of these results on subsequent decision making**
- **Use of health IT**

Clinical Reasoning

Clinical reasoning, including diagnostic decision making, is under-emphasized in current health care professional education and training (Graber et al., 2012; IOM, 2011a; Richardson, 2014; Stark and Fins, 2014; ten Cate, 2014; Trowbridge et al., 2013). This lack of focus on clinical reasoning and on the development of critical thinking skills throughout the education process is a contributor to diagnostic error (Brush, 2014; Durning, 2014; Richardson, 2007; ten Cate, 2014). A recent study found that a majority of the academic difficulties that medical students face "are of a cognitive nature and include difficulties in clinical reasoning" (Audétat et al., 2012, p. 217). Poor performance in clinical reasoning is generally discovered during later stages of training, which makes remediation more difficult (Audétat et al., 2012; Hauer et al., 2007). In recognition of the importance of clinical reasoning in health care professional education, the Medical College Aptitude Test (MCAT) recently added a critical analysis and reasoning skills section (AAMC, 2015a).

As discussed in Chapter 2, health care professionals have an ethical responsibility to improve clinical reasoning skills in order to improve diagnostic performance and avert diagnostic errors (Stark and Fins, 2014). Thus, educators need to ensure that students receive education and training opportunities that develop these skills—both fast system 1 processes and slow system 2 processes (Brush, 2014; Durning, 2014; Richardson, 2014; ten Cate, 2014). The development of clinical reasoning includes critical thinking skills such as analysis, evidence evaluation, and interpretation (Papp et al., 2014). Opportunities to improve clinical reasoning include instruction and practice on how to develop and refine a differential diagnosis and a focus on developing probabilistic reasoning skills (see Chapter 2) and also an understanding of likelihood ratios (Brush, 2014).[7] Students also need feedback and training in self-assessment and cognitive reflection in order to identify mistakes in their clinical reasoning and to assess their diagnostic performance. Without this, they may have trouble with calibration, or the development of an accurate sense of one's diagnostic abilities. Poor calibration contributes to clinician overconfidence and diagnostic errors (Berner and Graber, 2008; Croskerry and Norman, 2008; Meyer et al., 2013; Yang et al., 2012).

The success of diagnostic reasoning often depends on one's knowledge base of disease and the accompanying illness scripts[8] (Durning, 2014; Norman, 2014; ten Cate, 2014). Students need this wide knowledge base, especially to develop fast system 1 processes that rely on pattern recognition. However, there are concerns that the exposure that students receive to disease cases, actual or simulated, is inadequate to develop effective diagnostic decision making based on pattern recognition (Dhaliwal, 2014; Eva, 2005; Norman, 2014; ten Cate, 2014; Trowbridge et al., 2013). Early clinical experience, either through simulations or with patients, as well as an exposure to a variety of cases, including atypical cases, can help develop this knowledge base (Papa, 2014b; Richardson, 2014; ten Cate, 2014).

Equally important, students need to understand and become comfortable with the uncertainty that is inherent in the diagnostic process (Durning, 2014; Kassirer, 1989). Developing a better sense of and comfort with uncertainty may help clinicians avoid diagnostic errors related to premature closure as well as inappropriate use of diagnostic testing. Improved understanding of diagnostic uncertainty can help clinicians make decisions about whether further diagnostic testing or treatment is warranted. This could also facilitate improved collaboration with other health care professionals and better communication with patients and their families about the nature of a working diagnosis.

---

[7] The prior probability of a diagnosis is the probability assigned before new information regarding the patient is used to "update" the probability in order to arrive at the posterior probability. A likelihood ratio is defined as the percentage of diseased patients with a given test result divided by the percentage of well people with that same test result (Brush, 2014).

[8] Illness scripts are mental models of disease that include information about a disease, including potential causes of the disease, the pathophysiological process, and the signs and symptoms of the disease (Boshuizen and Schmidt, 2008).

Students also need exposure to easy-to-miss diagnoses and common causes of diagnostic error (Graber et al., 2012). This includes a focus on the work system factors that can contribute to diagnostic errors, such as communication and collaboration challenges among diagnostic team members; health IT tools that are not supportive of clinical reasoning activities; cultural, organizational, and physical environmental factors; and the impact of reporting, medical liability, and payment.

In addition, there needs to be a focus on heuristics (mental shortcuts) and biases, which play a role in clinical reasoning and present a major challenge to diagnosis (Croskerry, 2003, 2009, 2014; Eva and Norman, 2005; Kahneman, 2011; Klein, 1993) (see Chapter 2). Education and training that focuses on the cognitive heuristics and biases that can affect diagnosis and on how to counteract their effects are particularly important. Debiasing strategies, such as engaging in metacognition (i.e., critically thinking about one's thinking, reasoning, and decision making) have been proposed as a means to address the negative effect that heuristics can have on decision making. A number of debiasing strategies have been proposed, including considering the opposite, debiasing through awareness of bias, becoming aware of what one does not know, and others (Hirt and Markman, 1995; Hodges et al., 2001; Mumma and Steven, 1995; Mussweiler et al., 2000; Redelmeier, 2005). There is some debate about the effectiveness and feasibility of debiasing strategies (Norman, 2014; ten Cate, 2014); for example, monitoring every decision to ensure that no bias has occurred would be inefficient because heuristics work most of the time. However, because heuristics tend to fail in predictable ways, it is possible to determine the types of situations in which some heuristics are likely to lead to error.

For example, heuristic failure is likely to occur in the emergency medicine setting, given that this environment is highly complex, inconstant, and uncertain, and that emergency clinicians often work under time constraints that force them to rely heavily on heuristics (Croskerry, 2000a, 2002). Given the susceptibility of this environment to heuristics failure, several proposed solutions focus on the use of debiasing strategies in emergency medicine (Croskerry, 2000a, 2002; Pines, 2006). Additional strategies to reduce errors related to heuristics and biases include a greater focus on the development of expertise, offering clinicians more realistic training settings, providing decision support tools, and ensuring that the work system in which the diagnostic process occurs better supports decision making (Eva and Norman, 2005; Gigerenzer, 2000; Gigerenzer and Goldstein, 1996; Marewski and Gigerenzer, 2012; Weed and Weed, 2014; Wegwarth et al., 2009) (see Chapter 6). Because there is uncertainty regarding which strategies are best at reducing the impact of bias on diagnostic decision making, it is an area that needs further research (Croskerry et al., 2013a,b).

Several medical programs have begun offering clinical reasoning courses. For example, Dalhousie University offers a critical thinking course for medical students that teaches how decision making occurs, discusses cognitive biases and potential debiasing strategies, and provides students with tools for improved self-assessment and critical thinking development (Dalhousie University, 2015). Dalhousie also offers an online faculty development course to improve the education and training that medical students receive.

Developing clinical reasoning skills is important for practicing health care professionals who are beyond formal education and training settings. Continuing health care professional education can be leveraged to develop clinical reasoning skills as a lifelong competency. There are several continuing education opportunities available that focus on clinical reasoning and diagnosis, but a greater focus on them is needed (Cruz et al., 2009).

Teamwork and Communication

Despite widespread attention to the importance of teamwork skills, health care professionals are not adequately prepared to employ these skills in practice (IOM, 2014; Patel et al., 2009a; Pecukonis et al., 2008; Schmitt et al., 2011). The focus in this report on improving education and training in teamwork skills builds on earlier IOM work. For example, the study on continuing education concluded that professional development activities should ensure that health care professionals are proficient in the collaborative skills required for team-based care (IOM, 2010), and another study highlighted the need for transforming nursing education in order to prepare nurses to engage other health care professionals in a collaborative manner (IOM, 2011a). In addition, the IOM recently highlighted the importance of evaluating interprofessional education approaches and made recommendations on generating evidence to better identify successful interprofessional education practices (IOM, 2015).

Several leading organizations have concluded that interprofessional and teamwork training opportunities have been slow to materialize (Josiah Macy Jr. Foundation and Carnegie Foundation for the Advancement of Teaching, 2010). Barriers to teamwork and team-based education include "logistical challenges inherent in coordinating between two or more autonomous health professions schools, deep-rooted cultural differences between the health professions, differences in the educational curricula and pathways of the various health professions, and issues around program sustainability and funding" (Josiah Macy Jr. Foundation and Carnegie Foundation for the Advancement of Teaching, 2010, p. 3).

Academic institutions and training programs are beginning to offer more opportunities for health care professionals to improve their teamwork skills. As of 2012, 76 percent of medicals schools required students to participate in interprofessional education (AAMC, 2015b). The goals of the interprofessional education programs varied, but most aimed to familiarize students with the roles of other health care professionals (89 percent) and to teach students teamwork skills (76 percent) (AAMC, 2015b). Educational settings also varied, with schools offering training in classroom programs (77 percent), simulation center programs (60 percent), and clinical practice settings (44 percent) (AAMC, 2015b). For example, the University of Virginia's Center for Academic Strategic Partnerships for Interprofessional Research and Education offers workshops and clinical programs to improve teamwork skills and provides workshops for clinician–educators. Other programs offer courses taught jointly with students from both nursing and medical schools, provide interdisciplinary team-based training for the care of individuals with advanced illness, and use interactive interdisciplinary Web-based learning modules (Josiah Macy Jr. Foundation and Carnegie Foundation for the Advancement of Teaching, 2010). Academic centers have also been implementing simulation-based team training opportunities, which have shown promise in improving team performance and in the development of teamwork skills (Patel et al., 2009b). Although these efforts are encouraging, the committee concluded that a much greater emphasis on developing teamwork skills is needed. Rather than each program developing its own curriculum on an ad hoc basis, health care professional educators could collaborate in the development of curricula and training opportunities in teamwork.

An important teamwork skill in diagnosis is communication with patients, their families, and other health care professionals. Communication failures between health care professionals are recognized as a leading cause of patient harm and error, while poor communication between clinicians and patients is recognized as a barrier to accurate and timely diagnoses (Dingley et al., 2008; IHC, 2011). Although interpersonal communication skills are listed as a competency by the Accreditation Council for Graduate Medical Education (ACGME) and most medical specialty boards recognize communication as a core competency for practice, these skills may not be taught to students in a focused and standardized manner (Rider and Keefer, 2006). Health care professionals need to receive training in interpersonal communication skills to ensure that they can function effectively in teamwork settings. For example, one study found that students receiving communication training exhibited improved communication skills, such as relationship building and shared decision making (Yedidia et al., 2003). Effective communication training programs tend to last at least 1 day, to involve feedback, and to include role play and small group discussions (Berkhof et al., 2011). Tools to improve communication among health care professionals, such as the Situation-Background-Assessment-Recommendation Tool, help clinicians convey the most important information in an organized manner (Haig et al., 2006; Leonard et al., 2004) (see Box 4-8).

Health care professionals also need training in how to communicate openly and effectively with patients and their families. This training may include an emphasis on basic communication skills and also on

---

BOX 4-8
Situation-Background-Assessment-Recommendation Tool to Improve Communication Among Health Care Professionals

Before you call, be prepared! Be clear, concise, focus on the problem and only report what is relevant to the current situation!
Be sure you do the following:

- Assess the patient.
- Determine the appropriate person to call.
- Have the medical record available when you call.
- Review appropriate parts of the medical record (e.g., flow sheet, medication administration record, clinician notes/orders, labs).
- Use the following form to organize your conversation.

Situation: 5–10 second "punch line"—What is happening now? What are the chief complaints or acute changes?
This is _____. I'm calling about _____

Background: What factors led up to this event? Pertinent history (e.g., admitting diagnosis) and objective data (e.g., vital signs, labs) that support how patient got here.
The patient has_____

Assessment: What do you see? What do you think is going on? A diagnosis is not necessary; include the severity of the problem.
I think the problem is_____

Recommendation: What action do you propose? State what the patient needs (get a time frame).
I request that you_____

SOURCE: Adapted from Dingley et al., 2008.

topics such as communication with patients who are perceived as difficult, culturally and linguistically appropriate communication, interviewing techniques, history-taking skills, and delivering difficult diagnoses (AHRQ, 2015b; Smith and Longo, 2012). Other relevant strategies that could receive more attention include the teach-back method described in the patient engagement section of this chapter, encouraging questions from patients, and responding to patient emotions. In recognition of the importance of patient–clinician communication, a number of schools have implemented curricula designed to improve this communication (Georgetown University, 2015; University of Pittsburgh, 2015).

Outside of formal education settings, health care organizations can play a role in improving teamwork performance through team-based training practices (Salas et al., 2008). For example, a recent literature review found "moderate-to-high-quality evidence suggest[ing] team-training can positively impact healthcare team processes and, in turn, clinical processes and patient outcomes" (Weaver et al., 2014, p. 369). A training program designed by the Department of Defense and the Agency for Healthcare Research and Quality (AHRQ), Team Strategies and Tools to Enhance Performance and Patient Safety (TeamSTEPPS), has been used to improve teamwork in health care environments by increasing team awareness, clarifying roles and responsibilities, improving information sharing, and building efficient teams that optimize people and information to provide high quality care (AHRQ, 2015a; Straus et al., 2014). The system is at various stages of implementation in numerous facilities throughout the Military Health System (King et al., 2008). In recent years, AHRQ has launched a nationwide implementation program that trains master trainers to work with health care organizations interested in implementing TeamSTEPPS.

Diagnostic Testing

Diagnostic testing has become an integral component of the diagnostic process, yet medical school curricula have not kept pace with the advances in diagnostic testing and with how these advances affect diagnosis (Hallworth, 2011; Laposata and Dighe, 2007; Smith et al., 2010). A 2009 report from the Centers for Disease Control and Prevention on laboratory medicine noted that there is inadequate attention and emphasis on laboratory testing in the medical school curriculum, even though it plays a central role in medical practice (CDC, 2009). Another survey detailed the lack of emphasis on laboratory medicine within medical training programs: Although approximately 78 percent of medical schools require coursework in laboratory medicine, the median time dedicated to this topic is 12.5 hours, not including exposure to laboratory medicine gained through clinical rotations. However, training during clinical rotations is problematic because it is not standardized and may rely on clinician–educators who do not have an adequate background in laboratory medicine (Smith et al., 2010). Many of the processes within laboratory medicine—such as ordering the correct tests, understanding test performance characteristics (sensitivity and specificity), and interpreting tests results and, subsequently, making decisions—cannot be addressed using the teaching methods that many programs employ (Wilson, 2010).

The shortcomings in laboratory medicine education are well recognized by clinicians. According to several surveys, clinicians and students report feeling uncertain about which tests to order because of naming conventions, unfamiliarity with the available tests, and the rapid development of new diagnostic tests (Hickner et al., 2014; Laposata and Dighe, 2007). One of the largest sources of error in the test-ordering phase is health care professionals requesting an incorrect test (Laposata and Dighe, 2007). Clinicians order laboratory tests in 31.4 percent of primary care visits; however, they report uncertainty when ordering tests 14.7 percent of the time and confusion about interpreting results in 8.3 percent of the cases where they ordered tests (Hickner et al., 2014). There is also uncertainty among clinicians about applying test results to subsequent decision making, such as refining or expanding a differential diagnosis, determining the likelihood that a patient has a specific diagnosis on the basis of a positive or negative test result, deciding whether retesting or ordering new tests is appropriate, and beginning appropriate treatment. There are indications that students and practicing clinicians struggle with concepts like sensitivity and specificity and lack an understanding of how disease prevalence contributes to making decisions about a patient's diagnosis (Kroenke, 2013; Manrai et al., 2014; Ross, 2014). In a small survey of health care professionals, three-quarters of respondents failed to correctly calculate the positive predictive value of a test result for a specific disorder (Manrai et al., 2014). Similar surveys completed several decades ago found that many health care professionals had trouble applying statistical methods and understanding statistical concepts, suggesting that this may be a longstanding gap in health care professional education (Berwick et al., 1981; Casscells et al., 1978). Another study found that medical students are generally able to describe Bayes' theorem but are subsequently unable to apply this theorem to clinical practice (Bergus et al., 2004). These educational gaps negatively affect a clinician's ability to appropriately assign and update diagnostic probabilities in light of test findings.

In addition, there are concerns about an inadequate focus on anatomic pathology in medical education (Magid and Cambor, 2012). While aspects of anatomic pathology are covered in the medical school curriculum, the amount has decreased significantly over the years, particularly as medical schools have adopted integrated curricula (Talbert et al., 2009; Taylor et al., 2008). An inadequate understanding of anatomic pathology may negatively affect clinical decision making and the diagnostic process. For example, inadequate understanding of the mechanisms underlying inflammation might affect the ability to recognize diseases or disease processes and the selection of appropriate treatment to address inflammation. In addition, students may not understand the limitations of certain anatomic pathology tests (e.g., the limited sensitivity of Pap smears) and how to collect, prepare, and transport specimens (Magid and Cambor, 2011).

The use of medical imaging as a diagnostic tool has also increased substantially, and for many symptoms, medical imaging has become an integral part of the diagnostic process. Although many clinicians request medical imaging for their patients, the ordering of this imaging and the application of medical imaging interpretations to subsequent decision making are not emphasized in the medical school curriculum and subsequent training (Kondo and Swerdlow, 2013; Rubin and Blackham, 2015). Errors in imaging can occur during all phases of the process, from the ordering and selection of medical imaging to the interpretation of results and subsequent decision making. The majority of allopathic and osteopathic medical schools do not have a focused course on medical imaging, and medical imaging rotations are required in only 29 percent of medical schools (Rubin and Blackham, 2015). Typically, for most medical students medical imaging instruction is integrated into other coursework or clinical rotations in a very limited fashion (Kondo and Swerdlow, 2013; Rubin and Blackham, 2015). The teaching of important concepts in medical imaging, such as the scientific principles of imaging techniques, radiation safety, modality differences, and the use of contrast materials, is limited (Rubin and Blackham, 2015). A recent survey of fourth-year medical school students noted that the majority of students underestimated the risks associated with medical imaging techniques and were not informed about the American College of Radiology Appropriateness Criteria (Prezzia et al., 2013; Rubin and Blackham, 2015). Many medical schools do not follow the radiology-dedicated curriculum designed by the Alliance of Medical School Educators in Radiology (Rubin and Blackham, 2015).

Thus, health care professionals need improved education and training on the appropriate use of diagnostic tests and the application of these results to subsequent decision making. The committee recognizes that, given the growing number and complexity of the options available, it is not feasible to expect that clinicians will be familiarized with every available diagnostic test procedure. Therefore, in addition to improved education in diagnostic testing, improved collaboration among treating clinicians and pathologists and radiologists is warranted. Education and training focused on how to most effectively convey findings from pathologists and radiologists to treating clinicians may alleviate some of the challenges clinicians face with respect to understanding results and subsequent decision making.

Health IT

Health IT is an important component of the diagnostic process, including the involvement of EHRs, laboratory and medical imaging information systems, and decision support tools (see Chapter 5). As health IT becomes increasingly integrated into all aspects of health care, clinicians will likely rely more on it to facilitate diagnostic decision making and communication and collaboration among health care professionals and patients (Thibault, 2013). Thus, clinicians need to develop competencies in the use of health IT tools; however, many health care professionals do not receive adequate education and training in the use of health IT (Graber et al., 2012; McGowan et al., 2007). Individuals who lack competencies in health IT use will be unable to take advantage of these opportunities to improve diagnosis and reduce diagnostic error. Training health care professionals to work with health IT has been found to be a major challenge (NIST, 2010). In an effort to address this, the Office of the National Coordinator has been working with licensing bodies and medical societies to better integrate health IT into the medical education curriculum (Buntin et al., 2010). The Affordable Care Act includes provisions to incorporate health IT training into the education of primary care clinicians (Buntin et al., 2010). The IOM report *Health IT and Patient Safety* also emphasized the importance of improving workforce education and training on safe health IT use, using mechanisms such as formal education and postgraduate training as well as health care organization–facilitated training (IOM, 2012d).

Ensuring Competency in the Diagnostic Process

In addition to improving the content and teaching methods for health care professional education and training, oversight processes can help ensure that individuals achieve and maintain competency in the diagnostic process, including clinical reasoning, teamwork, communication, and the use of diagnostic testing and health IT. Health care professional oversight processes include education and training program accreditation, licensure, and certification. These oversight processes act as levers to induce change in the health care system: "Educational accreditation serves as a leverage point for the inclusion of particular educational content in a curriculum.

Licensure assesses that a student has understood and mastered formal curricula. Certification ensures that a practitioner maintains competence in a given area over time" (IOM, 2003a, p. 5). The committee received input suggesting that accreditation, licensure, and certification processes can be introduced to help ensure that health care professionals possess diagnostic competencies throughout the career trajectory (Brush, 2014; Papa, 2014a,b).

Organizations that accredit health care professional education and training programs (see Box 4-9) can use their accreditation requirements as a mechanism to ensure that these programs include appropriate curricular content to prepare students in the areas of the diagnostic process

---

BOX 4-9
Examples of Accreditation Organizations for
Health Care Professional Education and Training Programs

Accreditation Commission for Education in Nursing uses a core of standards to evaluate and accredit nursing education programs (ACEN, 2013).

Accreditation Council for Continuing Medical Education evaluates and accredits institutions and organizations offering continuing medical education for physicians and other health care professionals (ACCME, 2015).

Accreditation Council for Graduate Medical Education accredits graduate medical education programs (i.e., residency and fellowship programs) for physicians. Student performance on milestones or time-based competencies are used to assess graduate medical education programs (ACGME, 2015).

Accreditation Review Commission on Education for the Physician Assistant accredits physician assistant education programs (ARC-PA, 2015).

American Association of Colleges of Nursing's Commission on Collegiate Nursing Education accredits baccalaureate, graduate, and residency nursing programs (AACN, 2015).

American Osteopathic Association's (AOA's) Commission on Osteopathic College Accreditation accredits osteopathic medical schools, and the AOA Council on Continuing Medical Education accredits continuing medical education activities (AOA, 2015).

Liaison Committee on Medical Education, which is sponsored by the American Medical Association and the Association of American Medical Colleges, accredits medical education programs. For accreditation, programs must demonstrate that their graduates achieve the competencies necessary for subsequent training and for ensuring continuous learning and proficient practice (LCME, 2015).

that the committee has articulated. Accreditation organizations for all levels of health care professional education and training—that is, undergraduate, graduate, and continuing education—need to address diagnostic competencies. Many accreditation organizations already include skills important for diagnostic performance in their accreditation requirements, but these organizations can make competencies in the diagnostic process a larger priority within their requirements. For example, the IOM report *The Future of Nursing: Leading Change, Advancing Health* recommended that the "Commission on Collegiate Nursing Education [CCNE] and the National League for Nursing Accrediting Commission [NLNAC] should require that all nursing students demonstrate a comprehensive set of clinical performance competencies that encompass the knowledge and skills needed to provide care across settings and the lifespan" (IOM, 2011a, p. 282). Building on this recommendation, the CCNE and NLNAC could require nursing schools to offer interprofessional collaboration education and training opportunities focused specifically on the diagnostic process and the role of teams in achieving diagnostic accuracy. The Liaison Committee on Medical Education (LCME) and the ACGME include diagnostic competencies in accreditation requirements. For example, the LCME requires medical education programs to prepare students to "recognize and interpret symptoms and signs of disease" and "develop differential diagnoses and treatment plans" (LCME, 2015, p. 10). The ACGME and the American Board of Medical Specialties (ABMS) have identified six core competencies that all physicians should acquire during residency and fellowship programs and should maintain throughout practice (see Box 4-10) (ACGME, 2015). The ACGME is beginning to use milestones to evaluate performance on these competencies; several of these competencies are applicable to those the committee articulated (Nasca et al., 2012). For example, the ACGME requires that participating programs provide their students with opportunities to develop the skills necessary for lifelong, self-motivated learning; communication with patients, families, and other health care professionals; and a systems understanding of health care, including the importance of coordination and intra- and interprofessional teamwork (ACGME, 2015).

Organizations responsible for health care professional licensure and certification can help ensure that individual health care professionals have achieved and maintain competency in the skills essential for diagnosis. For example, the United States Medical Licensing Exam for physicians and the Uniform Licensure Requirements for practicing nurses could emphasize diagnostic competencies tailored to the scope of work of these professions (NCSBN, 2015). The ABMS, which grants board certification in more than 150 medical specialties and subspecialties, could ensure competencies in the diagnostic process both in initial board certification and

BOX 4-10

Six Core Competencies Developed by the American Board of Medical Specialties and the Accreditation Council for Graduate Medical Education

1. **Practice-Based Learning and Improvement:** Show an ability to investigate and evaluate patient care practices, appraise and assimilate scientific evidence, and improve the practice of medicine.
2. **Patient Care and Procedural Skills:** Provide care that is compassionate, appropriate, and effective treatment for health problems and to promote health.
3. **Systems-Based Practice:** Demonstrate awareness of and responsibility to the larger context and systems of health care. Be able to call on system resources to provide optimal care (e.g., coordinating care across sites or serving as the primary case manager when care involves multiple specialties, professions, or sites).
4. **Medical Knowledge:** Demonstrate knowledge about established and evolving biomedical, clinical, and cognate sciences and their application in patient care.
5. **Interpersonal and Communication Skills:** Demonstrate skills that result in effective information exchange and teaming with patients, their families, and professional associates (e.g., fostering a therapeutic relationship that is ethically sound, uses effective listening skills with nonverbal and verbal communication; working as both a team member and at times as a leader).
6. **Professionalism:** Demonstrate a commitment to carrying out professional responsibilities, adherence to ethical principles, and sensitivity to diverse patient populations.

SOURCES: ABMS, 2015; ACGME, 2015.

in the maintenance of certification efforts. For example, some specialty boards have begun assessing clinical reasoning skills through cognitive knowledge testing that requires clinicians to evaluate clinical scenarios in addition to content knowledge (Graber et al., 2012). Initial certification of health care professionals is important, but it may be insufficient to ensure sustained diagnostic competency throughout the career trajectory. Due to advances in the biomedical sciences, the knowledge required to maintain competency is rapidly growing; at the same time, health care professionals may also experience knowledge decay or the loss of previously learned knowledge (Cassel and Holmboe, 2008; IOM, 2013a; Su et al., 2000). Thus, many health care professional organizations, such as ABMS and the American Association of Physician Assistants, have developed renewal and maintenance of certification (MOC) programs (AAPA, 2015; ABMS, 2015). Though there has been controversy surrounding MOC, recent evidence suggests that it can improve performance (Iglehart and

Baron, 2012; O'Neill and Puffer, 2013; Teirstein, 2015). Meaningful and effective continuing education is important for all clinicians, and MOC efforts can ensure that clinicians have the appropriate competencies in the diagnostic process throughout the career trajectory. Many health care organizations now require MOC as a precondition for renewing staff privileges. Other licensure and certification organizations, including those for other health care professions, can also emphasize competency in the diagnostic process.

The committee concluded that oversight organizations, including accreditation organizations and professional licensure and certification bodies, can play an important role in improving diagnostic performance. **Thus, the committee recommends that health care professional certification and accreditation organizations should ensure that health care professionals have and maintain the competencies needed for effective performance in the diagnostic process, including**

- **Clinical reasoning**
- **Teamwork**
- **Communication with patients, their families, and other health care professionals**
- **Appropriate use of diagnostic tests and the application of these results on subsequent decision making**
- **Use of health IT**

RECOMMENDATIONS

Goal 1: Facilitate more effective teamwork in the diagnostic process among health care professionals, patients, and their families

Recommendation 1a: In recognition that the diagnostic process is a dynamic team-based activity, health care organizations should ensure that health care professionals have the appropriate knowledge, skills, resources, and support to engage in teamwork in the diagnostic process. To accomplish this, they should facilitate and support:
  - **Intra- and interprofessional teamwork in the diagnostic process.**
  - **Collaboration among pathologists, radiologists, other diagnosticians, and treating health care professionals to improve diagnostic testing processes.**

Recommendation 1b: Health care professionals and organizations should partner with patients and their families as diagnostic team members and facilitate patient and family engagement in the diag-

nostic process, aligned with their needs, values, and preferences. To accomplish this, they should:

- Provide patients with opportunities to learn about the diagnostic process.
- Create environments in which patients and their families are comfortable engaging in the diagnostic process and sharing feedback and concerns about diagnostic errors and near misses.
- Ensure patient access to electronic health records (EHRs), including clinical notes and diagnostic testing results, to facilitate patient engagement in the diagnostic process and patient review of health records for accuracy.
- Identify opportunities to include patients and their families in efforts to improve the diagnostic process by learning from diagnostic errors and near misses.

Goal 2: Enhance health care professional education and training in the diagnostic process

Recommendation 2a: Educators should ensure that curricula and training programs across the career trajectory:

- Address performance in the diagnostic process, including areas such as clinical reasoning; teamwork; communication with patients, their families, and other health care professionals; appropriate use of diagnostic tests and the application of these results on subsequent decision making; and use of health information technology.
- Employ educational approaches that are aligned with evidence from the learning sciences.

Recommendation 2b: Health care professional certification and accreditation organizations should ensure that health care professionals have and maintain the competencies needed for effective performance in the diagnostic process, including the areas listed above.

REFERENCES

AACH (American Academy on Communication in Healthcare). 2015. American Academy on Communication in Healthcare. www.aachonline.org (accessed March 16, 2015).

AACN (American Assocation of Colleges of Nursing). 2015. American Association of Colleges of Nursing. www.aacn.nche.edu (accessed May 10, 2015).

AAMC (Assocation of American Medical Colleges). 2015a. About the MCAT exam. www.aamc.org/students/applying/mcat/about (accessed March 18, 2015).

AAMC. 2015b. Curriculum inventory and reports: Interprofessional education. www.aamc. org/initiatives/cir (accessed March 18, 2015).

AAPA (American Academy of Physician Assistants). 2015. American Academy of Physician Assistants. www.aapa.org (accessed March 12, 2015).

ABIM (American Board of Internal Medicine). 2014. ABIM announces initiative to seek input on physician knowledge and skill assessment approaches. www.abim.org/news/abim-initiative-seek-input-on-physician-knowledge-skill-assessment-approaches.aspx (accessed July 24, 2015).

ABIM. 2015. Assessment 2020: Feedback in action. assessment2020.abim.org/projects (accessed July 24, 2015).

ABMS (American Board of Medical Specialties). 2015. Based on core competencies. www. abms.org/board-certification/a-trusted-credential/based-on-core-competencies (accessed July 24, 2015).

ACCME (Accreditation Council for Continuing Medical Education). 2015. Accreditation Council for Continuing Medical Education. www.accme.org (accessed March 12, 2015).

ACEN (Accreditation Commission for Education in Nursing). 2013. Accreditation Commission for Education in Nursing. www.acenursing.org/?refreshed (accessed June 5, 2015).

ACGME (Accreditation Council for Graduate Medical Education). 2015. Accreditation Council for Graduate Medical Education. www.acgme.org/acgmeweb (accessed March 12, 2015).

Adler-Milstein, J. 2015. America's health IT transformation: Translating the promise of electronic health records into better care. Paper presented at U.S. Senate Committee on Health, Education, Labor and Pensions, March 17.

Adler-Milstein, J., C. M. DesRoches, M. F. Furukawa, C. Worzala, D. Charles, P. Kralovec, S. Stalley, and A. K. Jha. 2014. More than half of U.S. hospitals have at least a basic EHR, but stage 2 criteria remain challenging for most. *Health Affairs* 33(9):1664–1671.

AHRQ (Agency for Healthcare Research and Quality). 2008. Transforming the morbidity and mortality conference into an instrument for systemwide improvement. In K. Henriksen, J. B. Battles, M. A. Keyes, and M. L. Grady (eds.), *Advances in patient safety: New directions and approaches (Vol. 2. Culture and redesign)* (pp. 357–363). AHRQ Publication No. 08-0034-2. Rockville, MD: Agency for Healthcare Research and Quality. www.ncbi. nlm.nih.gov/books/NBK43710/?report=reader#_NBK43710_pubdet (accessed July 2, 2015).

AHRQ. 2010a. *The roles of patient-centered medical homes and accountable care organizations in coordinating patient care.* AHRQ publication no. 11-M005-EF. Rockville, MD: Agency for Healthcare Research and Quality. http://pcmh.ahrq.gov/page/roles-patient-centered-medical-homes-and-accountable-care-organizations-coordinating-patient (accessed June 5, 2015).

AHRQ. 2010b. In conversation with. . . Pat Croskerry, MD, PhD. Web M&M morbidity and mortality rounds on the web. http://webmm.ahrq.gov/perspective.aspx?perspectiveID=87 (accessed July 24, 2015).

AHRQ. 2011. *Health literacy interventions and outcomes: An updated systematic review.* AHRQ Publication No. 11-E006. Rockville, MD: Agency for Healthcare Research and Quality.

AHRQ. 2012. *Improving patient safety systems for patients with limited english proficiency.* AHRQ Publication No. 12-0041. Rockville, MD: Agency for Healthcare Research and Quality. www.ahrq.gov/professionals/systems/hospital/lepguide/lepguide.pdf (accessed July 24, 2015).

AHRQ. 2013a. *2012 national healthcare disparities report.* AHRQ publication no. 13-0003. Rockville, MD: Agency for Healthcare Research and Quality.

AHRQ. 2013b. *2012 national healthcare quality report.* AHRQ publication no. 13-0002. Rockville, MD: Agency for Healthcare Research and Quality.

AHRQ. 2014a. Error disclosure. http://psnet.ahrq.gov/primer.aspx?primerID=2 (accessed March 16, 2015).

AHRQ. 2014b. Patient and family advisory councils. https://cahps.ahrq.gov/quality-improvement/improvement-guide/browse-interventions/Customer-Service/Listening-Posts/Advisory-Councils.html (accessed March 18, 2015).

AHRQ. 2014c. Patient centered medical home resource center. http://pcmh.ahrq.gov/page/defining-pcmh (accessed April 9, 2014).

AHRQ. 2015a. About TeamSTEPPS. http://teamstepps.ahrq.gov/about-2cl_3.htm (accessed March 26, 2015).

AHRQ. 2015b. Training to advance physicians' communication skills. https://cahps.ahrq.gov/quality-improvement/improvement-guide/browse-interventions/Communication/Physicians-Comm-Training/index.html (accessed March 26, 2015).

Ali, N. K., R. P. Ferguson, S. Mitha, and A. Hanlon. 2014. Do medical trainees feel confident communicating with low health literacy patients? *Journal of Community Hospital Internal Medicine Perspective* 4(2).

Allen, B., and W. T. Thorwarth. 2014. Comments from the American College of Radiology. Input submitted to the Committee on Diagnostic Error in Health Care, November 5 and December 29, 2014, Washington, DC.

Anderson, R. M., and M. M. Funnell. 2005. Patient empowerment: Reflections on the challenge of fostering the adoption of a new paradigm. *Patient Education and Counseling* 57(2):153–157.

AOA (American Osteopathic Association). 2015. American Osteopathic Association. www.osteopathic.org (accessed March 12, 2015).

ARC-PA (Accreditation Review Commission on Education for the Physician Assistant). 2015. Accreditation Review Commission on Education for the Physician Assistant. www.arc-pa.org (accessed March 12, 2015).

Arora, N. K., and C. A. McHorney. 2000. Patient preferences for medical decision making: Who really wants to participate? *Medical Care* 38(3):335–341.

ASCP (American Society for Clinical Pathology). 2014. Patient access to test results. www.ascp.org/Advocacy/Patient-Access-to-Test-Results.html (accessed March 16, 2015).

Audétat, M.-C., V. Dory, M. Nendaz, D. Vanpee, D. Pestiaux, N. Junod Perron, and B. Charlin. 2012. What is so difficult about managing clinical reasoning difficulties? *Medical Education* 46(2):216–227.

Baldwin, D. C., and R. A. W. Tsukuda. 1984. Interdisciplinary teams. In C. K. Cassel and J. R. Walsh (eds.), *Geriatric medicine: Volume III: Fundamentals of geriatric care* (pp. 421–435). New York: Springer-Verlag.

Beach, M. C., E. G. Price, T. L. Gary, K. A. Robinson, A. Gozu, A. Palacio, C. Smarth, M. W. Jenckes, C. Feuerstein, E. B. Bass, N. R. Powe, and L. A. Cooper. 2005. Cultural competence: A systematic review of health care provider educational interventions. *Medical Care* 43(4):356–373.

Bell, S., M. Anselmo, J. Walker, and T. Delbanco. 2014. Input submitted to the Committee on Diagnostic Error in Healthcare, December 2, 2014, Washington, DC.

Bergus, G., S. Vogelgesang, J. Tansey, E. Franklin, and R. Feld. 2004. Appraising and applying evidence about a diagnostic test during a performance-based assessment. *BMC Medical Education* 4:20.

Berkhof, M., H. J. van Rijssen, A. J. M. Schellart, J. R. Anema, and A. J. van der Beek. 2011. Effective training strategies for teaching communication skills to physicians: An overview of systematic reviews. *Patient Education and Counseling* 84(2):152–162.

Bernard, A. W., N. E. Kman, and S. Khandelwal. 2011. Feedback in the emergency medicine clerkship. *Western Journal of Emergency Medicine* 12(4):537–542.

Berner, E. S., and M. L. Graber. 2008. Overconfidence as a cause of diagnostic error in medicine. *American Journal of Medicine* 121(5 Suppl):S2–S23.

Berwick, D. M. 2011. Launching accountable care organizations—The proposed rule for the Medicare Shared Savings Program. *New England Journal of Medicine* 364(16):e32.

Berwick, D. M., H. V. Fineberg, and M. C. Weinstein. 1981. When doctors meet numbers. *The American Journal of Medicine* 71(6):991–998.

Bodenheimer, T. 2008. Coordinating care—A perilous journey through the health care system. *New England Journal of Medicine* 358(10):1064–1071.

Borrill, C. S., J. Carletta, A. J. Carter, J. F. Dawson, S. Garrod, A. Rees, A. Richards, D. Shapiro, and M. A. West. 2000. *The effectiveness of health care teams in the National Health Service.* Birmingham, UK: University of Aston in Birmingham.

Boshuizen, H. P. A., and H. G. Schmidt. 2008. The development of clinical reasoning expertise: Implications for teaching. In J. Higgs, M. Jones, S. Loftus, and N. Christensen (eds.), *Clinical reasoning in the health professions* (pp. 113–121). Oxford: Butterworth Heinemann/Elsevier.

Boulding, W., S. W. Glickman, M. P. Manary, K. A. Schulman, and R. Staelin. 2011. Relationship between patient satisfaction with inpatient care and hospital readmission within 30 days. *American Journal of Managed Care* 17(1):41–48.

Boult, C., A. F. Green, L. B. Boult, J. T. Pacala, C. Snyder, and B. Leff. 2009. Successful models of comprehensive care for older adults with chronic conditions: Evidence for the Institute of Medicine's "Retooling for an Aging America" report. *Journal of the American Geriatrics Society* 57(12):2328–2337.

Boyer, L., M. Williams, L. Callister, and E. Marshall. 2001. Hispanic women's perceptions regarding cervical cancer screening. *Journal of Obstetrics, Gynecologic, and Neonatal Nursing* 30(2):240–245.

Bruno, M. A., J. M. Petscavage-Thomas, M. J. Mohr, S. K. Bell, and S. D. Brown. 2014. The "open letter": Radiologists' reports in the era of patient web portals. *Journal of the American College of Radiology* 11(9):863–867.

Brush, J. E. 2014. Forming good habits to decrease diagnostic error: A case for likelihood ratios. Input submitted to the Committee on Diagnostic Error in Health Care, October 21, 2014, Washington, DC.

BSCF (Blue Shield of California Foundation). 2014. *Engaging California patients in major medical decisions.* San Francisco, CA: Blue Shield of California Foundation.

Buntin, M. B., S. H. Jain, and D. Blumenthal. 2010. Health information technology: Laying the infrastructure for national health reform. *Health Affairs* 29(6):1214–1219.

Bushe, G. R., and A. Chu. 2011. Fluid teams: Solutions to the problems of unstable team membership. *Organizational Dynamics* 40(3):181–188.

Butcher, L. 2014. The patient portal to the future. Healthcare Financial Management Association. www.hfma.org/Leadership/Archives/2014/Spring/The_Patient_Portal_to_the_Future (accessed May 11, 2015).

Campbell, C., I. Silver, J. Sherbino, O. ten Cate, and E. S. Holmboe. 2010. Competency-based continuing professional development. *Medical Teacher* 32(8):657–662.

Casscells, W., A. Schoenberger, and T. B. Graboys. 1978. Interpretation by physicians of clinical laboratory results. *New England Journal of Medicine* 299(18):999–1001.

Cassel, C. K., and E. S. Holmboe. 2008. Professionalism and accountability: The role of specialty board certification. *Transactions of the American Clinical and Climatological Association* 119:295–304.

Castro, A., and E. Ruiz. 2009. The effects of nurse practitioner cultural competence on Latina patient satisfaction. *Journal of the American Academy of Nurse Practitioners* 21(5):278–286.

CDC (Centers for Disease Control and Prevention). 2009. Patient-centered care and laboratory medicine: National status report: 2008–2009 update.

CDC. 2014. Early Release of Selected Estimates Based on Data from the National Health Information Survey, January-September 2014: Usual place to go for medical care. www. cdc.gov/nchs/data/nhis/earlyrelease/earlyrelease201503_02.pdf (accessed May 7, 2015).

CFAH (Center for Advancing Health). 2014a. Be a prepared patient. www.cfah.org/prepared-patient (accessed March 18, 2015).

CFAH. 2014b. Center for Advancing Health engagement behavior framework. www.cfah.org/engagement/research/engagement-behavior-framework (accessed April 3, 2014).

CFAH. 2014c. What does it take for all Americans to find good health care and make the most of it? www.cfah.org/about/about-us (accessed April 3, 2014).

CFAH. 2015. Patient engagement. www.cfah.org/engagement (accessed March 16, 2015).

CFAR (Center for Applied Research), J. Tomasik, and C. Fleming. 2015. Lessons from the field: Promising interprofessional collaboration practices. White Paper, Robert Wood Johnson Foundation. www.rwjf.org/content/dam/farm/reports/reports/2015/rwjf418568 (accessed June 5, 2015).

Chang, J. H., E. Vines, H. Bertsch, D. L. Fraker, B. J. Czerniecki, E. F. Rosato, T. Lawton, E. F. Conant, S. G. Orel, L. Schuchter, K. R. Fox, N. Zieber, J. H. Glick, and L. J. Solin. 2001. The impact of a multidisciplinary breast cancer center on recommendations for patient management: The University of Pennsylvania experience. Cancer 91(7):1231–1237.

Cifra, C. L., K. L. Jones, J. A. Ascenzi, U. S. Bhalala, M. M. Bembea, J. C. Fackler, and M. R. Miller. 2014. The morbidity and mortality conference as an adverse event surveillance tool in a paediatric intensive care unit. BMJ Quality & Safety 23(11):930–938.

Cifra, C. L., K. L. Jones, J. A. Ascenzi, U. S. Bhalala, M. M. Bembea, D. E. Newman-Toker, J. C. Fackler, and M. R. Miller. 2015. Diagnostic errors in a PICU: Insights from the morbidity and mortality conference. Pediatric Critical Care Medicine: A Journal of the Society of Critical Care Medicine and the World Federation of Pediatric Intensive and Critical Care Societies 16(5):468–476.

CMS (Centers for Medicare & Medicaid Services). 2013. Pioneer accountable care organizations succeed in improving care, lowering costs. Baltimore, MD: Department of Health and Human Services. www.cms.gov/Newsroom/MediaReleaseDatabase/Press-releases/2013-Press-releases-items/2013-07-16.html (accessed June 5, 2015).

Cohen, P., A. L. Tan, and A. Penman. 2009. The multidisciplinary tumor conference in gynecologic oncology—Does it alter management? International Journal of Gynecological Cancer 19(9):1470–1472.

Cooke, M., D. M. Irby, and B. C. O'Brien. 2010. Summary of educating physicians: A call for reform of medical school and residency. San Francisco, CA: Jossey–Bass.

Cosgrove, D. M., M. Fisher, P. Gabow, G. Gottlieb, G. C. Halvorson, B. C. James, G. S. Kaplan, J. B. Perlin, R. Petzel, G. D. Steele, and J. S. Toussaint. 2013. Ten strategies to lower costs, improve quality, and engage patients: The view from leading health system CEOs. Health Affairs 32(2):321–327.

Coulter, A., S. Parsons, and J. Askham. 2008. Where are the patients in decision-making about their own care? Copenhagen, Denmark, June 25–27: World Health Organization Regional Office for Europe.

Cox, E. D., K. A. Nackers, H. N. Young, M. A. Moreno, J. F. Levy, and R. M. Mangione-Smith. 2012. Influence of race and socioeconomic status on engagement in pediatric primary care. Patient Education and Counseling 87(3):319–326.

Crabtree, B. F., P. A. Nutting, W. L. Miller, K. C. Stange, E. E. Stewart, and C. R. Jaén. 2010. Summary of the National Demonstration Project and recommendations for the patient-centered medical home. Annals of Family Medicine 8(Suppl 1):S80–S90.

Croskerry, P. 2000a. The cognitive imperative: Thinking about how we think. Academic Emergency Medicine 7(11):1223–1231.

Croskerry, P. 2000b. The feedback sanction. *Academic Emergency Medicine* 7(11):1232–1238.

Croskerry, P. 2002. Achieving quality in clinical decision making: Cognitive strategies and detection of bias. *Academic Emergency Medicine* 9(11):1184–1204.

Croskerry, P. 2003. The importance of cognitive errors in diagnosis and strategies to minimize them. *Academic Medicine* 78(8):775–780.

Croskerry, P. 2009. A universal model of diagnostic reasoning. *Academic Medicine* 84(8): 1022–1028.

Croskerry, P. 2013. From mindless to mindful practice—Cognitive bias and clinical decision making. *New England Journal of Medicine* 368(26):2445–2448.

Croskerry, P. 2014. Bias: A normal operating characteristic of the diagnosing brain. *Diagnosis* 1(1):23–27.

Croskerry, P., and G. Norman. 2008. Overconfidence in clinical decision making. *American Journal of Medicine* 121(5 Suppl):S24–S29.

Croskerry, P., G. Singhal, and S. Mamede. 2013a. Cognitive debiasing 1: Origins of bias and theory of debiasing. *BMJ Quality and Safety* 22(Suppl 2):ii58–ii64.

Croskerry, P., G. Singhal, and S. Mamede. 2013b. Cognitive debiasing 2: Impediments to and strategies for change. *BMJ Quality and Safety* 22(Suppl 2):ii65–ii72.

Cruz, D. M., C. M. Pimenta, and M. Lunney. 2009. Improving critical thinking and clinical reasoning with a continuing education course. *Journal of Continuing Education in Nursing* 40(3):121–127.

Dalhousie University. 2015. Dalhousie University Medical School critical thinking program. http://medicine.dal.ca/departments/core-units/DME/critical-thinking.html (accessed March 26, 2015).

Danforth, K. N., A. E. Smith, R. K. Loo, S. J. Jacobsen, B. S. Mittman, and M. H. Kanter. 2014. Electronic clinical surveillance to improve outpatient care: Diverse applications within an integrated delivery system. *eGEMS* 2(1):1056.

Deber, R. B., N. Kraetschmer, S. Urowitz, and N. Sharpe. 2007. Do people want to be autonomous patients? Preferred roles in treatment decision-making in several patient populations. *Health Expectations* 10(3):248–258.

Delbanco, T., J. Walker, S. K. Bell, J. D. Darer, J. G. Elmore, N. Farag, H. J. Feldman, R. Mejilla, L. Ngo, J. D. Ralston, S. E. Ross, N. Trivedi, E. Vodicka, and S. G. Leveille. 2012. Inviting patients to read their doctors' notes: A quasi-experimental study and a look ahead. *Annals of Internal Medicine* 157(7):461–470.

Dentzer, S. 2012. One payer's attempt to spur primary care doctors to form new medical homes. *Health Affairs* 31(2):341–349.

Dhaliwal, G. 2014. Blueprint for diagnostic excellence. Presentation to the Committee on Diagnostic Error in Health Care, November 21, 2014, Washington, DC.

Dineen, B. R., and R. A. Noe. 2003. The impact of team fluidity and its implications for human resource management research and practice. In J. J. Martocchio and G. R. Ferris (eds.), *Research in personnel and human resources management, Vol. 22* (pp. 1–37). Oxford, England: Elsevier Science Ltd.

Dingley, C. D., K. Daugherty, M. K. Derieg, and R. Persing. 2008. Improving patient safety through provider communication strategy enhancements. In K. Henriksen, J. B. Battles, M. A. Keyes, and M. L. Grady (eds.), *Advances in patient safety: New directions and alternative approaches (Vol. 3: Performance and tools)* (pp. 90-107). AHRQ publication no. 08-0034-3. Rockville, MD: Agency for Healthcare Research and Quality. www.ahrq.gov/professionals/quality-patient-safety/patient-safety-resources/resources/advances-in-patient-safety-2/vol3/Advances-Dingley_14.pdf (accessed June 5, 2015).

Dunn, R., J. S. Beaudry, and Klavas.Angela. 2002. Survey of research on learning styles. *California Journal of Science Education* 2(2):75–98.

Durning, S. J. 2014. Submitted input. Input submitted to the Committee on Diagnostic Error in Health Care, October 24, 2014, Washington, DC.

Durso, L. E., and I. H. Meyer. 2013. Patterns and predictors of disclosure of sexual orientation to healthcare providers among lesbians, gay men, and bisexuals. *Sexuality Research and Social Policy* 10(1): 35-42.

Dyche, L., and D. Swiderski. 2005. The effect of physician solicitation approaches on ability to identify patient concerns. *Journal of General Internal Medicine* 20(3):267–270.

Edmondson, A. C. 2012. *Teaming: How organizations learn, innovate, and compete in the knowledge economy*. San Francisco: Jossey-Bass.

Entwistle, V. A., D. McCaughan, I. S. Watt, Y. Birks, J. Hall, M. Peat, B. Williams, J. Wright, and Patient Involvement in Patient Safety Group. 2010. Speaking up about safety concerns: Multi-setting qualitative study of patients' views and experiences. *Quality and Safety in Health Care* 19:1–7.

Etchegaray, J. M., M. J. Ottosen, L. Burress, W. M. Sage, S. K. Bell, T. H. Gallagher, and E. J. Thomas. 2014. Structuring patient and family involvement in medical error event disclosure and analysis. *Health Affairs (Millwood)* 33(1):46–52.

Eva, K. W. 2005. What every teacher needs to know about clinical reasoning. *Medical Education* 39(1):98–106.

Eva, K. W., and G. R. Norman. 2005. Heuristics and biases—A biased perspective on clinical reasoning. *Medical Education* 39(9):870–872.

Evans, M. 2013. Doctors argue for decision aids to promote patient engagement. *Modern Healthcare*. www.modernhealthcare.com/article/20131127/MAGAZINE/311309982 (accessed April 4, 2014).

FamilyDoctor.org. 2014. Health information on the web: Finding reliable information. http://familydoctor.org/familydoctor/en/healthcare-management/self-care/health-information-on-the-web-finding-reliable-information.printerview.all.html (accessed March 16, 2015).

Feinberg School of Medicine. 2015. Education: MD curriculum at Feinburg. www.feinberg.northwestern.edu/education/curriculum/index.html (accessed March 16, 2015).

Flores, G. 2006. Language barriers to health care in the United States. *New England Journal of Medicine* 355(3):229–231.

Foglia, M. B., and K. I. Fredriksen-Goldsen. 2014. Health disparities among LGBT older adults and the role of nonconscious bias. *Hastings Center Report* 44(s4):S40–S44.

Fowler, F. 2011. Patients want to be involved. http://informedmedicaldecisions.org/wp-content/uploads/2011/05/Perspectives_Patient_Involvement.pdf (accessed June 5, 2015).

Fox, S., and M. Duggan. 2013. Health online 2013. www.pewinternet.org/2013/01/15/health-online-2013 (accessed March 18, 2015).

Frampton, S. B., S. Horowitz, and B. J. Stumpo. 2009. Open medical records. *The American Journal of Nursing* 109(8):59–63.

Friesen, M. A., A. Herbst, J. W. Turner, K. G. Speroni, and J. Robinson. 2013. Developing a patient-centered ISHAPED handoff with patient/family and parent advisory councils. *Journal of Nursing Care and Quality* 28(3):208–216.

Frosch, D. L., S. G. May, K. A. S. Rendle, C. Tietbohl, and G. Elwyn. 2012. Authoritarian physicians and patients' fear of being labeled "difficult" among key obstacles to shared decision making. *Health Affairs (Millwood)* 31(5):1030–1038.

Furukawa, M. F., J. King, V. Patel, C. J. Hsiao, J. Adler–Milstein, and A. K. Jha. 2014. Despite substantial progress in EHR adoption, health information exchange and patient engagement remain low in office settings. *Health Affairs* 33(9):1672–1679.

Gallagher, T. H., A. D. Waterman, A. G. Ebers, V. J. Fraser, and W. Levinson. 2003. Patients' and physicians' attitudes regarding the disclosure of medical errors. *JAMA* 289(8):1001–1007.
Gandhi, T. K. 2014. Focus on diagnostic errors: Understanding and prevention. Presentation to the Committee on Diagnostic Error in Health Care, August 7, 2014, Washington, DC.
Gandhi, T. K., and T. H. Lee. 2010. Patient safety beyond the hospital. *New England Journal of Medicine* 363(11):1001–1003.
Gandhi, T. K., A. Kachalia, E. J. Thomas, A. L. Puopolo, C. Yoon, T. A. Brennan, and D. M. Studdert. 2006. Missed and delayed diagnoses in the ambulatory setting: A study of closed malpractice claims. *Annals of Internal Medicine* 145(7):488–496.
Georgetown University. 2015. First year curriculum module: Physician–patient communication. https://som.georgetown.edu/medicaleducation/curriculum/firstyearmodules/modules/ppc (accessed March 26, 2015).
Gertler, S. A., Z. Coralic, A. Lopez, J. C. Stein, and U. Sarkar. 2014. Root cause analysis of ambulatory adverse drug events that present to the emergency department. *Journal of Patient Safety*. February 27. Epub ahead of print.
Gigerenzer, G. 2000. *Adaptive thinking: Rationality in the real world*. New York: Oxford University Press.
Gigerenzer, G., and D. G. Goldstein. 1996. Reasoning the fast and frugal way: Models of bounded rationality. *Psychology Review* 103(4):650–669.
Glickman, S. W., W. Boulding, M. Manary, R. Staelin, M. T. Roe, R. J. Wolosin, E. M. Ohman, E. D. Peterson, and K. A. Schulman. 2010. Patient satisfaction and its relationship with clinical quality and inpatient mortality in acute myocardial infarction. *Circulation: Cardiovascular Quality and Outcomes* 3(2):188–195.
Govern, P. 2013. Diagnostic management efforts thrive on teamwork. http://news.vanderbilt.edu/2013/03/diagnostic-management-efforts-thrive-on-teamwork (accessed February 11, 2015).
Graber, M., R. Wachter, and C. Cassel. 2012. Bringing diagnosis into the quality and safety equations. *JAMA* 308(12):1211–1212.
Graedon, T., and J. Graedon. 2014. Let patients help with diagnosis. *Diagnosis* 1(1):49–51.
Gruman, J. C. 2013. An accidental tourist finds her way in the dangerous land of serious illness. *Health Affairs* 32(2):427–431.
Hager, M., S. Russell, and S. W. Fletcher. 2008. *Continuing education in the health professions: Improving healthcare through lifelong learning, Proceedings of a conference sponsored by the Josiah Macy Jr. Foundation*. Bermuda. New York: Josiah Macy Jr. Foundation. www.josiahmacyfoundation.org (accessed June 5, 2015).
Haig, K. M., S. Sutton, and J. Whittington. 2006. SBAR: A shared mental model for improving communication between clinicians. *Joint Commission Journal on Quality and Patient Safety* 32(3):167–175.
Hallworth, M. J. 2011. The "70% claim": What is the evidence base? *Annals of Clinical Biochemistry* 48(6):487–488.
Haskell, H. W. 2014. What's in a story? Lessons from patients who have suffered diagnostic failure. *Diagnosis* 1(1):53–54.
Hauer, K. E., A. Teherani, K. M. Kerr, P. S. O'Sullivan, and D. M. Irby. 2007. Student performance problems in medical school clinical skills assessments. *Academic Medicine* 82(10 Suppl):S69–S72.
Hautz, W. E., J. E. Kämmer, S. K. Schauber, C. D. Spies, and W. Gaissmaier. 2015. Diagnostic performance by medical students working individually or in teams. *JAMA* 313(3):303–304.

Health Affairs. 2010. Patient-centered medical homes: Health affairs policy brief. *Health Affairs*. September 14. http://healthaffairs.org/healthpolicybriefs/brief_pdfs/ healthpolicybrief_25.pdf (accessed June 5, 2015).

HealthIT.gov. 2015. Patient ability to electronically view, download & transmit (VDT) health information. www.healthit.gov/providers-professionals/achieve-meaningful-use/ core-measures-2/patient-ability-electronically-view-download-transmit-vdt-health- information (accessed March 15, 2015).

Hekelman, F. P., E. Vanek, K. Kelly, and S. Alemagno. 1993. Characteristics of family physi- cians' clinical teaching behaviors in the ambulatory setting: A descriptive study. *Teach- ing and Learning in Medicine: An International Journal* 5(1):18–23.

Hendrich, A., C. K. McCoy, J. Gale, L. Sparkman, and P. Santos. 2014. Ascension Health's demonstration of full disclosure protocol for unexpected events during labor and de- livery shows promise. *Health Affairs* 33(1):139–145.

Henriksen, K., and J. Brady. 2013. The pursuit of better diagnostic performance: A human factors perspective. *BMJ Quality and Safety* 22(Suppl 2):ii1–ii5.

HHS (Department of Health and Human Services). 2013. Usual source of care: Women's health USA: An illustrated collection of current and historical data, published annually. http://mchb.hrsa.gov/whusa13/health-services-utilization/p/usual-source-care.html (accessed May 7, 2015).

HHS. 2014. HHS strengthens patients' right to access lab test reports. www.hhs.gov/news/ press/2014pres/02/20140203a.html (accessed June 5, 2015).

HHS. 2015. What are the national CLAS standards? www.thinkculturalhealth.hhs.gov/ Content/clas.asp#clas_standards (accessed May 11, 2015).

Hickner, J., P. J. Thompson, T. Wilkinson, M. Epner, M. Shaheen, A. M. Pollock, J. Lee, C. C. Duke, B. R. Jackson, and J. R. Taylor. 2014. Primary care physicians' challenges in ordering clinical laboratory tests and interpreting results. *Journal of the American Board of Family Medicine* 27(2):268–274.

Hines, L. E., and J. E. Murphy. 2011. Potentially harmful drug–drug interactions in the elderly: A review. *The American Journal of Geriatric Pharmacotherapy* 9(6):364–377.

Hirsh, D. A., E. S. Holmboe, and O. ten Cate. 2014. Time to trust: Longitudinal integrated clerkships and entrustable professional activities. *Academic Medicine* 89(2):201–204.

Hirt, E., and K. Markman. 1995. Multiple explanation: A consider-an-alternative strategy for debiasing judgments. *Journal of Personality and Social Psychology* 69:1069–1086.

Hodges, B., G. Regehr, and D. Martin. 2001. Difficulties in recognizing one's own incompe- tence: Novice physicians who are unskilled and unaware of it. *Academic Medicine* 76(10 Suppl):S87–S89.

Holmboe, E. S., and S. J. Durning. 2014. Assessing clinical reasoning: moving from in vitro to in vivo. *Diagnosis* 1(1):111–117.

Holmboe, E. S., J. Sherbino, D. M. Long, S. R. Swing, and J. R. Frank. 2010. The role of assess- ment in competency-based medical education. *Medical Teacher* 32(8):676–682.

HRSA (Health Resources and Services Administration). 2015. Teaching health center gradu- ate medical education (THCGME). http://bhpr.hrsa.gov/grants/teachinghealthcenters (accessed March 16, 2015).

Iglehart, J. K. 2011. Assessing an aco prototype—Medicare's physician group practice dem- onstration. *New England Journal of Medicine* 364(3):198–200.

Iglehart, J. K., and R. B. Baron. 2012. Ensuring physicians' competence—Is maintenance of certification the answer? *New England Journal of Medicine* 367(26):2543–2549.

IHC (Institute for Healthcare Communication). 2011. Impact of communication in health- care. http://healthcarecomm.org/about-us/impact-of-communication-in-healthcare (accessed March 26, 2015).

IHC. 2015. Institute for Healthcare Communication. www.healthcarecomm.org (accessed March 16, 2015).

IMDF (Informed Medical Decisions Foundation). 2014. What is shared decision making? www.informedmedicaldecisions.org/what-is-shared-decision-making (accessed March 18, 2015).

IOM (Institute of Medicine). 2001. *Crossing the quality chasm: A new health system for the 21st century*. Washington, DC: National Academy Press.

IOM. 2003a. *Health professions education: A bridge to quality*. Washington, DC: The National Academies Press.

IOM. 2003b. *Unequal treatment: Confronting racial and ethnic disparties in health care*. Washington, DC: The National Academies Press.

IOM. 2004. *Health literacy: A prescription to end confusion*. Washington, DC: The National Academies Press.

IOM. 2008. *Retooling for an aging America: Building the health care workforce*. Washington, DC: The National Academies Press.

IOM. 2010. *Redesigning continuing education in the health professions*. Washington, DC: The National Academies Press.

IOM. 2011a. *The future of nursing: Leading change, advancing health*. Washington, DC: The National Academies Press.

IOM. 2011b. *The health of lesbian, gay, bisexual, and transgender people: Building a foundation for better understanding*. Washington, DC: The National Academies Press.

IOM. 2011c. *Relieving pain in America: A blueprint for transforming prevention, care, education, and research*. Washington, DC: The National Academies Press.

IOM. 2012a. *10 attributes of a health literate organization: Discussion paper*. Washington, DC: Institute of Medicine

IOM. 2012b. *Communicating with patients on health care evidence: Discussion paper*. Washington, DC: Institute of Medicine.

IOM. 2012c. *Core principles and values of effective team-based health care: Discussion paper*. Washington, DC: Institute of Medicine.

IOM. 2012d. *Health IT and patient safety: Building safer systems for better care*. Washington, DC: The National Academies Press.

IOM. 2012e. *The mental health and substance use workforce for older adults: In whose hands?* Washington, DC: The National Academies Press.

IOM. 2013a. *Best care at lower cost: The path to continuously learning health care in America*. Washington, DC: The National Academies Press.

IOM. 2013b. *Delivering high-quality cancer care: Charting a new course for a system in crisis*. Washington, DC: The National Academies Press.

IOM. 2014. *Graduate medical education that meets the nation's health needs*. Washington, DC: The National Academies Press.

IOM. 2015. *Measuring the impact of interprofessional education on collaborative practice and patient outcomes*. Washington, DC: The National Academies Press.

Jarvis-Selinger, S., D. D. Pratt, and G. Regehr. 2012. Competency is not enough: Integrating identity formation into the medical education discourse. *Academic Medicine* 87(9):1185–1190.

The Joint Commission. 2007. "What did the doctor say?" Improving health literacy to protect patient safety. www.jointcommission.org/What_Did_the_Doctor_Say/default.aspx (accessed May 11, 2015).

The Joint Commission. 2014. Sentinel event data: Root causes by event type 2004-2q2014. www.jointcommission.org/Sentinel_Event_Statistics (accessed February 4, 2015).

The Joint Commission. 2015. Speak Up initiatives. www.jointcommission.org/speakup.aspx (accessed March 16, 2015).

Josiah Macy Jr. Foundation. 2011. *Ensuring an effective physician workforce for the United States: Recommendations for graduate medical education to meet the needs of the public, the second of two conferences—The content and format of GME, chaired by Debra Weinstein, M.D. May, 2011, Atlanta, GA.* New York: Josiah Macy Jr. Foundation.

Josiah Macy Jr. Foundation. 2014. *Partnering with patients, families, and communities: An urgent imperative for health care, Conference recommendations.* New York: Josiah Macy Jr. Foundation. www.macyfoundation.org/publications/publication/partnering-with-patients-families-and-communities-an-urgent-imperative-for (accessed June 5, 2015).

Josiah Macy Jr. Foundation and Carnegie Foundation for the Advancement of Teaching. 2010. *Educating nurses and physicians: Towards new horizons. Advancing inter-professional education in academic health centers, Conference summary.* New York: Josiah Macy Jr. Foundation. www.macyfoundation.org/docs/macy_pubs/JMF_Carnegie_Summary_Web Version_%283%29.pdf (accessed June 5, 2015).

Julavits, H. 2014. Diagnose this! How to be your own best doctor. *Harper's* April:25–35.

Kachalia, A., K. G. Shojania, T. P. Hofer, M. Piotrowski, and S. Saint. 2003. Does full disclosure of medical errors affect malpractice liability? The jury is still out. *Joint Commission Journal on Quality and Patient Safety* 29(10):503–511.

Kahneman, D. 2011. *Thinking, fast and slow.* New York: Farrar, Straus and Giroux.

Kaiser Permanente. 2012. Smart partners about your health, edited by K. Permanente. http://c.ymcdn.com/sites/www.npsf.org/resource/collection/930A0426-5BAC-4827-AF94-1CE1624CBE67/SMART-Partners-Guide1.pdf (accessed June 26, 2015).

Kak, N., B. Burkhalter, and M. Cooper. 2001. *Measuring the competence of healthcare providers.* Bethesda, MD: Published for USAID by the Center for Human Services, Quality Assurance Project.

Kanter, M. 2014. Diagnostic errors—Patient safety. Presentation to the committee on Diagnostic Error in Health Care, August 7, 2014, Washington, DC.

Kassirer, J. P. 1989. Our stubborn quest for diagnostic certainty. A cause of excessive testing. *New England Journal of Medicine* 320(22):1489–1491.

Keating, N. L., M. B. Landrum, E. B. Lamont, S. R. Bozeman, L. N. Shulman, and B. J. McNeil. 2012. Tumor boards and the quality of cancer care. *Journal of the National Cancer Institute.* doi: 10.1093/jnci/djs502. http://jnci.oxfordjournals.org/content/early/2012/12/24/jnci.djs502 (accessed June 5, 2015).

Kern, C. 2014. ACOs face barriers to implementing health IT. www.healthitoutcomes.com/doc/acos-face-barriers-to-implementing-health-it-0001 (accessed March 25, 2015).

Keroack, M. A., B. J. Youngberg, J. L. Cerese, C. Krsek, L. W. Prellwitz, and E. W. Trevelyan. 2007. Organizational factors associated with high performance in quality and safety in academic medical centers. *Academic Medicine* 82(12):1178–1186.

King, H. B., J. Battles, D. P. Baker, A. Alonso, E. Salas, J. Webster, L. Toomey, and M. Salisbury. 2008. TeamSTEPPS™: Team strategies and tools to enhance performance and patient safety. In K. Henriksen, J. B. Battles, M. A. Keyes, and M. L. Grady (eds.), *Advances in patient safety: New directions and alternative approaches (Vol. 3: Performance and tools).* AHRQ publication no. 00-0034-3. Rockville, MD: Agency for Healthcare Research and Quality. www.ahrq.gov/professionals/quality-patient-safety/patient-safety-resources/resources/advances-in-patient-safety-2/vol3/Advances-King_1.pdf (accessed June 5, 2015).

Klein, G. 1993. Sources of error in naturalistic decision making tasks. *Proceedings of the Human Factors and Ergonomics Society, 37th Annual Meeting* 368–371.

Klein, J. G. 2005. Five pitfalls in decisions about diagnosis and prescribing. *BMJ* 330(7494):781–783.

Kondo, K. L., and M. Swerdlow. 2013. Medical student radiology curriculum: What skills do residency program directors believe are essential for medical students to attain? *Academic Radiology* 20(3):263–271.

Kroenke, K. 2013. Diagnostic testing and the illusory reassurance of normal results: Comment on "Reassurance after diagnostic testing with a low pretest probability of serious disease." *JAMA Internal Medicine* 173(6):416–417.

Kroft, S. H. 2014. Statement of Steven H. Kroft, American Society for Clinical Pathology (ASCP). Presentation to the Committee on Diagnostic Error in Health Care, April 28, 2014, Washington, DC.

Laposata, M., and A. Dighe. 2007. "Pre-pre" and "post-post" analytical error: High-incidence patient safety hazards involving the clinical laboratory. *Clinical Chemistry and Laboratory Medicine* 45(6):712–719.

LCME (Liaison Committee on Medical Education). 2015. Functions and structure of a medical school: Standards for accreditation of medical education programs leading to the M.D. Degree. Liaison Committee on Medical Education. www.lcme.org/publications. htm#standards-section (accessed July 24, 2015).

Leonard, M., S. Graham, and D. Bonacum. 2004. The human factor: The critical importance of effective teamwork and communication in providing safe care. *Quality and Safety in Health Care* 13(suppl 1):i85–i90.

Levinson, W., A. Kao, A. Kuby, and R. A. Thisted. 2005. Not all patients want to participate in decision making. *Journal of General Internal Medicine* 20(6):531–535.

Lie, D. A., E. Lee-Rey, A. Gomez, S. Bereknyei, and C. H. Braddock, 3rd. 2011. Does cultural competency training of health professionals improve patient outcomes? A systematic review and proposed algorithm for future research. *Journal of General Internal Medicine* 26(3):317–325.

Lipson, J. G., H. M. Weinstein, E. A. Gladstone, and R. H. Sarnoff. 2003. Bosnian and Soviet refugees' experiences with health care. *Western Journal of Nursing Research* 25(7):854–871.

Longtin, Y., H. Sax, L. L. Leape, S. E. Sheridan, L. Donaldson, and D. Pittet. 2010. Patient participation: Current knowledge and applicability to patient safety. *Mayo Clinic Proceedings* 85(1):53–62.

Lucian Leape Institute. 2014. *Safety is personal: Partnering with patients and families for the safest care. Report of the Roundtable on Consumer Engagement in Patient Safety.* Boston, MA: National Patient Safety Foundation.

Lujan, H. L., and S. E. DiCarlo. 2006. First-year medical students prefer multiple learning styles. *Advances in Physiological Education* 30(1):13–16.

Lurie, S. J. 2012. History and practice of competency-based assessment. *Medical Education* 46(1):49–57.

Magid, M. S., and C. L. Cambor. 2011. The integration of pathology into the clinical years of undergraduate medical education: a survey and review of the literature. *Human Pathology* 43(4):567–576.

Malone, D. C., D. S. Hutchins, H. Haupert, P. Hansten, B. Duncan, R. C. Van Bergen, S. L. Solomon, and R. B. Lipton. 2005. Assessment of potential drug–drug interactions with a prescription claims database. *American Journal of Health-System Pharmacy* 62(19):1983–1991.

Manrai, A. K., G. Bhatia, J. Strymish, I. S. Kohane, and S. H. Jain. 2014. Medicine's uncomfortable relationship with math: Calculating positive predictive value. *JAMA Internal Medicine* 174(6):991–993.

Marcus, E. 2003. Cases: When a patient is lost in the translation. *The New York Times*, April 8.

Marewski, J. N., and G. Gigerenzer. 2012. Heuristic decision making in medicine. *Dialogues in Clinical Neuroscience* 14(1):77–89.

Marvel, M. K., R. M. Epstein, K. Flowers, and H. B. Beckman. 1999. Soliciting the patient's agenda: Have we improved? *JAMA* 281(3):283–287.

Mayer, R. E. 2010. Applying the science of learning to medical education. *Medical Education* 44(6):543–549.

Mayo Clinic. 2015. Patient care and health information. www.mayoclinic.org/patient-care-and-health-information (accessed March 26, 2015).

Mazor, K. M., D. W. Roblin, S. M. Greene, C. A. Lemay, C. L. Firneno, J. Calvi, C. D. Prouty, K. Horner, and T. H. Gallagher. 2012. Toward patient-centered cancer care: Patient perceptions of problematic events, impact, and response. *Journal of Clinical Oncology* 30(15):1784–1790.

Mazzocco, K., D. B. Petitti, K. T. Fong, D. Bonacum, J. Brookey, S. Graham, R. E. Lasky, J. B. Sexton, and E. J. Thomas. 2009. Surgical team behaviors and patient outcomes. *American Journal of Surgery* 197(5):678–685.

McDonald, K. M. 2014. The diagnostic field's players and interactions: From the inside out. *Diagnosis* 1(1):55–58.

McDonald, K. M., C. L. Bryce, and M. L. Graber. 2013. The patient is in: Patient involvement strategies for diagnostic error mitigation. *BMJ Quality and Safety* 22(2):30–36.

McGaghie, W. C., S. B. Issenberg, E. R. Cohen, J. H. Barsuk, and D. B. Wayne. 2011. Does simulation-based medical education with deliberate practice yield better results than traditional clinical education? A meta-analytic comparative review of the evidence. *Academic Medicine* 86(6):706–711.

McGowan, J., M. Passiment, and H. M. Hoffman. 2007. Educating medical students as competent users of health information technologies: The MSOP data. *Studies in Health Technologies and Informatics* 129(Pt 2):1414–1418.

McLaughlin, J. E., M. T. Roth, D. M. Glatt, N. Gharkholonarehe, C. A. Davidson, L. M. Griffin, D. A. Esserman, and R. J. Mumper. 2014. The flipped classroom: A course redesign to foster learning and engagement in a health professions school. *Academic Medicine* 89(2):236–243.

MedPAC (Medicare Payment Advisory Commission). 2010. Shared decision making and its implications for Medicare. In MedPAC, *Report to the Congress: Aligning incentives in medicine* (pp. 191–210). Washington, DC: MedPAC. www.medpac.gov/documents/reports/Jun10_Ch07.pdf?sfvrsn=0 (accessed June 5, 2015).

Mello, M. M., R. C. Boothman, T. McDonald, J. Driver, A. Lembitz, D. Bouwmeester, B. Dunlap, and T. Gallagher. 2014. Communication-and-resolution programs: The challenges and lessons learned from six early adopters. *Health Affairs* 33(1):20–29.

Meyer, A. N. D., V. L. Payne, D. W. Meeks, R. Rao, and H. Singh. 2013. Physicians' diagnostic accuracy, confidence, and resource requests: a vignette study. *JAMA Internal Medicine* 173(21):1952–1958.

Milan, F. B., L. Dyche, and J. Fletcher. 2011. "How am I doing?" Teaching medical students to elicit feedback during their clerkships. *Medical Teacher* 33(11):904–910.

Morcke, A., T. Dornan, and B. Eika. 2013. Outcome (competency) based education: An exploration of its origins, theoretical basis, and empirical evidence. *Advances in Health Sciences Education* 18(4):851–863.

Mulley, A. G., C. Trimble, and G. Elwyn. 2012. Stop the silent misdiagnosis: Patients' preferences matter. *BMJ* 345(1).

Mumma, G., and W. Steven. 1995. Procedural debiasing of primary/anchoring effects in clinical-like judgments. *Journal of Clinical Psychology* 51(6):841–853.

Mussweiler, T., F. Strack, and T. Pfeiffer. 2000. Overcoming the inevitable anchoring effect: Considering the opposite compensates for selective accessibility. *Personality and Social Psychology Bulletin* 26(9):1142–1150.

Myers, L. 2013. Medical student perspective: Memory mountain: A more pleasurable route. www.acponline.org/medical_students/impact/archives/2013/07/perspect (accessed March 16, 2015).

Nasca, T. J., I. Philibert, T. Brigham, and T. C. Flynn. 2012. The next GME accreditation system—Rationale and benefits. *New England Journal of Medicine* 366(11):1051–1056.

National Commission on Physician Payment Reform. 2013. *Report of the National Commission on Physician Payment Reform*. Washington, DC: National Commission on Physician Payment Reform.

Naylor, M. D., K. D. Coburn, E. T. Kurtzman, H. Buck, J.Van Cleave, and C. Cott. 2010. *Inter-professional team-based primary care for chronically ill adults: State of the science.* Unpublished white paper presented at the ABIM Foundation Meeting to Advance Team-Based Care for the Chronically Ill in Ambulatory Settings, March 24–25, 2010, Philadelphia, PA.

NCI (National Cancer Institute). 2015. NCI dictionary of cancer terms: Tumor board review. www.cancer.gov/dictionary?cdrid=322893 (accessed March 16, 2015).

NCSBN (National Council of State Boards of Nursing). 2015. National Council of State Boards of Nursing. www.ncsbn.org/index.htm (accessed June 5, 2015).

Newman, E. A., A. B. Guest, M. A. Helvie, M. A. Roubidoux, A. E. Chang, C. G. Kleer, K. M. Diehl, V. M. Cimmino, L. Pierce, D. Hayes, L. A. Newman, and M. S. Sabel. 2006. Changes in surgical management resulting from case review at a breast cancer multidisciplinary tumor board. *Cancer* (107):2346–2351.

Newman-Toker, D. E., K. M. McDonald, and D. O. Meltzer. 2013. How much diagnostic safety can we afford, and how should we decide? A health economics perspective. *BMJ Quality and Safety* 22(Suppl 2):ii11–ii20.

NIST (National Institute of Standards and Technology), J. Redish, and S. Lowry. 2010. *Usability in health IT: Technical strategy, research, and implementation.* Rockville, MD: National Institute of Standards and Technology. Summary of Workshop and Usability in Health IT, Washington, DC, July 13.

NLM (National Library of Medicine). 2012a. Evaluating Internet health information: A tutorial from the National Library of Medicine. www.nlm.nih.gov/medlineplus/webeval/webeval.html (accessed March 16, 2015).

NLM. 2012b. MedlinePlus guide to healthy Web surfing. www.nlm.nih.gov/medlineplus/healthywebsurfing.html (accessed February 11, 2015).

NNLM (National Network of Libraries of Medicine). 2013. Prevalence of low health literacy. nnlm.gov/outreach/consumer/hlthlit.html#A3 (accessed April 4, 2014).

NORC. 2014. Demonstrating the effectiveness of patient feedback in improving the accuracy of medical records. Chicago, IL: NORC. www.healthit.gov/sites/default/files/20120831_odrfinalreport508.pdf (accessed June 5, 2015).

Norman, G. 2014. Diagnostic errors. Input submitted to the Committee on Diagnostic Error in Health Care, October 24, 2014, Washington, DC.

Nouri, S. S., and R. E. Rudd. 2015. Health literacy in the "oral exchange": An important element of patient–provider communication. *Patient Education and Counseling* 98(5):565–571.

NPSF (National Patient Safety Foundation). 2015a. Ask me 3. www.npsf.org/?page=askme3 (accessed March 25, 2015).

NPSF. 2015b. RCA^2: Improving root cause analyses and actions to prevent harm. http://c.ymcdn.com/sites/www.npsf.org/resource/resmgr/PDF/RCA2_first-online-pub_061615.pdf?hhSearchTerms=%22rca%22 (accessed July 6, 2015).

NPSF and SIDM (Society to Improve Diagnosis in Medicine). 2014. Checklist for getting the right diagnosis. www.npsf.org/?page=rightdiagnosis and http://c.ymcdn.com/sites/www.npsf.org/resource/collection/930A0426-5BAC-4827-AF94-1CE1624CBE67/Checklist-for-Getting-the-Right-Diagnosis.pdf (accessed June 26, 2015).

Nutter, D., and M. Whitcomb. 2001. *The AAMC Project on the Clinical Education of Medical Students.* Washington, DC: Association of American Medical Colleges.

OHSU (Oregon Health & Science University). 2014. A bold new curriculum aligns physician education with our health care future. School of Medicine, Oregon Health & Science University. www.ohsu.edu/xd/education/schools/school-of-medicine/about/curriculum-transformation/upload/SoM-Curriculum-transformation-interactive-12.pdf (accessed July 23, 2015).

O'Mahony, S., E. Mazur, P. Charney, Y. Wang, and J. Fine. 2007. Use of multidisciplinary rounds to simultaneously improve quality outcomes, enhance resident education, and shorten length of stay. *Journal of General Internal Medicine* 22(8):1073–1079.

O'Malley, A. S., G. R. Cohen, and J. M. Grossman. 2010. Electronic medical records and communication with patients and other clinicians: Are we talking less? Center for Studying Health System Change, Issue Brief No. 131:1–4. www.hschange.com/CONTENT/1125 (accessed June 5, 2015).

O'Neill, T. R., and J. C. Puffer. 2013. Maintenance of certification and its association with the clinical knowledge of family physicians. *Academic Medicine* 88(6):780–787.

OpenNotes. 2015. What is OpenNotes? www.myopennotes.org/about-opennotes (accessed January 2, 2015).

Paez, K., J. Allen, M. Beach, K. Carson, and L. Cooper. 2009. Physician cultural competence and patient ratings of the patient–physician relationship. *Journal of General Internal Medicine* 24(4):495–498.

Papa, F. J. 2014a. Learning sciences principles that can inform the construction of new approaches to diagnostic training. *Diagnosis* 1(1):125–129.

Papa, F. J. 2014b. A response to the IOM's ad hoc Committee on Diagnostic Error in Health Care. Input submitted to the Committee on Diagnostic Error in Health Care, October 24, 2014, Washington, DC.

Papp, K. K., G. C. Huang, L. M. Lauzon Clabo, D. Delva, M. Fischer, L. Konopasek, R. M. Schwartzstein, and M. Gusic. 2014. Milestones of critical thinking: A developmental model for medicine and nursing. *Academic Medicine* 89(5):715–720.

Patel, V., N. A. Yoskowitz, and J. F. Arocha. 2009a. Towards effective evaluation and reform in medical education: A cognitive and learning sciences perspective. *Advances in Health Sciences Education* 14(5):791–812.

Patel, V., N. A. Yoskowitz, J. F. Arocha, and E. H. Shortliffe. 2009b. Cognitive and learning sciences in biomedical and health instructional design: A review with lessons for biomedical informatics education. *Journal of Biomedical Informatics* 42(1):176–197.

Pawlik, T. M., D. Laheru, R. H. Hruban, J. Coleman, C. L. Wolfgang, K. Campbell, S. Ali, E. K. Fishman, R. D. Schulick, J. M. Herman, and the Johns Hopkins Multidisciplinary Pancreas Clinic Team. 2008. Evaluating the impact of a single-day multidisciplinary clinic on the management of pancreatic cancer. *Annals of Surgical Oncology* 15(8):2081–2088.

Pecukonis, E., O. Doyle, and D. L. Bliss. 2008. Reducing barriers to interprofessional training: Promoting interprofessional cultural competence. *Journal of Interprofessional Care* 22(4):417–428.

Peters, E., J. Hibbard, P. Slovic, and N. Dieckmann. 2007. Numeracy skill and the communication, comprehension, and use of risk–benefit information. *Health Affairs* 26(3):741–748.

Pines, J. M. 2006. Profiles in patient safety: Confirmation bias in emergency medicine. *Academic Emergency Medicine* 13:90–94.

Porter, M. E. 2010. What is value in health care? *New England Journal of Medicine* 363(26):2477–2481.

Porter, M. E., and T. H. Lee. 2013. The strategy that will fix health care. *Harvard Business Review* 91(10):50–70.

Press, M. J. 2014. Instant replay—A quarterback's view of care coordination. *New England Journal of Medicine* 371(6):489–491.

Prezzia, C., G. Vorona, and R. Greenspan. 2013. Fourth-year medical student opinions and basic knowledge regarding the field of radiology. *Academic Radiology* 20(3):272–283.

Price-Wise, G. 2008. Language, culture, and medical tragedy: The case of Willie Ramirez. http://healthaffairs.org/blog/2008/11/19/language-culture-and-medical-tragedy-the-case-of-willie-ramirez (accessed May 11, 2015).

Priyanath, A., J. Feinglass, N. C. Dolan, C. Haviley, and L. A. Venta. 2002. Patient satisfaction with the communication of mammographic results before and after the Mammography Quality Standards Reauthorization Act of 1998. *American Journal of Roentgenology* 178(2):451–456.

Puhl, R., and K. D. Brownell. 2001. Bias, discrimination, and obesity. *Obesity Research* 9(12):788–805.

Rao, V. M., and D. C. Levin. 2012. The overuse of diagnostic imaging and the Choosing Wisely Initiative. *Annals of Internal Medicine* 157(8):574–576.

Redelmeier, D. A. 2005. The cognitive psychology of missed diagnoses. *Annals of Internal Medicine* 142(2):115–120.

Rhoades, D. R., K. F. McFarland, W. H. Finch, and A. O. Johnson. 2001. Speaking and interruptions during primary care office visits. *Family Medicine* 33(7):528–532.

Richardson, W. S. 2007. We should overcome the barriers to evidence-based clinical diagnosis! *Journal of Clinical Epidemiology* 60(3):217–227.

Richardson, W. S. 2014. Twenty suggestions that could improve clinical diagnosis and reduce diagnostic error. Input submitted to the Committee on Diagnostic Error in Health Care, October 24, 2014, Washington, DC.

Rider, E. A., and C. H. Keefer. 2006. Communication skills competencies: Definitions and a teaching toolbox. *Medical Education* 40(7):624–629.

Rittenhouse, D. R., S. M. Shortell, and E. S. Fisher. 2009. Primary care and accountable care—Two essential elements of delivery-system reform. *New England Journal of Medicine* 361(24):2301–2303.

Roades, C. 2013. The new imperative of patient engagement for hospitals and health systems. Health Affairs Blog. http://healthaffairs.org/blog/2013/02/15/the-new-imperative-of-patient-engagement-for-hospitals-and-health-systems (accessed April 9, 2014).

Rolfe, I. E., and R. W. Sanson-Fisher. 2002. Translating learning principles into practice: A new strategy for learning clinical skills. *Medical Education* 36(4):345–352.

Ronda, G., J. Grispen, M. Ickenroth, G.–J. Dinant, N. De Vries, and T. Van der Weijden. 2014. The effects of a Web-based decision aid on the intention to diagnostic self-testing for cholesterol and diabetes: A randomized controlled trial. *BMC Public Health* 14(1):1–12.

Ross, J. S. 2014. Editor's note: Ensuring correct interpretation of diagnostic test results. *JAMA Internal Medicine* 174(6):993.

Rubin, Z., and K. Blackham. 2015. The state of radiologic teaching practice in preclinical medical education: Survey of American medical, osteopathic, and podiatric schools. *Journal of the American College of Radiology* 12(4):403–408.

Ryan, C. 2013. Language use in the United States: 2011, American community survey reports. www.census.gov/prod/2013pubs/acs-22.pdf (accessed July 25, 2015).

Safran, D. G., M. Kosinski, A. R. Tarlov, W. H. Rogers, D. H. Taira, N. Lieberman, and J. E. Ware. 1998. The primary care assessment survey: Tests of data quality and measurement performance. *Medical Care* 36(5):728–739.

Salas, E., D. DiazGranados, S. J. Weaver, and H. King. 2008. Does team training work? Principles for health care. *Academic Emergency Medicine* 15(11):1002–1009.

Santoso, J. T., B. Schwertner, R. L. Coleman, and E. V. Hannigan. 2004. Tumor board in gynecologic oncology. *International Journal of Gynecological Cancer* 14(2):206–209.

Sarkar, U., D. Bonacum, W. Strull, C. Spitzmueller, N. Jin, A. Lopez, T. D. Giardina, A. N. Meyer, and H. Singh. 2012. Challenges of making a diagnosis in the outpatient setting: A multi-site survey of primary care physicians. *BMJ Quality and Safety* 21(8):641–648.

Sarkar, U., B. Simchowitz, D. Bonacum, W. Strull, A. Lopez, L. Rotteau, and K. Shojania. 2014. A qualitative analysis of physician perspectives on missed and delayed outpatient diagnosis: The focus on system-related factors. *Joint Commission Journal on Quality and Patient Safety* 40(10):461–470.

Sawyer, R. K. (ed.). 2006. *The Cambridge handbook of the learning sciences.* New York: Cambridge University Press.

Sawyer, R. K. 2008. *Optimising learning: Implications of learning sciences research.* Paris: OECD. www.oecd.org/edu/ceri/40805146.pdf (accessed June 5, 2015).

Say, R., M. Murtagh, and R. Thomson. 2006. Patients' preference for involvement in medical decision making: A narrative review. *Patient Education and Counseling* 60(2):102–114.

SCAI (Society for Cardiovascular Angiography and Interventions). 2014. SCAI expands auc calculator app to support clinical decision making for diagnostic catheterization and imaging for heart failure: Society for Cardiovascular Angiography and Interventions. www.scai.org/Press/detail.aspx?cid=edaf8ad9-4d7a-4147-ac4f-4d62585b7f56#.VY2FbLHD9zN (accessed June 25, 2015).

Scalese, R., V. Obeso, and S. B. Issenberg. 2008. Simulation technology for skills training and competency assessment in medical education. *Journal of General Internal Medicine* 23(Suppl 1):46–49.

Schiff, G. D. 2008. Minimizing diagnostic error: The importance of follow-up and feedback. *American Journal of Medicine* 121(5):S38–S42.

Schiff. G. D. 2014a. Presentation to IOM Committee on Diagnostic Error in Health Care, August 7, 2014, Washington, DC.

Schiff, G. D. 2014b. Diagnosis and diagnostic errors: Time for a new paradigm. *BMJ Quality and Safety* 23(1):1–3.

Schiff, G. D., O. Hasan, S. Kim, R. Abrams, K. Cosby, B. L. Lambert, A. S. Elstein, S. Hasler, M. L. Kabongo, N. Krosnjar, R. Odwazny, M. F. Wisniewski, and R. A. McNutt. 2009. Diagnostic error in medicine: Analysis of 583 physician-reported errors. *Archives of Internal Medicine* 169(20):1881–1887.

Schiff, G., P. Griswold, B. R. Ellis, A. L. Puopolo, N. Brede, H. R. Nieva, F. Federico, N. Leydon, J. Ling, D. Wachenheim, L. L. Leape, and M. Biondolillo. 2014. Doing right by our patients when things go wrong in the ambulatory setting. *Joint Commission Journal on Quality and Patient Safety/Joint Commission Resources* 40(2):91–96.

Schillinger, D., J. Piette, K. Grumbach, F. Wang, C. Wilson, C. Daher, K. Leong-Grotz, C. Castro, and A. B. Bindman. 2003. Closing the loop: Physician communication with diabetic patients who have low health literacy. *Archives of Internal Medicine* 163(1):83–90.

Schmitt, M., A. Blue, C. A. Aschenbrener, and T. R. Viggiano. 2011. Core competencies for interprofessional collaborative practice: Reforming health care by transforming health professionals' education. *Academic Medicine* 86(11):1351.

Schoen, C., R. Osborn, M. M. Doty, M. Bishop, J. Peugh, and N. Murukutla. 2007. Toward higher-performance health systems: Adults' health care experiences in seven countries, 2007. *Health Affairs* 26(6):w717–w734.

Schulman, K. A., J. A. Berlin, W. Harless, J. F. Kerner, S. Sistrunk, B. J. Gersh, R. Dubé, C. K. Taleghani, J. E. Burke, S. Williams, J. M. Eisenberg, W. Ayers, and J. J. Escarce. 1999. The effect of race and sex on physicians' recommendations for cardiac catheterization. *New England Journal of Medicine* 340(8):618–626.

Schwartz, M. B., H. O'Neal Chambliss, K. D. Brownell, S. N. Blair, and C. Billington. 2003. Weight bias among health professionals specializing in obesity. *Obesity Research* 11(9):1033–1039.

Seegmiller, A. C., A. S. Kim, C. A. Mosse, M. A. Levy, M. A. Thompson, M. K. Kressin, M. H. Jagasia, S. A. Strickland, N. M. Reddy, E. R. Marx, K. J. Sinkfield, H. N. Pollard, W. D. Plummer, W. D. Dupont, E. K. Shultz, R. S. Dittus, W. W. Stead, S. A. Santoro, and M. M. Zutter. 2013. Optimizing personalized bone marrow testing using an evidence-based, interdisciplinary team approach. *American Journal of Clinical Pathology* 140(5):643–650.

Semigran, H. L., J. A. Linder, C. Gidengil, and A. Mehrotra. 2015. Evaluation of symptom checkers for self diagnosis and triage: Audit study. *BMJ* 351:h3480.

Sequist, T., E. Schneider, M. Anastario, E. Odigie, R. Marshall, W. Rogers, and D. Safran. 2008. Quality monitoring of physicians: Linking patients' experiences of care to clinical quality and outcomes. *Journal of General Internal Medicine* 23(11):1784–1790.

Shojania, K. G., I. Silver, and W. Levinson. 2012. Continuing medical education and quality improvement: A match made in heaven? *Annals of Internal Medicine* 156(4):305–308.

Shumate, M., R. Ibrahim, and R. Levitt. 2010. Dynamic information retrieval and allocation flows in project teams with discontinuous membership. *European Journal of International Management* 4(6):556–575.

SIDM (Society to Improve Diagnosis in Medicine). 2015. Patient Toolkit. www.improve diagnosis.org/?page=PatientToolkit (accessed August 27, 2015).

SIDM and NPSF (National Patient Safety Foundation). 2014. Reducing diagnostic error: Nurses and clinical staff: Ten things I could do tomorrow. http://c.ymcdn.com/sites/www. npsf.org/resource/collection/0716DBAD-99BB-460E-9837-1E357423C51C/Reducing-Diagnostic-Error-Nurses-and-Clinical-Staff-Ten-Things-I-Could-Do-Tomorrow.pdf (accessed May 11, 2015).

Singh, H. 2014. Building a robust conceptual foundation for defining and measuring diagnostic errors. Presentation to the Committee on Diagnostic Error in Health Care, August 7, 2014, Washington, DC.

Smith, B. R., M. Aguero-Rosenfeld, J. Anastasi, B. Baron, A. Berg, J. L. Bock, S. Campbell, K. P. Crookston, R. Fitzgerald, M. Fung, R. Haspel, J. G. Howe, J. Jhang, M. Kamoun, S. Koethe, M. D. Krasowski, M. L. Landry, M. B. Marques, H. M. Rinder, W. Roberts, W. E. Schreiber, S. L. Spitalnik, C. A. Tormey, P. Wolf, and Y. Y. Wu. 2010. Educating medical students in laboratory medicine: A proposed curriculum. *American Journal of Clinical Pathology* 133(4):533–542.

Smith, T. J., and D. L. Longo. 2012. Talking with patients about dying. *New England Journal of Medicine* 367(17):1651.

Soni, K., and G. Dhaliwal. 2012. Misleading complaint: Commentary by Krishan Soni, M.D., M.B.A., and Gurpreet Dhaliwal, M.D. http://webmm.ahrq.gov/case.aspx?caseID=273 (accessed June 5, 2015).

Sorbero, M. E., D. O. Farley, S. Mattke, and S. L. Lovejoy. 2008. *Outcome measures for effective teamwork in inpatient care: Final report.* Santa Monica, CA: RAND Corporation.

Spain, E. 2014. Do doctors spend too much time looking at computer screen? Gazing at electronic health records diverts doctors' attention from patients. Northwestern University, January 23. www.northwestern.edu/newscenter/stories/2014/01/do-doctors-spend-too-much-time-looking-at-computer-screen.html (accessed June 5, 2015).

Starfield, B. 2000. Is U.S. health really the best in the world? *JAMA* 284(4):483–485.

Stark, M., and J. J. Fins. 2014. The ethical imperative to think about thinking: Diagnostics, metacognition, and medical professionalism. *Cambridge Quarterly of Healthcare Ethics* 23(4):386–396.

Stevenson, F. A. 2003. General practitioners' views on shared decision making: A qualitative analysis. *Patient Education and Counseling* 50(3):291–293.

Straus, C. M., E. M. Webb, K. L. Kondo, A. W. Phillips, D. M. Naeger, C. W. Carrico, W. Herring, J. A. Neutze, G. R. Haines, and G. D. Dodd, 3rd. 2014. Medical student radiology education: Summary and recommendations from a national survey of medical school and radiology department leadership. *Journal of the American College of Radiology* 11(6):606–610.

Stremikis, K., C. Schoen, and A. K. Fryer. 2011. *A call for change: The 2011 Commonwealth Fund survey of public views of the U.S. health system.* Commonwealth Fund issue brief. www.commonwealthfund.org/~/media/Files/Publications/Issue%20Brief/2011/Apr/1492_Stremikis_public_views_2011_survey_ib.pdf (accessed June 5, 2015).

Su, E., T. A. Schmidt, N. C. Mann, and A. D. Zechnich. 2000. A randomized controlled trial to assess decay in acquired knowledge among paramedics completing a pediatric resuscitation course. *Academic Emergency Medicine* 7(7):779–786.

Sutcliffe, K. M., E. Lewton, and M. M. Rosenthal. 2004. Communication failures: An insidious contributor to medical mishaps. *Academic Medicine* 79(2):186–194.

Swain, M., and V. Patel. 2014. Patient access to test results among clinical laboratories. ONC Data Brief No. 13:1-9. Washington, DC: Office of the National Coordinator for Health Information Technology. www.healthit.gov/sites/default/files/onc-data-brief-13-labsurveydatabrief.pdf (accessed June 5, 2015).

Talbert, M. L., E. R. Ashwood, N. A. Brownlee, J. R. Clark, R. E. Horowitz, R. B. Lepoff, A. Neumann, C. N. Otis, S. Z. Powell, and T. M. Sodeman. 2009. Resident preparation for practice: a white paper from the College of American Pathologists and Association of Pathology Chairs. *Archives of Pathology & Laboratory Medicine* 133(7):1139–1147.

Taylor, C. R., B. R. DeYoung, and M. B. Cohen. 2008. Pathology education: quo vadis?. *Human Pathology* 39(11):1555–1561.

Teherani, A., D. M. Irby, and H. Loeser. 2013. Outcomes of different clerkship models: Longitudinal integrated, hybrid, and block. *Academic Medicine* 88(1):35–43.

Teirstein, P. S. 2015. Boarded to death—Why maintenance of certification is bad for doctors and patients. *New England Journal of Medicine* 372(2):106–108.

ten Cate, O. 2014. Advice to the Institute of Medicine Committee on Diagnostic Error. Input submitted to the Committee on Diagnostic Error in Health Care, November 25, 2014, Washington, DC.

Thibault, G. E. 2013. Reforming health professions education will require culture change and closer ties between classroom and practice. *Health Affairs* 32(11):1928–1932.

Torre, D. M., B. J. Daley, J. L. Sebastian, and D. M. Elnicki. 2006. Overview of current learning theories for medical educators. *American Journal of Medicine* 119(10):903–907.

Trowbridge, R. 2014. Diagnostic performance: Measurement and feedback. Presentation to the Committee on Diagnostic Error in Health Care, August 7, 2014, Washington, DC.

Trowbridge, R., G. Dhaliwal, and K. Cosby. 2013. Educational agenda for diagnostic error reduction. *BMJ Quality and Safety* 22(Suppl 2):ii28–ii32.

University of Pittsburgh. 2015. Institute for Doctor–Patient Communication. www.dom.pitt.edu/dgim/IDPC/about.html (accessed March 26, 2015).

Vashdi, D. R., P. A. Bamberger, and M. Erez. 2013. Can surgical teams ever learn? The role of coordination, complexity, and transitivity in action team learning. *Academy of Management Journal* 56(4):945–971.

Walker, J., J. D. Darer, J. G. Elmore, and T. Delbanco. 2014. The road toward fully transparent medical records. *New England Journal of Medicine* 370(1):6–8.

Weaver, S. J., S. M. Dy, and M. A. Rosen. 2014. Team-training in healthcare: A narrative synthesis of the literature. *BMJ Quality and Safety* 23(5):359–372.

Weed, L. L., and L. Weed. 2014. Diagnosing diagnostic failure. *Diagnosis* 1(1):13–17.

Wegwarth, O., W. Gaissmaier, and G. Gigerenzer. 2009. Smart strategies for doctors and doctors-in-training: Heuristics in medicine. *Medical Education* 43(8):721–728.

Weingart, S. N. 2013. Patient engagement and patient safety. Agency for Healthcare Quality and Research. http://webmm.ahrq.gov/perspective.aspx?perspectiveID=136 (accessed February 7, 2014).

Weingart, S. N., O. Pagovich, D. Z. Sands, J. M. Li, M. D. Aronson, R. B. Davis, D. W. Bates, and R. S. Phillips. 2005. What can hospitalized patients tell us about adverse events? Learning from patient-reported incidents. *Journal of General Internal Medicine* 20(9):830–836.

WHO (World Health Organization). 2010. *Framework for action on interprofessional education and collaborative practice*. Geneva: World Health Organization.

Wilson, M. L. 2010. Educating medical students in laboratory medicine. *American Journal of Clinical Pathology* 133(4):525–528.

Wilson-Stronks, A., and E. Galvez. 2007. *Hospitals, language, and culture: A snapshot of the nation, exploring cultural and linguistic services in the nation's hospitals*. The Joint Commission. www.jointcommission.org/assets/1/6/hlc_paper.pdf (accessed June 5, 2015).

Xyrichis, A., and E. Ream. 2008. Teamwork: A concept analysis. *Journal of Advanced Nursing* 61(2):232–241.

Yang, H., C. Thompson, and M. Bland. 2012. The effect of clinical experience, judgment task difficulty and time pressure on nurses' confidence calibration in a high fidelity clinical simulation. *BMC Medical Informatics and Decision Making* 12(1):113.

Yedidia, M. J., C. C. Gillespie, E. Kachur, M. D. Schwartz, J. Ockene, A. E. Chepaitis, C. W. Snyder, A. Lazare, and M. Lipkin, Jr. 2003. Effect of communications training on medical student performance. *JAMA* 290(9):1157–1165.

Zhi, M., E. L. Ding, J. Theisen-Toupal, J. Whelan, and R. Arnaout. 2013. The landscape of inappropriate laboratory testing: A 15-year meta-analysis. *PLoS ONE* 8(11):e78962.

Zimmerman, T. M., and G. Amori. 2007. Including patients in root cause and system failure analysis: Legal and psychological implications. *Journal of Healthcare Risk Management* 27(2):27–34.

5

Technology and Tools in the Diagnostic Process

A wide variety of technologies and tools are involved in the diagnostic process (see Figure 5-1), but the primary focus of the chapter is on health information technology (health IT) tools. Health IT covers a broad range of technologies used in health care, including electronic health records (EHRs), clinical decision support, patient engagement tools, computerized provider order entry, laboratory and medical imaging information systems, health information exchanges, and medical devices. Health IT plays key roles in various aspects of the diagnostic process: capturing information about a patient that informs the diagnostic process, including the clinical history and interview, physical exam, and diagnostic testing results; shaping a clinician's workflow and decision making in the diagnostic process; and facilitating information exchange.

The committee concluded that health IT has the potential to impact the diagnostic process in both positive and negative ways. When health IT tools support diagnostic team members and tasks in the diagnostic process and reflect human-centered design principles, health IT has the potential to improve diagnosis and reduce diagnostic errors. Despite this potential, however, there have been few demonstrations that health IT actually improves diagnosis in clinical practice (El-Kareh et al., 2013). Indeed, many experts are concerned that current health IT tools are not effectively facilitating the diagnostic process and may be contributing to diagnostic errors (Basch, 2014; Berenson et al., 2011; El-Kareh et al., 2013; Kuhn et al., 2015; Ober, 2015; ONC, 2014b; Verghese, 2008). This chapter discusses the design of health IT for the diagnostic process, the interoperability of patient health information, patient safety issues related to

The Work System

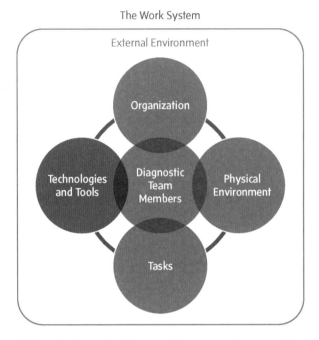

FIGURE 5-1 Technologies and tools are an important element of the work system in which the diagnostic process occurs.

the use of health IT, and the potential for health IT to aid in the measurement of diagnostic errors. The committee makes one recommendation aimed at ensuring that health IT tools and technologies facilitate timely and accurate diagnoses. In addition, this chapter briefly reviews the use of mobile health (mHealth) and telemedicine in the diagnostic process. Other technologies, such as diagnostic testing, are discussed in Chapter 2.

This content builds on earlier Institute of Medicine (IOM) work, including the report *Health IT and Patient Safety: Building a Safer Health System* (IOM, 2012a). That report emphasized that health IT functions within the context of a larger sociotechnical system involving the technology itself, the people who work within the system, the workflow (or actions and procedures clinicians are anticipated to perform as they deliver care), the organization using the technology, and the external environment. Box 5-1 includes the recommendations from the 2012 report; this chapter's text references these recommendations where relevant.

DESIGN OF HEALTH IT FOR THE DIAGNOSTIC PROCESS

The design of health IT has the potential to support the diagnostic process. In particular, by supporting the individuals involved in the diagnostic process and the tasks they perform, health IT may improve diagnostic performance and reduce the potential for diagnostic errors. The increasing complexity of health care has required health care professionals to know and apply vast amounts of information, and these demands are outstripping human cognitive capacity and contributing to challenges in diagnosis (see Chapter 2). El-Kareh et al. (2013, p. ii40) asserted that "[u]naided clinicians often make diagnostic errors" because they are "[v]ulnerable to fallible human memory, variable disease presentation, clinical disease processes plagued by communication lapses, and a series of well-documented 'heuristics,' biases and disease-specific pitfalls." It is widely recognized that health IT has the potential to help health care professionals address or mitigate these human limitations.

Although health IT interventions are not appropriate for every quality-of-care challenge, there are opportunities to improve diagnosis through appropriate use of health IT. For instance, a well-designed health IT system can facilitate timely access to information; communication among health care professionals, patients, and their families; clinical reasoning and decision making; and feedback and follow-up in the diagnostic process (El-Kareh et al., 2013; Schiff and Bates, 2010). Table 5-1 describes a number of opportunities to reduce diagnostic errors through the use of health IT. The range of these suggestions is broad; some are pragmatic opportunities for intervention and others are more visionary, given the limitations of today's health IT tools.

A number of researchers have identified patient safety risks that may result from poorly designed health IT tools (Harrington et al., 2011; IOM, 2012a; Meeks et al., 2014; Sittig and Singh, 2012; Walker et al., 2008). In recognition of these risks, the 2012 IOM report described the key attributes of safe health IT, including (IOM, 2012a, p. 78):

- Easy retrieval of accurate, timely, and reliable native and imported data;
- A system the user wants to interact with;
- Simple and intuitive data displays;
- Easy navigation;
- Evidence at the point of care to aid decision making;
- Enhancements to workflow, automating mundane tasks, and streamlining work, never increasing physical or cognitive workload;

BOX 5-1
Recommendations from *Health IT and Patient*
Safety: Building a Safer Health System

Recommendation 1: The Secretary of Health and Human Services (HHS) should publish an action and surveillance plan within 12 months that includes a schedule for working with the private sector to assess the impact of health IT [health information technology] on patient safety and minimizing the risk of its implementation and use. The plan should specify:

  a. The Agency for Healthcare Research and Quality (AHRQ) and the National Library of Medicine (NLM) should expand their funding of research, training, and education of safe practices as appropriate, including measures specifically related to the design, implementation, usability, and safe use of health IT by all users, including patients.
  b. The Office of the National Coordinator (ONC) for Health Information Technology should expand its funding of processes that promote safety that should be followed in the development of health IT products, including standardized testing procedures to be used by manufacturers and health care organizations to assess the safety of health IT products.
  c. The ONC and AHRQ should work with health IT vendors and health care organizations to promote post-deployment safety testing of EHRs [electronic health records] for high-prevalence, high-impact EHR-related patient safety risks.
  d. Health care accrediting organizations should adopt criteria relating to EHR safety.
  e. AHRQ should fund the development of new methods for measuring the impact of health IT on safety using data from EHRs.

Recommendation 2: The Secretary of HHS should ensure insofar as possible that health IT vendors support the free exchange of information about health IT experiences and issues and not prohibit sharing of such information, including details (e.g., screenshots) relating to patient safety.

Recommendation 3: The ONC should work with the private and public sectors to make comparative user experiences across vendors publicly available.

Recommendation 4: The Secretary of HHS should fund a new Health IT Safety Council to evaluate criteria for assessing and monitoring the safe use of health IT and the use of health IT to enhance safety. This council should operate within an existing voluntary consensus standards organization.

Recommendation 5: All health IT vendors should be required to publicly register and list their products with the ONC, initially beginning with EHRs certified for the meaningful use program.

Recommendation 6: The Secretary of HHS should specify the quality and risk management process requirements that health IT vendors must adopt, with a particular focus on human factors, safety culture, and usability.

Recommendation 7: The Secretary of HHS should establish a mechanism for both vendors and users to report health IT–related deaths, serious injuries, or unsafe conditions.

    a. Reporting of health IT–related adverse events should be mandatory for vendors.

    b. Reporting of health IT–related adverse events by users should be voluntary, confidential, and nonpunitive.

    c. Efforts to encourage reporting should be developed, such as removing the perceptual, cultural, contractual, legal, and logistical barriers to reporting.

Recommendation 8: The Secretary of HHS should recommend that Congress establish an independent federal entity for investigating patient safety deaths, serious injuries, or potentially unsafe conditions associated with health IT. This entity should also monitor and analyze data and publicly report results of these activities.

Recommendation 9a: The Secretary of HHS should monitor and publicly report on the progress of health IT safety annually beginning in 2012. If progress toward safety and reliability is not sufficient as determined by the Secretary, the Secretary should direct the Food and Drug Administration (FDA) to exercise all available authorities to regulate EHRs, health information exchanges, and personal health records.

Recommendation 9b: The Secretary should immediately direct FDA to begin developing the necessary framework for regulation. Such a framework should be in place if and when the Secretary decides the state of health IT safety requires FDA regulation as stipulated in Recommendation 9a above.

Recommendation 10: HHS, in collaboration with other research groups, should support cross-disciplinary research toward the use of health IT as part of a learning health care system. Products of this research should be used to inform the design, testing, and use of health IT. Specific areas of research include

    a. User-centered design and human factors applied to health IT,

    b. Safe implementation and use of health IT by all users,

    c. Sociotechnical systems associated with health IT, and

    d. Impact of policy decisions on health IT use in clinical practice.

SOURCE: IOM, 2012a.

TABLE 5-1 Opportunities to Reduce Diagnostic Error Through
Electronic Clinical Documentation

Role for Electronic Documentation	Goals and Features of Redesigned Systems
Providing access to information	Ensure ease, speed, and selectivity of information searches; aid cognition through aggregation, trending, contextual relevance, and minimizing of superfluous data.
Recording and sharing assessments	Provide a space for recording thoughtful, succinct assessments, differential diagnoses, contingencies, and unanswered questions; facilitate sharing and review of assessments by both patient and other clinicians.
Maintaining dynamic patient history	Carry forward information for recall, avoiding repetitive patient querying and recording while minimizing copying and pasting.
Maintaining problem lists	Ensure that problem lists are integrated into workflow to allow for continuous updating.
Tracking medications	Record medications that the patient is actually taking, patient responses to medications, and adverse effects in order to avert misdiagnoses and ensure timely recognition of medication problems.
Tracking tests	Integrate management of diagnostic test results into note workflow to facilitate review, assessment, and responsive action as well as documentation of these steps.
Ensuring coordination and continuity	Aggregate and integrate data from all care episodes and fragmented encounters to permit thoughtful synthesis.
Enabling follow-up	Facilitate patient education about potential red-flag symptoms; track follow-up.
Providing feedback	Automatically provide feedback to clinicians upstream, facilitating learning from outcomes of diagnostic decisions.
Providing prompts	Provide checklists to minimize reliance on memory and directed questioning to aid in diagnostic thoroughness and problem solving.
Providing placeholder for resumption of work	Delineate clearly in the record where clinician should resume work after interruption, preventing lapses in data collection and thought process.
Calculating Bayesian probabilities	Embed calculator into notes to reduce errors and minimize biases in subjective estimation of diagnostic probabilities.
Providing access to information sources	Provide instant access to knowledge resources through context-specific "infobuttons" triggered by keywords in notes that link user to relevant textbooks and guidelines.

TABLE 5-1 Continued

Role for Electronic Documentation	Goals and Features of Redesigned Systems
Offering second opinion or consultation	Integrate immediate online or telephone access to consultants to answer questions related to referral triage, testing strategies, or definitive diagnostic assessments.
Increasing efficiency	More thoughtful design, workflow integration, and distribution of documentation burden could speed up charting, freeing time for communication and cognition.

SOURCE: Schiff and Bates, 2010. *New England Journal of Medicine,* G. Schiff and D. W. Bates. Can electronic clinical documentation help prevent diagnostic errors? 362(12):1066–1069. 2010. Massachusetts Medical Society. Reprinted with permission from Massachusetts Medical Society.

- Easy transfer of information to and from other organizations and clinicians; and
- No unanticipated downtime.

If health IT products do not have these features, it may be difficult for users to effectively interact with the technology, contributing to work-arounds (alternate pathways to achieve a particular functionality) or unsafe uses of the technology, as well as errors associated with the correct use of the technology. Although many of these risks apply to health care broadly, the committee concluded that health IT risks are particularly concerning for the diagnostic process. Poor design, poor implementation, and poor use of health IT can impede the diagnostic process at various junctures throughout the process. For instance, a confusing or cluttered user interface could contribute to errors in information integration and interpretation that result in diagnostic errors. Poor integration of health IT tools into clinical workflow may create cognitive burdens for clinicians that take time away from clinical reasoning activities.

To ensure that health IT supports patients and health care professionals in the diagnostic process, collaboration between the federal government, the health IT industry, and users is warranted. The 2012 IOM report concluded that the safety of health IT is a shared responsibility and described the ways in which health IT vendors, users, governmental agencies, health care organizations, and others can collaborate to improve the safety of health IT. Users include a wide variety of clinicians (such as treating health care professionals, clinicians with diagnostic testing expertise, pharmacists, and others), as well as patients and their families (HIMSS, 2014). For example, by working with users, health IT vendors can improve safety during all phases of the design of their products, from requirements gathering to product testing. In addition, the report called on the Office of the National Coordinator for Health Information Technology (ONC) to expand funding for processes that promote safety in the development of health IT products (IOM, 2012a). **In line with these recommendations, the committee recommends that health IT vendors and ONC should work together with users to ensure that health IT used in the diagnostic process demonstrates usability, incorporates human factors knowledge, integrates measurement capability, fits well within clinical workflow, provides clinical decision support, and facilitates the timely flow of information among patients and health care professionals involved in the diagnostic process.** Collaboration among health IT vendors, ONC, and users can help to identify best practices in the design, implementation, and use of health IT products used in the diagnostic process. Further research in designing health IT for the diagnostic process is also needed (see Chapter 8). The sections below describe the importance of these various features in the design of health IT for the diagnostic process. The committee did not want to impose specific requirements for how this recommendation is implemented, because the approach would be too proscriptive. The committee's recommendation emphasizes that collaboration is needed among the health IT vendor community, ONC, and users, and it outlines the essential characteristics of health IT to improve diagnosis and reduce diagnostic errors.

Usability and Human Factors

The potential benefits of health IT for improving diagnosis cannot be realized without usable, useful health IT systems. Usability has been defined as "the extent to which a product can be used by specified users to achieve specified goals with effectiveness, efficiency, and satisfaction in a specified context of use" (ISO, 1998). According to the Healthcare Information Management Systems Society (HIMSS), a system exhibits good usability when it is "easy to use and effective. It is intuitive, forgiving of mistakes and allows one to perform necessary tasks quickly, efficiently and with a minimum of mental effort. Tasks which can be performed by the software . . . are done in the background, improving accuracy and freeing up the user's cognitive resources for other tasks" (HIMSS, 2009, p. 3).

Recent discussions of usability have focused on the importance of incorporating design principles that take human factors[1] into account

---

[1] Human factors (or ergonomics) is defined as "the scientific discipline concerned with the understanding of interactions among humans and other elements of a system, and the

(Middleton et al., 2013). A number of terms have been used to describe the optimal design approach, including human-centered design, user-centered design, use-centered design, and participatory design. The committee opted for the more inclusive term, human-centered design, to describe how the involvement of all stakeholders, rather than just users, is affected by the health IT system. A human-centered design approach balances the requirements of the technical system of computers and software with those of the larger sociotechnical system (Gasson, 2003). Although some health IT vendors have adopted human-centered design principles, the practice is not universal (AHRQ, 2010). Furthermore, usability challenges may only become evident after the system has been implemented or after it has been in widespread use. Accordingly, it is important to make continuous improvements to the design, implementation, and use of health IT (Carayon et al., 2008). Opportunities to assess the effects of technology on the diagnostic process are discussed in Chapter 3.

Although clinicians have reported a high level of use and satisfaction with certain health IT features, such as electronic prescribing (Makam et al., 2013), a number of challenges with usability remain, and the National Institute of Standards and Technology has indicated that usability is often overlooked in the adoption of EHR systems (NIST, 2015). Health IT that is not designed and implemented to support the diagnostic process can increase vulnerability to diagnostic errors. The American Medical Association (AMA) recently released a statement that health IT is misaligned with the cognitive and workflow requirements of medicine and listed eight priorities for improving the usability of EHRs (AMA, 2014) (see Box 5-2). Future research on health IT usability will be important (see Chapter 8).

As mentioned in Box 5-2, a major issue related to health IT is how it will affect the patient–clinician relationship. The hope is that health IT will enhance patient and clinician communication and collaboration by, for example, facilitating patient access to health information (see Chapter 4). However, this needs to be facilitated by health IT tools that assist patients and their families in engaging in the diagnostic process (such as patient access to clinical notes; see Recommendation 1). Patient portals provide patients with access to their medical information, but poor usability—including navigational problems and unmet expectations about functionality—can hinder adoption of such tools among patients (Greenhalgh, 2010). Additional patient-facing health IT tools include mHealth applica-

profession that applies theory, principles, data and methods to design in order to optimize human well-being and overall system performance. Practitioners of ergonomics and ergonomists contribute to the design and evaluation of tasks, jobs, products, environments and systems in order to make them compatible with the needs, abilities and limitations of people" (IEA, 2000).

BOX 5-2
American Medical Association's Improving Care:
Priorities to Improve Electronic Health Record (EHR) Usability

- **Enhance physicians' ability to provide high-quality patient care.** Effective communication and engagement between patients and physicians should be of central importance in EHR design. The EHR should fit seamlessly into the practice and not distract physicians from patients.

- **Support team-based care.** EHR design and configuration must (1) facilitate clinical staff to perform work as necessary and to the extent their licensure and privileges permit and (2) allow physicians to dynamically allocate and delegate work to appropriate members of the care team as permitted by institutional policies.

- **Promote care coordination.** EHRs should have an enhanced ability to automatically track referrals and consultations as well as to ensure that the referring physician is able to follow the patient's progress/activity throughout the continuum of care.

- **Offer product modularity and configurability.** Modularity of technology will result in EHRs that offer the flexibility necessary to meet individual practice requirements. Application program interfaces can be an important contributor to this modularity.

- **Reduce cognitive workload.** EHRs should support medical decision making by providing concise, context-sensitive, and real-time data uncluttered by extraneous information. EHRs should manage information flow and adjust for context, environment, and user preferences.

- **Promote data liquidity.** EHRs should facilitate connected health care—interoperability across different venues such as hospitals, ambulatory care settings, laboratories, pharmacies and post-acute and long-term-care settings. This means not only being able to export data but also to properly incorporate external data from other systems into the longitudinal patient record. Data sharing and open architecture must address EHR data "lock in."

- **Facilitate digital and mobile patient engagement.** Whether for health and wellness or the management of chronic illnesses, interoperability between a patient's mobile technology and the EHR will be an asset.

- **Expedite user input into product design and post-implementation feedback.** An essential step to user-centered design is incorporating end-user feedback into the design and improvement of a product. EHR technology should facilitate this feedback.

SOURCE: Copyright 2014 American Medical Association. All Rights Reserved.

tions, such as symptom checkers, but concerns about their validity are ongoing (see section on mHealth) (Jutel and Lupton, 2015; Semigran et al., 2015). In addition, there are concerns that clinicians may be unwilling or not know how to act on information collected by patients though mHealth, wearable technologies, or other forums (Dwoskin and Walker, 2014; Ramirez, 2012).

Furthermore, there are also significant concerns that "technology is cleaving the sacred bond between doctor and patient" and that the EHR distracts clinicians from patient-centered care (Wachter, 2015, p. 27). One article suggested that the EHR has negatively affected the clinician–patient bond by prioritizing the computer above the patient. In this view, the patient is no longer the most important thing in the examining room because the machine, rather than the patient, has become the center of the clinician's focus (Ober, 2015). Verghese described this phenomenon as the emergence of the iPatient (or the EHR as a surrogate for a real patient), arguing that there is a real danger to reducing the attention paid to the patient: "If one eschews the skilled and repeated examination of the real patient, then simple diagnoses and new developments are overlooked, while tests, consultations, and procedures that might not be needed are ordered" (Verghese, 2008).

An important component of usability is whether it supports teamwork in the diagnostic process. Health IT has the potential to strengthen intra- and interprofessional teamwork by providing structural support for enhanced collaboration among the health care professionals involved in the diagnostic process. There is evidence that EHRs facilitate primary care teamwork via enhanced communication, redefined team roles, and improved delegation (O'Malley et al., 2015). However, this is not the case across the board; the AMA has noted that many EHR systems "are not well configured to facilitate team-based care and require physicians to enter data or perform tasks that other team members should be empowered to complete" (AMA, 2014, p. 5).

Reducing the cognitive burdens on clinicians is another key feature of usable health IT systems. Health IT has the potential to support clinicians in the diagnostic process by managing information flow and filtering and presenting information in a way that facilitates decision making. A thoughtfully designed user interface has the potential to help clinicians develop a more complete view of a patient's condition by capturing and presenting all of the patient's health information in one place.

In particular, the problem list feature of EHRs can help clinicians to quickly see a patient's most important health problem; it is a way of organizing a patient's health information within the health record. The problem list derives from the problem-oriented medical record, developed by

Lawrence Weed (Jacobs, 2009). "Problem-oriented" has two interrelated meanings (Weed and Weed, 2011, p. 134):

- the information in the medical record is organized by the patient problem to which the information relates (as distinguished from the traditional arrangement by source, with doctors' notes in one place, nurses' notes in another, lab data in another, etc.), and
- problems are defined in terms of the patient's complete medical needs rather than providers' beliefs or specialty orientation (thus, for example, the record should cover not just the "chief complaint" but all identified medical needs, and those needs should be defined in terms of the problems requiring solution, not in terms of providers' diagnostic hypotheses or treatment plans).

The problem list includes all past and present diagnoses, as well as the time of occurrence and whether the problem was resolved, and links to further information on each entry in the list (AHIMA, 2011; Weed, 1968). Although studies have shown that use of high-quality problem lists is associated with better patient care (Hartung, 2005; Simborg et al., 1976), variability in the structure and content of problem lists has limited its effectiveness in improving patient care (AHIMA, 2011; Holmes et al., 2012). There is a move to standardize the structure and content of problem lists in EHRs through the use of diagnostic and problem codes (AHIMA, 2011). To encourage this change, meaningful use criteria require that participants maintain an up-to-date, coded problem list for at least 80 percent of their patients (AHIMA, 2011).

Unfortunately, poorly designed health IT systems, such as those with confusing user interfaces and disorganized patient information, may contribute to cognitive overload rather than easing the cognitive burden on clinicians. Poorly designed systems can detract from clinician efficiency and impede information integration and interpretation in the diagnostic process. A recent analysis of the graphical display of diagnostic test results in EHRs found that few of the current EHRs meet evidence-based criteria for how to improve comprehension of such information (Sittig et al., 2015). For example, one EHR system graphed diagnostic testing results in reverse chronological order; none of the EHRs in the analysis had graphs with y-axis labels that displayed both the name of the variable and the units of measurement. Human factors engineering approaches, such as a heuristic evaluation or an assessment of how well a particular interface design complies with established design principles for usability, could help identify usability problems and guide the design of user interfaces (CQPI, 2015). One key feature of an effective user interface is simplicity. "Simplicity in design refers to everything from lack of visual clutter and concise information display to inclusion of only functionality that is needed to effectively accomplish tasks" (HIMSS, 2009). Clinicians have expressed dissatisfaction about EHR screens being too busy due to a high degree of display clutter (or the high density of objects). In their review, Moacdieh and Sarter (2015) found: "Displays described as cluttered have been shown to degrade the ability to monitor and detect signal changes, to delay visual search, to increase memory load, to instill confidence in wrong judgments, to lead to confusion, and to negatively affect situational awareness, reading, and linguistic processing" (p. 61).

Another principle of usability is efficiency (HIMSS, 2009). Inefficient health IT tools may impede diagnosis by adding to clinicians' work burdens, leaving them with less time for the cognitive work involved in diagnosis and communicating with patients and the other health care professionals who are involved in the patients' care. Clinicians need to be able to complete a task without having to undergo extra steps, such as clicking, scrolling, or switching between a keyboard and mouse; however, many health IT tools are cumbersome to navigate. One study of emergency department clinicians found that inputting information consumed more of their time than any other activity, including patient care (Hill et al., 2013). By counting computer mouse "clicks," the researchers found that it took 6 clicks to order an aspirin tablet, 8 clicks to order a chest X-ray, 15 clicks to provide a patient with one prescription, and 40 clicks to document the exam of a hand and wrist injury. Hill and colleagues (2013) estimated that a clinician could make 4,000 clicks in one 10-hour shift. EHRs may also present clinicians with more alerts than they can effectively manage. For example, many comprehensive EHR systems automatically generate alerts in response to abnormal diagnostic testing results, but Singh and colleagues (2013) found that information overload may contribute to clinicians missing test results. Almost 70 percent of clinicians surveyed said that they received more alerts than they could effectively manage, and almost 30 percent of clinicians reported that they had personally missed alerts that resulted in patient care delays.

Makam and colleagues (2013) found that clinicians spend an appreciable amount of time using EHRs outside of their clinic hours. Almost half of the clinicians they surveyed reported that completing EHR documentation for each scheduled half-day clinic session required 1 or more extra hours of work, and 30 percent reported that they spent at least 1 extra hour communicating electronically with patients, even though they may not get paid for this time. Howard and colleagues (2013, p. 107) found mixed results on work burden when they studied small, independent, community-based primary care practices: "EHR use reduced some clinician work (i.e., prescribing, some lab-related tasks, and communication within the office), while increasing other work (i.e., charting, chronic disease and preventive care tasks, and some lab-related tasks)."

Measurement Capability

Health IT can also be used to measure diagnostic errors by leveraging the vast amounts of patient data contained in health IT databases (Shenvi and El-Kareh, 2014; Singh et al., 2007b, 2012). For instance, algorithms can be developed that periodically scan EHRs for diagnostic errors or clinical scenarios that suggest a diagnostic error has occurred. An example of the former would be cases of patients with newly diagnosed pulmonary embolism who were seen in the 2 weeks preceding diagnosis by an outpatient or emergency department clinician with symptoms that may have indicated pulmonary embolism (e.g., cough, shortness of breath, chest pain). An example of the latter may be patients who are hospitalized or seen in the emergency department within 2 weeks of an unscheduled outpatient visit, which may be suggestive of a failure to correctly diagnosis the patient at the first visit (Singh et al., 2007b, 2012; Sittig and Singh, 2012). In both of these instances, health IT systems need to incorporate user-friendly platforms that enable health care organizations to measure diagnostic errors or surrogate measures. For health IT systems that are used by multiple health care organizations or across multiple settings (inpatient and outpatient), common platforms for measuring diagnostic errors will permit comparisons of diagnostic error rates across organizations and settings. Improving the identification of diagnostic errors is an important recommendation of this committee (see Chapter 6), and health IT vendors should facilitate efforts to do so by developing tools that enable organizations to more easily determine the rates of diagnostic errors, especially those that are common and that have serious implications for patients (e.g., pulmonary embolism, acute myocardial infarction, and stroke).

Fit Within Clinical Workflow

The diagnostic process is not a single task, but rather a series of tasks that involve multiple people across the health care continuum. Clinical workflow, or the sequence of physical and cognitive tasks performed by various people within and between work environments, affects the diagnostic process at many junctures (Carayon et al., 2010). A critical element of workflow is health IT: Effective integration of health IT into the clinical workflow is essential for preventing diagnostic errors. However, integrating health IT into the clinical workflow is made more difficult by the wide range of workflows used by different individuals participating in the diagnostic process, both within one setting and across care settings. According to HIMSS, there are more than 50 physician specialties, and each of these specialties has its own software needs, including the unique software needs of the other health care professionals involved in that specialty (e.g., nurses, pharmacists, physical therapists, respiratory therapists, and medical dieticians). Each specialty may have different tasks that require a range of software interface designs (HIMSS, 2009). Furthermore, the actual clinical workflow does not always follow a formal, linear process; for example, orders may need to be executed before the proper administrative data, such as a patient's social security number, is entered or even known (Ash et al., 2004). As a result, health IT systems need both flexibility and modularity so that they can be tailored to specific workflow needs. Additionally, the time spent implementing and maintaining health IT systems may negatively impact workflow and even contribute to error (IOM, 2012a). For instance, EHR systems may become temporarily inaccessible because of software updates or network failure.

Clinical Documentation

Clinical documentation is central to patient care and often occupies a significant amount of clinicians' time (Hripcsak et al., 2011). Clinical documentation has been defined as "the process of recording historical data, observations, assessments, interventions, and care plans in an individual's health record. The purpose of documentation is to facilitate clinical reasoning and decision making by clinicians and promote communication and coordination of care among members of the care team" (Kuperman and Rosenbloom, 2013, p. 6). Beyond supporting patient care, clinical documentation also needs to meet requirements outside of the clinical care setting, including billing, accreditation, legal, and research purposes (Hripcsak and Vawdrey, 2013). Clinical documentation is used to justify the level of service billed to insurers, to collect information for research or quality improvement purposes, and to inform a legal record in case of litigation (Rosenbloom et al., 2011). For example, the electronic documentation of clinical decisions and activity, including both user-entered data and metadata, "may affect the course of malpractice litigation by increasing the availability of documentation with which to defend or prove a malpractice claim" (Magnalmurti et al., 2010, p. 2063). Payment and liability concerns, in combination with the growth in EHRs, have resulted in extensive and growing clinical documentation—sometimes referred to as "note bloat"—that has led to a situation in which key information in a patient's medical record can be obscured (Kuhn et al., 2015). A number of clinicians have expressed concern that clinical documentation is not promoting high-quality diagnosis and is instead primarily centered around billing and legal requirements, forcing clinicians to "focus on ticking boxes rather than on thoughtfully documenting their clinical thinking" (Schiff and Bates, 2010, p. 1066). In addition, research has shown that electronic documentation adds to clinicians' work burden: Intensive care unit residents and physicians spend substantially more time on clinical review and documentation after EHR implementation (Carayon et al., 2015). For example, extensive clinical documentation for justifying payment, facilitated by the copy and paste feature of EHRs, can contribute to cognitive overload and impede clinical reasoning. Chapter 7 further elaborates on how documentation guidelines for billing interfere with the diagnostic process and presents the committee's recommendation for how to better align documentation guidelines with clinical reasoning activities.

A major goal of using data collected within EHRs for legal, billing, and population-wide health management has led to a profusion of structured clinical documentation formats within health IT tools. However, structured documentation may cause problems for clinicians because they "value different factors when writing clinical notes, such as narrative expressivity, amenability to the existing workflow, and usability" (Rosenbloom et al., 2011, p. 181). Clinicians need to be able to record information efficiently and in ways that render it useful to other health care professionals involved in caring for a patient. Research has found "that in a shared context, concise, unconstrained, free-text communication is most effective for coordinating work around a complex task" (Ash et al., 2004, p. 106). There are also concerns that overly structured data entry has impacted clinicians' cognitive focus and abilities to focus on and attend to relevant information in the EHR (Ash et al., 2004).

Tools, such as speech recognition technology, have been developed to assist clinicians with clinical documentation, with varying degrees of success. Though several studies have found that voice recognition technology can improve the turnaround time of results reporting (Johnson et al., 2014; Prevedello et al., 2014; Singh and Pal, 2011), there are a number of issues associated with this technology that make it difficult to implement or may negatively impact the diagnostic process. This includes high implementation costs, the need for extensive user training, decreased report quality due to technology-related errors, and workflow interruptions (Bhan et al., 2008; de la Cruz, 2014; Fratzke et al., 2014; Houston and Rupp, 2000; Hoyt and Yoshihashi, 2010; Johnson et al., 2014; Quint et al., 2008).

Another technology that may help address the challenges of clinical documentation is natural language processing (Hripcsak and Vawdrey, 2013). Natural language processing extracts data from free text, converting clinicians' notes and narratives into structured, standardized formats. When the task is sufficiently constrained and when there is sufficient time to train the system, natural language processing systems can extract information with minimal effort and very high performance (Uzuner et al., 2008). Health IT vendors have begun to incorporate natural language processing software into EHRs. Additional technologies, particularly data mining, hold promise for improving clinical documentation in the future. Data mining "relies on the collective experience of all previous notes to steer how data should be entered in a new note" (Hripcsak and Vawdrey, 2013, p. 2). These technologies also hold promise for improving clinical decision support, discussed below.

Clinical Decision Support in Diagnosis

Health IT has the potential to support the diagnostic process through clinical decision support (CDS) tools. CDS provides clinicians and patients "with knowledge and person-specific information [that is] intelligently filtered or presented at appropriate times, to enhance health and health care" (HealthIT.gov, 2013). A number of studies have shown that clinical decision support systems can improve the rates of certain desirable clinician behaviors such as appropriate test ordering, disease management, and patient care (Carayon et al., 2010; Lobach and Hammond, 1997; Meigs et al., 2003; Roshanov et al., 2011; Sequist et al., 2005).

Diagnostic decision support tools can provide support to clinicians and patients throughout each stage of the diagnostic process, such as during information acquisition, information integration and interpretation, the formation of a working diagnosis, and the making of a diagnosis (Del Fiol et al., 2008; Zakim et al., 2008). Box 5-3 categorizes health IT tools according to the tasks they assist with in the diagnostic process (El-Kareh et al., 2013). Tools such as infobuttons can be integrated into EHRs and provide links to relevant online information resources, such as medical textbooks, clinical practice guidelines, and appropriateness criteria; there is evidence that infobuttons can help clinicians answer questions at the point of care and that they lead to a modest increase in the efficiency of information delivery (Del Fiol et al., 2008). CDS can also facilitate the ordering of the diagnostic tests that help clinicians develop accurate and timely diagnoses. In its input to the committee, the American College of Radiology stated that structured decision support for image ordering and reporting is critical for reducing diagnostic errors (Allen and Thorwarth, 2014). The Protecting Access to Medicare Act, passed in 2014, includes a provision that requires clinicians to use specified criteria when ordering advanced imaging procedures and directs the Department of Health and Human Services to identify CDS tools to help clinicians order these imaging procedures.[2] Given the growth of molecular testing and advanced

---

[2] Protecting Access to Medicare Act of 2014: www.congress.gov/bill/113th-congress/house-bill/4302 (accessed December 6, 2015).

BOX 5-3
Categories Describing Different Steps in Diagnosis
Targeted by Diagnostic Health Information Technology Tools

- Tools that assist in information gathering
- Cognition facilitation by enhanced organization and display of information
- Aids to the generation of a differential diagnosis
- Tools and calculators to assist in weighing diagnoses
- Support for the intelligent selection of diagnostic tests/plan
- Enhanced access to diagnostic reference information and guidelines
- Tools to facilitate reliable follow-up, assessment of patient course, and response
- Tools/alerts that support screening for the early detection of disease in asymptomatic patients
- Tools that facilitate diagnostic collaboration, particularly with specialists
- Systems that facilitate feedback and insight into diagnostic performance

SOURCE: El-Kareh et al., 2013. Reproduced from Use of health information technology to reduce diagnostic error. R. El-Kareh, O. Hasan, and G. Schiff. *BMJ Quality and Safety* 22(Suppl 2):ii40–ii51, with permission from BMJ Publishing Group Ltd.

---

imaging techniques, the importance of clinical decision support in aiding decisions involving this aspect of the diagnostic process is likely to increase.

Although decision support technologies have been around for quite some time (Weed and Weed, 2011; Weed and Zimny, 1989), there is still much room for progress. Questions about the validity and utility of diagnostic decision support tools still remain. A number of studies have assessed the performance of diagnostic decision support tools. Researchers such as Ramnarayan et al. (2003) have developed scores to measure the impact of diagnostic decision support on the quality of clinical decision making. These scores assess the performance of diagnostic decision support tools based on how often the "correct" diagnosis is produced by either the decision support system or by the clinicians after using the decision support; the scores also take into account the rank of the correct diagnosis on the list of differential diagnoses. There may be problems with these criteria, however; for example, rare diagnoses may be less likely to be considered because of a lower ranking. A review of four differential diagnosis generators found these tools to be "subjectively assistive and functional for clinical diagnosis and education" (Bond et al., 2012, p. 214). On a five-point scale (5 when the actual diagnosis was suggested on the first screen or in the first 20 suggestions, and 0 when no suggestions were close to the clinical diagnosis), the differential diagnosis generators received scores ranging from 1.70 to 3.45. Additional studies suggest that diagnostic decision support tools have the potential to improve the accuracy of diagnosis (Graber and Mathew, 2008; Kostopoulou et al., 2015; Ramnarayan et al., 2006, 2007). However, the studies assessing diagnostic decision support tools were conducted in highly controlled research settings; further research is needed to understand the performance of diagnostic decision support tools in clinical practice (see Chapter 8).

Though relatively early in its development, the application of new computational methods, such as artificial intelligence and natural language processing, has the potential to improve clinical decision support (Arnaout, 2012). For instance, these approaches can analyze large amounts of complex patient data (such as patient notes, diagnostic testing results, genetic information, as well as clinical and molecular profiles) and compare the results to "thousands of other patient EHRs to identify similarities and associations, thus, elucidating trends in disease course and management" (Castaneda, 2015, p. 12).

In addition to these efforts involving generalized decision support tools, there are also ongoing efforts to use decision support in radiology. One such decision support tool is computer-aided detection (CAD), which is designed to help radiologists during imaging interpretation by analyzing images for patterns associated with underlying disease (e.g., breast cancer during mammography screening). Despite the broad acceptance and use of CAD, there is mixed evidence demonstrating its effectiveness (Rao et al., 2010). Although CAD is not yet mature, the technology holds promise for improving detection.

Challenges with the usability and acceptability of diagnostic decision support have hindered adoption of these tools in clinical practice (Berner, 2014). For these tools to be useful, they need to be used only when appropriate, to be understandable, and to enable clinicians to quickly determine the level of urgency and relevancy. Decision support needs to function within the workflow and physical environment of the diagnostic process, which may include distractions and interruptions. If decision support tools are to be optimally designed, it will be necessary to consider tailoring the support to different users based on such factors as experience and workload. For example, a highly trained or highly experienced user may be better able to navigate a computer interface that is cumbersome than a less experienced user.[3] And the more experienced clinicians may need support to avoid pitfalls in diagnosis due to the use of system 1 processes, whereas more novice clinicians may need access to additional information to support system 2 processes. Research on how clinicians use

---

[3] Although a cumbersome interface may also be challenging to an experienced user.

technology may provide insight into the ways that human–automation interactions may be contributing to errors. EHR systems log users' actions through both user-entered data (i.e., timing of events and who performed them) and metadata. EHRs can also measure the rate at which clinicians override alerts and medication-dose defaults.

In addition, there are a number of potential patient safety risks associated with decision support. A systematic review found that an over-reliance on decision support has the potential to reduce independent clinician judgment and critical thinking (Goddard et al., 2012). A decision support tool could provide incorrect advice if it has incomplete information or applies outdated treatment guidelines (AHLA, 2013). This may place a clinician in a position in which he or she believes that the decision support is correct and therefore discounts his or her own assessment of the issue. Although Friedman and colleagues (1999) found that the use of clinical decision support was associated with a modest increase in diagnostic accuracy, in 6 percent of cases, clinicians overrode their own correct decisions due to erroneous advice from the decision support system. Informational content, as well as the presentation of information in decision support, can lead to adverse events. Adverse events relating to informational content are grouped around three themes: (1) changing roles and/or elimination of clinicians and staff, (2) the currency of CDS content, and (3) inaccurate or misleading CDS content. Adverse events relating to presentation of information are grouped by: (a) the rigidity of systems, (b) sources of alert fatigue, and (c) sources of potential errors (Ash et al., 2007).

Timely Flow of Information

The timely and effective exchange of information among health care professionals and patients is critical to improving diagnosis, and breakdowns in that communication are a major contributor to adverse events, including diagnostic errors (Gandhi et al., 2000; Poon et al., 2004; Schiff, 2005; Singh et al., 2007a). Health IT has the potential to reduce communication breakdowns, including breakdowns in intra- and interpersonal communication, in communication among patients and health care professionals, and in information exchange (e.g., the reporting of test results) (Singh et al., 2008). As discussed in Chapter 4, improved patient access to EHRs, including diagnostic testing results and clinical notes, can promote improved engagement in the diagnostic process and facilitate more timely information flow between and among patients and health care professionals. Health IT can also assist with the tracking of test results and follow-up (see Chapter 6). For example, the AMA (2014) concluded that EHRs can support care coordination if they "automatically track referrals and consultations as well as ensure that the referring physician is easily able to follow the patient's progress/activity throughout the continuum of care" (p. 5).

However, health IT tools may not be facilitating optimal communication among health care professionals, and they may even contribute to communication breakdowns. For example, Parkash and colleagues (2014) found that EHRs may not alert clinicians when surgical pathology reports have been amended, which may result in an incorrect diagnosis that is based on the original pathology report, an incorrect treatment plan, and the potential for serious consequences for a patient. A lack of interoperability (discussed below) can also prevent the timely flow of information among health care professionals.

Furthermore, another effect of health IT tools may be a reduction in informal, in-person collaborations between clinicians that can facilitate insights into the diagnostic process. In-person consultation between treating clinicians and the radiology department was common prior to the computerization of radiology and the introduction of the picture archiving communications system (Wachter, 2015). With the transition to filmless radiology systems, there has been a decrease in in-person consultations with the radiology department (Reiner et al., 1999).

An example of the importance of the timely flow of information is illustrated by the delayed diagnosis of Ebola in a Dallas emergency department (see Box 5-4). As the committee was deliberating in 2014, the most widespread outbreak yet seen of the Ebola virus occurred (CDC, 2015). Although the epidemic was primarily localized to several West African countries, the United States experienced its first case of Ebola virus in September 2014, a highly publicized example of diagnostic error. The committee included this case because it demonstrates the complex etiology of diagnostic error, including the roles that health IT and interprofessional communication play in conveying information in the diagnostic process.

INTEROPERABILITY OF HEALTH IT

Another health IT–related challenge in the diagnostic process is the lack of interoperability, or the inability of different IT systems and software applications to communicate, exchange data, and use the information that has been exchanged (HIMSS, 2014). It is not unusual for the diagnostic process to occur over a protracted period of time, with multiple clinicians across different care settings involved in the process. A free flow of information is critical to ensuring accurate and timely diagnoses because in order for health care professionals to develop a complete picture of a patient's health problem, all relevant health information needs to be available and accessible. A lack of interoperability can impede the

BOX 5-4
A Case of Diagnostic Error:
Delayed Diagnosis of Ebola Virus Infection

Case History

Thomas Eric Duncan traveled from Liberia to the United States in September 2014. He visited a Texas area emergency department on September 25, presenting with nonspecific symptoms, including fever, nausea, abdominal pain, and a severe headache, symptoms that can be attributed to a number of common acute illnesses (Upadhyay et al., 2014). Mr. Duncan informed the triage nurse of his recent travel from Africa (Dunklin and Thompson, 2014). The electronic health record (EHR) indicated that Mr. Duncan arrived with a fever of 100°F, which spiked to 103°F, and then dropped to 101°F prior to discharge (*Dallas Morning News*, 2014; Energy & Commerce Committee, 2014; Upadhyay et al., 2014). The physician who evaluated Mr. Duncan during this visit was not aware of his travel history (*Dallas Morning News*, 2014). Mr. Duncan underwent a series of tests, including a computed tomographic scan, and was released with a diagnosis of sinusitis, but a later evaluation found that the imaging results were not consistent with this diagnosis (Upadhyay et al., 2014). Mr. Duncan returned to the hospital on September 28 via ambulance (Energy & Commerce Committee, 2014; Upadhyay et al., 2014). On September 30 he was confirmed to have the Ebola virus (Energy & Commerce Committee, 2014), and on October 8 Mr. Duncan died from this infection. The hospital accepted responsibility for the diagnostic error (Upadhyay et al., 2014).

The chief clinical officer of Texas Health Resources stated in testimony to the U.S. Congress, "Unfortunately, in our initial treatment of Mr. Duncan, despite our best intentions and a highly skilled medical team, we made mistakes. We did not correctly diagnose his symptoms as those of Ebola. We are deeply sorry" (Energy & Commerce Committee, 2014).

Discussion

Current evidence suggests that patients seen in the emergency department are at high risk of experiencing diagnostic errors because of the range of conditions seen, the time pressures involved, and complexity of the work system environment (Campbell et al., 2007). As illustrated in this case of diagnostic error, a number of factors typically contribute to many adverse safety events (Graber, 2013).

Patient history and physical exam often suggest the correct diagnosis (Peterson et al., 1992). In this example, Mr. Duncan's travel history was especially relevant to his medical condition (*Dallas Morning News*, 2014). Although the travel history was obtained by the nurse, the physician examining Mr. Duncan told the *Dallas Morning News* that the "travel information was not easily visible in my standard workflow" (*Dallas Morning News*, 2014). Communication breakdowns likely contributed to this diagnostic error: The travel history may not have been communicated or communicated adequately among the patient and his care team. Additionally, the significance of this information may not have been considered during the diagnostic process (Dunklin and Thompson, 2014; Upadhyay et al., 2014). Without knowledge of the travel history, the physician chose a much more common condition as the possible explanation (Dunklin and Thompson, 2014).

Although most diagnostic errors involve common conditions, this case illustrates the problem of diagnosing rare diseases (zebras), when much more common diseases (horses) could explain similar symptoms. There is no easy solution to this problem. The challenge has been well described in Atul Gawande's book *Complications*, when he compared a necrotizing fasciitis diagnosis with cellulitis. In considering such a rare diagnosis, he said, "I felt a little foolish considering the diagnosis—it was a bit like thinking the Ebola virus had walked into the ER" (Gawande, 2002, p. 233).

Understanding the information flow and communication breakdowns in this case is a more challenging task (Upadhyay et al., 2014). The nurse documented the travel history in the nursing note, which was not considered by the physician. This raised a number of questions:

- Was documentation in the EHR sufficient to convey this information?
- When is verbal communication of key facts necessary?
- Was the EHR designed appropriately to support sharing of important information?
- Are the notes in EHRs too hard to locate and share in the typical workflow of a busy emergency department?
- Are notes valued appropriately by members of the care team?
- Does the format of a nursing note (template versus unstructured) influence how key information is communicated?

After the diagnostic error of Ebola occurred, Texas Presbyterian implemented a number of organizational and technological changes intended to reduce the risk of similar errors in the future. A public statement outlining the lessons learned and responses to this diagnostic error included

- "Upgraded medical record software to highlight travel risks
- New triage procedures initiated to quickly identify at-risk individuals
- A triage procedure to move high-risk patients immediately from the emergency department
- A final step for cleared patients: 30 minutes prior to discharge, vital signs will be rechecked. If anything is abnormal, the physician will be notified
- Increased emphasis on face-to-face communication." (Watson, 2014)

Teaching Points

1. Although diagnostic errors typically involve common conditions, patients with unusual or rare conditions are at high risk for diagnostic error if their symptoms mimic those of more common conditions.
2. The etiology of a diagnostic error is typically multifactorial. The various contributions of the work system, including the cognitive characteristics of clinicians and the complex interactions between them, can best be understood by adopting a human factors perspective.
3. Breakdowns in information flow and communication are some of the most common factors identified in cases of diagnostic error, just as they are in other major patient safety adverse events.
4. Although EHR technology provides many advantages to the diagnostic process, it can also cause a predisposition to certain types of errors, such as ineffective search for important information.

diagnostic process because it can limit or delay access to the data available for clinical decision making. When health care systems do not exchange data, clinical information may be inaccurate or inadequate. For instance, one version of a patient's EHR may exist on the primary clinical information system while a variety of outdated or partial versions of the record are present in other places. Furthermore, the record on the primary clinical information system may not necessarily be complete.

Given the importance of the free flow of information to diagnosis, ONC can play a critical role in improving interoperability. The vision that ONC has articulated for the interoperability of health IT is of an "ecosystem that makes the right data available to the right people at the right time across products and organizations in a way that can be relied upon and meaningfully used by recipients" (ONC, 2014a, p. 2). By 2024, ONC anticipates that individuals, clinicians, communities, and researchers will have access to a variety of interoperable products. However, the progress toward achieving health information exchange and interoperability has been slow (CHCF, 2014). For example, office-based exchange of information remains low; a study conducted by Furukawa et al. (2014) found that only 14 percent of the clinicians surveyed reported sharing data with clinicians outside their organization. Recognizing that progress in interoperability is critical to improving the diagnostic process, the committee calls on ONC to more rapidly require that health IT systems meet interoperability requirements. **Thus, the committee recommends that ONC should require health IT vendors to meet standards for interoperability among different health IT systems to support effective, efficient, and structured flow of patient information across care settings to facilitate the diagnostic process by 2018.** This recommendation is in line with the recent legislation that repealed the sustainable growth rate, which included a provision that declared it a national objective to "achieve widespread exchange of health information through interoperable certified [EHR] technology nationwide by December 31, 2018."[4] The law requires the Secretary of Health and Human Services (HHS) to develop metrics to evaluate progress on meeting this objective by July 2016. Furthermore, the legislation stipulates that if interoperability has not been achieved by 2018, the Secretary is required to submit a report to Congress in 2019 that identifies the barriers and makes recommendations for federal government action to achieve interoperability, including adjusting payments for not being meaningful EHR users and criteria for decertifying certified EHR technology products.

Improved interoperability across different health care organizations—as well as across laboratory and radiology information systems—is criti-

_____
[4] Medicare Access and CHIP Reauthorization Act of 2015. P.L. 114-10 (April 16, 2015).

cal to improving the diagnostic process. Challenges to interoperability include the inconsistent and slow adoption of standards, particularly among organizations that are not subject to EHR certification programs, as well as a lack of incentives, including a business model that generates revenue for health IT vendors via fees associated with transmitting and receiving data (Adler-Milstein, 2015; CHCF, 2014). The IOM report *Health IT and Patient Safety: Building a Safer Health System* recognized interoperability as a key feature of safely functioning health IT and noted that interoperability needs to be in place across the entire health care continuum: "Currently, laboratory data have been relatively easy to exchange because good standards exist such as Logical Observation Identifiers Names and Codes (LOINC) and are widely accepted. However, important information such as problem lists and medication lists (which exist in some health IT products) are not easily transmitted and understood by the receiving health IT product because existing standards have not been uniformly adopted" (IOM, 2012a, p. 86). Although laboratory data may be relatively easy to exchange, a recent report noted that the lack of incentives (or penalties) for organizations that are not subject to the EHR certification process under the Medicare and Medicaid EHR Incentive Programs (such as clinical laboratories) also contributes to poor interoperability (CHCF, 2014).

Additionally, the interface between EHRs and laboratory and radiology information systems typically has limited clinical information, and the lack of sufficiently detailed information makes it difficult for a pathologist or radiologist to determine the proper context for interpreting findings or to decide whether diagnostic testing is appropriate (Epner, 2015). For example, one study found that important non-oncological conditions (such as Crohn's disease, human immunodeficiency virus, and diabetes) were not mentioned in 59 percent of radiology orders and the presence of cancer was not mentioned in 8 percent of orders, demonstrating that the complete patient context is not getting received (Obara et al., 2015). Insufficient clinical information can be problematic as radiologists and pathologists often use this information to inform their interpretations of diagnostic testing results and suggestions for next steps (Alkasab et al., 2009; Obara et al., 2015). In addition, the Centers for Disease Control and Prevention's Clinical Laboratory Improvement Advisory Committee (CLIAC) expressed concern over the patient safety risks regarding the interoperability of laboratory data and display discrepancies in EHRs (CDC, 2014; CLIAC, 2012). They recommended that laboratory health care professionals collaborate with other stakeholders to "develop effective solutions to reduce identified patient safety risks in and improve the safety of EHR systems" regarding laboratory data (CDC, 2014, p. 3). There have been some efforts to improve the transmission of clinical context with diagnostic testing orders; for example, a quality improvement initiative in the outpatient and emergency department settings was able to improve the consistency with which radiology orders were accompanied by a complete clinical history (Hawkins et al., 2014).

Another emerging challenge is the interoperability between EHRs and patient-facing health IT, such as physical activity data, glucose monitoring, and other health-related applications (see section on mHealth) (Marceglia et al., 2015; Otte-Trojel et al., 2014).[5]

Economic incentives are another barrier to achieving interoperability. Current market conditions create business incentives for information blocking, that is, "when persons or entities knowingly and unreasonably interfere with the exchange or use of electronic health information" (ONC, 2015, p. 8). A variety of persons or entities may engage in information blocking practices, but most complaints of information blocking are related to the actions of health IT developers. Health IT vendors may "charge fees that make it cost-prohibitive for most customers to send, receive, or export electronic health information stored in EHRs, or to establish interfaces that enable such information to be exchanged" (ONC, 2015, p. 15). For instance, clinicians may pay $5,000 to $50,000 each to secure the right to set up connections that allow them to transmit information regularly to laboratories, health information exchanges, or governments (Allen, 2015). Additional fees may be charged each time a clinician sends, receives, or even searches for (or "queries") data (ONC, 2015). Health care organizations are also capable of engaging in information blocking. For instance, larger hospital systems that already capture a large proportion of patients' clinical information internally may be less motivated to join health information exchanges. In such instances, "information is seen as a tool to retain patients within their system, not as a tool to improve care" (Tsai and Jha, 2014, p. 29).

Issues related to data security and privacy will need to be considered as interoperability and health information exchange increases. The personal information stored within health IT systems needs to be secure. However, these data also need to be easily available when patients move from one system to another. Transparency will become increasingly important as interoperability improves and as data aggregation for quality improvement and population health management becomes more common. The ONC recognizes that it will be important to "support greater transparency for individuals regarding business practices of entities that use their data, particularly those that are not covered by the HIPAA [Health Insurance Portability and Accountability Act] Privacy and Security Rules" (ONC, 2014a, p. 5).

---

[5] Interoperability is one challenge surrounding patient-facing technologies; there are also other important considerations, such as vetting the quality of patient-reported data.

SAFETY OF HEALTH IT IN DIAGNOSIS

Patient safety risks related to the use of health IT in the diagnostic process are an important concern because there is growing recognition that health IT can result in adverse events (IOM, 2012a; ONC, 2014b; Walker et al., 2008), including sentinel events that result in permanent patient harm or death (The Joint Commission, 2015b). Such health IT safety risks have been described in the context of a sociotechnical system, in which the system components (including technology, people, workflow, organizational factors, and external environment) can dynamically interact and contribute to adverse events (IOM, 2012a; Sittig and Singh, 2010). A number of health IT–related patient safety risks may affect the diagnostic process and the occurrence of diagnostic errors. For example, challenges with the usability of EHRs have led to work-arounds from their intended use; although many of these work-arounds are benign, there is the potential for negative effects on patient safety and diagnosis (Ash et al., 2004; Friedman et al., 2014; IOM, 2012a; Koppel et al., 2008). Clinical documentation in the EHR and the use of the copy and paste functionality of EHRs are areas of increased concern. While the use of copy and paste functionality may increase efficiency by saving time that would otherwise be spent retyping or reentering information, it carries with it a number of risks, including redundancy that contributes to lengthy notes and cognitive overload as well as the spreading of inaccurate, outdated, or incomprehensible information (AHIMA, 2014; The Joint Commission, 2015a; Kuhn et al., 2015). New safety risks may also include errors related to entering and retrieving information (such as juxtaposition errors), errors in communication and coordination (mistaking information entry into an EHR system as a successful communication act), and health IT system maintainability (Ash et al., 2004). For instance, a pathologist may assume that the entry of new test results into an EHR system means that the results have been communicated to the clinician, even though this may not be the case (documentation in the EHR is not necessarily equivalent to communication).

Unfortunately, contractual provisions, intended to protect vendors' intellectual property interests and liability from the unsafe use of health IT products, limit the free exchange of information about health IT–related patient safety risks (IOM, 2012a). Specifically, "some vendors require contract clauses that force [health IT] system purchasers to adopt vendor-defined policies that prevent the disclosure of errors, bugs, design flaws, and other [health IT]-software-related hazards" (Goodman et al., 2011, p. 77). These contractual barriers may propagate safety risks and pose significant challenges to the use of data for future patient safety and quality improvement research (IOM, 2012a). In recognition of these challenges, the American Medical Informatics Association board of directors convened a task force to help resolve issues surrounding vendor–user contracts and made a number of suggestions for improving health IT contract language (see Box 5-5). Westat prepared a report for ONC that provides an overview of the key contract terms for health care organizations to be aware of when negotiating agreements with health IT vendors (Westat, 2013).

BOX 5-5
Recommendations from an American Medical Informatics Association Special Task Force on Health Information Technology Contracts

1. Contracts should not contain language that prevents system users, including clinicians and others, from using their best judgment about what actions are necessary to protect patient safety. This includes freedom to disclose system errors or flaws, whether introduced or caused by the vendor, the client, or any other third party. Disclosures made in good faith should not constitute violations of [health information technology (health IT)] contracts. This recommendation neither entails nor requires the disclosure of trade secrets or of intellectual property.
2. Hospitals, physician purchasers, and other users should understand that commercial products' screen designs and descriptions of software-supported workflows represent corporate assets developed at a cost to software vendors. Unless doing so would prematurely prevent disclosure of flaws, users should consider obligations to protect vendors' intellectual property and proprietary materials when disclosing (potential) flaws. Users should understand and accept their obligation to notify vendors before disclosing such features, and be aware of the range of remedies available to both the purchaser and the vendor in addressing safety issues. Equally, or more important, users should consider obligations to protect patient safety via such disclosures.
3. Because vendors and their customers share responsibility for patient safety, contract provisions should not attempt to circumvent fault and should recognize that both vendors and purchasers share responsibility for successful implementation. For example, vendors should not be absolved from harm resulting from system defects, poor design or usability, or hard-to-detect errors. Similarly, purchasers should not be absolved from harm resulting from inadequate training and education, inadequate resourcing, customization, or inappropriate use.
4. While vendors have legitimate corporate interests and duties (e.g., to shareholders), contract language should make explicit a commitment by all parties to patient care and safety, and, as applicable, to biomedical research and public health.
5. Vendors should be protected from claims in which a facility (hospital, medical office, practitioner, etc.) causes errors that cannot reasonably be attributed to a defect in the design or manufacture of a product, or to vendor-related problems in installation, updating, or configuration processes. Similarly, vendors should

In line with the movement toward more transparency, the IOM report on patient safety and health IT recommended that the Secretary of HHS "should ensure insofar as possible that health IT vendors support the free exchange of information about health IT experiences and issues and not prohibit sharing of such information, including details (e.g., screenshots) relating to patient safety" (IOM, 2012a, p. 7). **The committee endorses**

not be held responsible for circumstances in which users make foolish or intentional errors.

6. "Hold harmless" clauses in contracts between electronic health application vendors and purchasers or clinical users, if and when they absolve the vendors of responsibility for errors or defects in their software, are unethical. Some of these clauses have stated in the past that [health IT] vendors are not responsible for errors or defects, even after vendors have been informed of problems.

7. A collaborative system or process of third- or neutral-party dispute resolution should be developed. Contracts should contain language describing a process for timely and, as appropriate, transparent conflict resolution.

8. Contracts should make explicit a mechanism by which users/clients can communicate problems to the company; and vendors should have a mechanism for dealing with such problems (compare in this regard the processes in place for adverse event and device failure tracking by implantable medical device manufacturers).

9. Contracts should require that system defects, software deficiencies, and implementation practices that threaten patient safety should be reported, and information about them be made available to others, as appropriate. Vendors and their customers, including users, should report and make available salient information about threats to patient safety resulting from software deficiencies, implementation errors, and other causes. This should be done in a way easily accessible to customers and to potential customers. This information, when provided to customers, should be coupled with applicable suggested fixes, and should not be used to penalize those making the information available. Disclosure of information should not create legal liability for good-faith reporting. Large [health IT] systems undergo thousands of revisions when looked at on a feature-by-feature basis. Requirements that the vendor notify every customer of every single feature change on a real-time basis would have the unintended result of obscuring key safety risks, as customers would have to bear the expense of analyzing thousands of notifications about events which are typically rare. Therefore, vendors should notify customers as soon as possible about any product or configuration issues (1) of which they are aware and (2) which pose a risk to patients.

SOURCE: K. W. Goodman, E. S. Berner, M. A. Dente, B. Kaplan, R. Koppel, D. Rucker, D. Z. Sands, and P. Winkelstein, Challenges in ethics, safety, best practices, and oversight regarding HIT vendors, their customers, and patients: A report of an AMIA special task force, *Journal of the American Medical Informatics Association*, 2011,18(1):77–81, by permission of the American Medical Informatics Association.

this recommendation and further recommends that the Secretary of HHS should require health IT vendors to permit and support the free exchange of information about real-time user experiences with health IT design and implementation that adversely affect the diagnostic process. Health IT users can discuss patient safety concerns related to health IT products used in the diagnostic process in appropriate forums. Such forums include the forthcoming ONC Patient Safety Center or patient safety organizations (see Chapter 7) (RTI International, 2014; Sittig et al., 2014a). In addition, the Agency for Healthcare Research and Quality has developed a Common Format reporting form for health IT adverse events and ONC is beginning to evaluate patient safety events related to health IT (ONC, 2014b).

Because the safety of health IT is critical for improvements to the diagnostic process, health IT vendors need to proactively monitor their products in order to identify potential adverse events, which could contribute to diagnostic errors and challenges in the diagnostic process (Carayon et al., 2011). To ensure that their products are unlikely to contribute to diagnostic errors and adverse events, vendors need to have independent third-party evaluations performed on whichever of their health IT products are used in the diagnostic process. **Thus, the committee recommends that the Secretary of HHS should require health IT vendors to routinely submit their products for independent evaluation and notify users about potential adverse effects on the diagnostic process related to the use of their products.** Health IT vendors may consider using self-assessment tools, such as the SAFER guides, to prepare for the evaluations (Sittig et al., 2014b). If health IT products have the potential to contribute to diagnostic errors or have other adverse effects on the diagnostic process, health IT vendors have a responsibility to communicate this information to their customers in a timely manner.

OTHER DIAGNOSTIC TECHNOLOGIES

In addition to health IT, several emerging technologies, such as telemedicine/telehealth and mHealth/wearable technologies, present opportunities to improve the diagnostic process. This section examines the use of these technologies by health care professionals and patients to improve the diagnostic process.[6]

---

[6] The use of emerging technologies in diagnosis and treatment raises a number of regulatory, legal, and policy issues that are beyond the scope of this discussion (such as privacy and security concerns, payment, credentialing, licensure, program integrity, liability, and others).

Telemedicine and Telehealth

Although the definitions vary, telemedicine and telehealth generally refer to the delivery of care, consultations, and information using communications technology (American Telemedicine Association, 2015). A 2012 IOM workshop defined both telemedicine and telehealth, saying that they "describe the use of medical information exchanged from one site to another via electronic communications to improve the patient's health status. Although evolving, telemedicine is sometimes associated with direct patient clinical services and telehealth is sometimes associated with a broader definition of remote health care services" (IOM, 2012b, p. 3). Telemedicine encompasses an increasing array of applications and services, such as "two-way video, e-mail, smart phones, wireless tools, and other forms of telecommunication technology" (American Telemedicine Association, 2015).

Telemedicine typically is used in two settings: (1) between a clinician and a patient who is in a different location or (2) between two clinicians for consultations. The transmission of images, data, and sound can take place either synchronously (real-time), where the consulting clinician participates in the examination of the patient while diagnostic information is collected and transmitted, or asynchronously (anytime), through store-and-forward technology that transmits digital information for the consulting clinician to review at a later time.

As new payment and care delivery models are being implemented and evaluated, there is a growing recognition of the potential for technological capabilities to improve patient accessibility to health care services and also to improve care coordination and affordability. Telemedicine can create additional options for how individuals receive health care, while lessening the dependence on traditional in-person methods of receiving medical treatment. Telemedicine arrangements have emerged in a number of medical specialties (e.g., radiology, pathology, dermatology, ophthalmology, cardiology, neurology, geriatrics, and psychiatry), certain hospital service lines (e.g., home health and dentistry), and certain patient populations (e.g., prison inmates).

Telemedicine poses a number of challenges in the diagnostic process that may differ from those in traditional health care visits. For example, in the absence of a prior patient–clinician relationship, a clinician may not know enough details about the patient's history to ask pertinent questions, which may lead clinicians to overutilize diagnostic testing (Huff, 2014). In addition, telemedicine approaches can limit a clinician's ability to perform a comprehensive physical exam; certain medical conditions cannot be diagnosed effectively via a telemedicine encounter (Robison, 2014). There is also the potential for technological failures and transmission errors during a telemedicine encounter that can impair the diagnostic process and medical evaluation (Carranza et al., 2010). It is important that both patients and clinicians fully understand the telemedicine process and its associated limitations and risks, including the scope of the diagnostic health care services that can be delivered safely through this medium. Additionally, health care professionals may need to document their findings differently in the absence of face-to-face interactions, given the absence of a comprehensive physical exam. Clinicians participating in telemedicine need to be attuned to care continuity and coordination issues and to effectively convey to their patients who has accountability over their care and whom they should contact for follow-up. Finally, health care professionals will need to keep abreast of professional standards of care and the relevant state laws that create heightened requirements for a particular telemedicine activity and which may affect the diagnostic process.

The following text provides an overview of telemedicine applications in radiology, pathology, and neurology.

Teleradiology

Teleradiology has been a forerunner in telemedicine arrangements "with on-call emergency reporting being used in over 70 percent of radiology practices in the United States and general teleradiology by 'nighthawk services' around the world" (Krupinski, 2014, p. 5). In these arrangements, outsourced, off-hour radiology interpretations are provided by physicians credentialed in the United States who are either located within the United States or abroad. Continuous developments in picture archiving and communication systems and radiology information systems have strengthened the overall teleradiology process, including image capture, storage, processing, and reporting. In response to such developments, there has been an increase in the sub-specialization of radiologists along systems- and disease-related specialties. Greater sub-subspecialization has led to increased expansion and utilization of teleradiology in major urban as well as rural and medically underserved areas (Krupinski, 2014).

Telepathology

Telepathology is currently being used in select locations for a variety of clinical applications, including the diagnosis of frozen section specimens, primary histopathological diagnoses, second opinion diagnoses, and subspecialty pathology consultations, although telemedicine approaches could also be considered for clinical pathology purposes (Dunn et al., 2009; Graham et al., 2009; Kayser et al., 2000; Massone et al., 2007). Telepathology involves a hub-site pathologist that can access a remote-site microscope and has the ability to control the movement of the slide and adjust magnification, focus, and lighting while the images are viewed on a computer screen (Dunn et al., 2009). Because the field selection is accomplished by the consultant, the information obtained, except for digital imaging capabilities, is functionally the same as the consultant would obtain using a microscope in his or her own office. By providing immediate access to off-site pathologists as well as direct access to subspecialty pathologists, telepathology has the potential to improve both diagnostic accuracy and speed (turnaround time) for the patients at the remote site. Moreover, a telepathology consultation allows the local pathologist and consulting pathologist to examine the case at the same time, which could improve the educational potential of the interaction because the local pathologist can observe firsthand the diagnostic approach employed by the consulting pathologist (Low, 2013).

Teleneurology

One application of telemedicine in neurology is telestroke, a widespread and growing practice model (Krupinski, 2014; Silva et al., 2012). Successful management of acute ischemic stroke is extremely time-dependent, which makes it particularly important to have technological tools that can facilitate acute stroke evaluation and management in rural areas and other areas underserved by neurologists and thus improve post-stroke outcomes (Rubin and Demaerschalk, 2014).

A recent Mayo Clinic study explored the efficiency of remote neurological assessments in diagnosing concussions in football players on the sidelines of games in rural Arizona. For the study, an off-site neurologist used a portable unit to perform neurological exams on players who had suffered possible head injuries and recommended whether the players were safe to return to the field (Vargas et al., 2012). These types of innovations may help facilitate the diagnostic process, especially for time-sensitive medical conditions.

mHealth and Wearable Technologies

mHealth applications[7] and wearable technologies[8] are transforming health care delivery for both health care professionals and patients, and

---

[7] Mobile applications are software programs that have been developed to run on a computer or mobile device to accomplish a specific purpose.

[8] Electronics embedded in watchbands, clothing, contact lenses, or other wearable equipment.

they have the potential to influence the diagnostic process. The recent proliferation of mHealth applications has resulted in a broad and evolving array of mHealth applications that are available to both clinicians and patients. mHealth applications are often designed to assist clinicians at the point of care and include drug reference guides, medical calculators, clinical practice guidelines, textbooks, literature search portals, and other decision support aids. Other mHealth applications are designed specifically for patients and facilitate the gathering of diagnostic data or assist patients in coordinating care by keeping track of their medical conditions, diagnostic tests, and treatments.

mHealth applications may augment traditional health care professional education by providing opportunities for interactive teaching and more personalized educational experiences for students. They also have the potential to support clinical decision making at the point of care (Boulos et al., 2014). A systematic review found an increase in the appropriateness of diagnostic and treatment decisions when mobile devices were used for clinical decision support, but the researchers who performed the study noted that the evidence was limited; thus, more research will be needed to draw reliable conclusions concerning whether and how these mobile devices help and in what circumstances and how they should be used (Divall et al., 2013). Other mHealth applications designed for clinicians may serve as an alternative to traditional health IT tools and have the potential to improve diagnosis in emergency or low-resource settings. For example, tablets could be used to view medical images, and recent evidence suggests that they are comparable to conventional picture archiving and communications systems or liquid-crystal display monitor systems in diagnosing several conditions, although further research is needed (Johnson et al., 2012; McLaughlin et al., 2012; Park et al., 2013). Smartphones have been used in conjunction with specialized attachments to make certain laboratory-based diagnostics more accessible (Laksanasopin et al., 2015). For example, an adaptor with electrocardiogram electrodes may transmit electrical data that can be used to detect abnormal heart rhythms (Lau et al., 2013). Future generations of such technologies may be even more advanced; there is an ongoing Qualcomm Tricorder XPRIZE in which teams are competing to build a device that can accurately diagnose 16 health conditions and assess five vital signs in real time (XPRIZE, 2015).

In response to an increasing demand from patients for self-monitoring tools, a plethora of patient-centered mHealth applications have become available. They can perform a variety of functions related to such lifestyle factors as weight management, activity levels, and smoking cessation. Patients may also leverage certain mHealth applications to actively participate in the diagnostic process, such as consumer symptom checkers, which offer patients access to targeted searches based on their symptoms and enable patients to compile their own differential diagnoses, print out the results, and compare their findings with their clinicians' findings. Other mHealth applications for patients, such as wearable technologies, are intended to facilitate data collection, and they offer an additional source of patient data which may improve clinicians' ability to diagnose certain conditions. For example, patients with diabetes may synchronize a glucometer attachment to their mobile device to track blood glucose and upload the data through an Internet connection (Cafazzo et al., 2012).

Despite the potential for mHealth applications to improve diagnosis, a number of challenges remain. In particular, the quality of mobile applications can be quite variable, and there are concerns about the accuracy and safety of these applications, especially about how well they conform to evidence-based recommendations (Chomutare et al., 2011; Powell et al., 2014). For example, Semigran and colleagues (2015, p. h3480) evaluated available symptom trackers for patients and concluded that "symptom checkers had deficits in both triage and diagnosis." The evaluation found that the symptom checkers identified the correct diagnosis first in 34 percent of the cases, and they listed the correct diagnosis within the top 20 list in 58 percent of the cases (Semigran et al., 2015). Jutel and Lupton (2015, p. 94) call for further research of these applications given their variable development and quality—"the sheer number and constant proliferation of medical apps in general pose difficulties for regulatory agencies to maintain oversight of their quality and accuracy"—as well the impact of these applications on the patient–clinician relationship.

Furthermore, there is a lack of data that support or identify the best practices for their use, including integrating such technologies with EHRs, patient monitoring systems, and other health IT infrastructure (Mosa et al., 2012). Issues related to usability and health literacy will also need to be addressed in order to ensure that mHealth applications effectively meet user needs and facilitate the diagnostic process. The rapid pace of innovation and the evolving regulatory framework for mHealth are other challenges (Cortez et al., 2014).

RECOMMENDATION

Goal 3: Ensure that health information technologies support patients and health care professionals in the diagnostic process

Recommendation 3a: Health information technology (health IT) vendors and the Office of the National Coordinator for Health Information Technology (ONC) should work together with users to ensure that health IT used in the diagnostic process demonstrates

usability, incorporates human factors knowledge, integrates measurement capability, fits well within clinical workflow, provides clinical decision support, and facilitates the timely flow of information among patients and health care professionals involved in the diagnostic process.

Recommendation 3b: ONC should require health IT vendors to meet standards for interoperability among different health IT systems to support effective, efficient, and structured flow of patient information across care settings to facilitate the diagnostic process by 2018.

Recommendation 3c: The Secretary of Health and Human Services should require health IT vendors to:
- Routinely submit their products for independent evaluation and notify users about potential adverse effects on the diagnostic process related to the use of their products.
- Permit and support the free exchange of information about real-time user experiences with health IT design and implementation that adversely affect the diagnostic process.

REFERENCES

Adler-Milstein, J. 2015. America's health IT transformation: Translating the promise of electronic health records into better care. Paper presented before the U.S. Senate Committee on Health, Education, Labor and Pensions, March 17. www.help.senate.gov/imo/media/doc/Adler-Milstein.pdf (accessed June 5, 2015).

AHIMA (American Health Information Management Association). 2011. Problem List Guidance in the EHR. *Journal of AHIMA* 82(9):52–58.

AHIMA. 2014. Appropriate use of the copy and paste functionality in electronic health records. www.ahima.org/topics/ehr (accessed March 27, 2015).

AHLA (American Health Lawyers Association). 2013. Minimizing EHR-related serious safety events. www.mmicgroup.com/resources/industry-news-and-updates/2013/369-ahla-resource-to-minimize-ehr-related-serious-safety-events (accessed July 29, 2015).

AHRQ (Agency for Healthcare Research and Quality). 2010. Electronic Health Record Usability: Vendor Practices and Perspectives. AHRQ Publication No. 09(10)-0091-3-EF. Rockville, MD: Agency for Healthcare Research and Quality.

Alkasab, Tarik K., Jeannette Ryan Alkasab, and Hani H. Abujudeh. 2009. Effects of a computerized provider order entry system on clinical histories provided in emergency department radiology requisitions. *Journal of the American College of Radiology* 6(3):194–200.

Allen, A. 2015. Doctors say data fees are blocking health reform. *Politico*, February 23. www.politico.com/story/2015/02/data-fees-health-care-reform-115402.html (accessed June 6, 2015).

Allen, B., and W. T. Thorwarth. 2014. Comments from the American College of Radiology. Input submitted to the Committee on Diagnostic Error in Health Care, November 5 and December 29, 2014, Washington, DC.

AMA (American Medical Assocation). 2014. Improving care: Priorities to improve electronic health record usability. www.ama-assn.org/ama/pub/about-ama/strategic-focus/enhancing-professional-satisfaction-and-practice-sustainability.page (accessed February 9, 2015).

American Telemedicine Association. 2015. What is telemedicine? www.americantelemed.org/about-telemedicine/what-is-telemedicine#.VWHni0b9x7x (accessed May 24, 2015).

Arnaout, R. 2012. Elementary, my dear doctor watson. *Clinical Chemistry* 58(6):986–988.

Ash, J. S., M. Berg, and E. Coiera. 2004. Some unintended consequences of information technology in health care: The nature of patient care information system-related errors. *Journal of the American Medical Informatics Association* 11(2):104–112.

Ash, J. S., D. F. Sittig, E. M. Campbell, K. P. Guappone, and R. H. Dykstra. 2007. Some unintended consequences of clinical decision support systems. *AMIA Annual Symposium Proceedings* 26–30.

Basch, P. 2014. ONC's 10-year roadmap towards interoperability requires changes to the meaningful use program. http://healthaffairs.org/blog/2014/11/03/oncs-10-year-roadmap-towards-interoperability-requires-changes-to-the-meaningful-use-program (accessed March 27, 2015).

Berenson, R. A., P. Basch, and A. Sussex. 2011. Revisiting E&M visit guidelines—A missing piece of payment reform. *New England Journal of Medicine* 364(20):1892–1895.

Berner, E. S. 2014. What can be done to increase the use of diagnostic decision support systems? *Diagnosis* 1(1):119–123.

Bhan, S. N., C. L. Coblentz, and S. H. Ali. (2008). Effect of voice recognition on radiologist reporting time. *Canadian Association of Radiologists Journal* 59(4):203–209.

Bond, W. F., L. M. Schwartz, K. R. Weaver, D. Levick, M. Giuliano, and M. L. Graber. 2012. Differential diagnosis generators: An evaluation of currently available computer programs. *Journal of General Internal Medicine* 27(2):213–219.

Boulos, M. N., A. C. Brewer, C. Karimkhani, D. B. Buller, and R. P. Dellavalle. 2014. Mobile medical and health apps: State of the art, concerns, regulatory control and certification. *Online Journal of Public Health Informatics* 5(3):229.

Cafazzo, J. A., M. Casselman, N. Hamming, D. K. Katzman, and M. R. Palmert. 2012. Design of an mHealth app for the self-management of adolescent type 1 diabetes: A pilot study. *Journal of Medical Internet Research* 14(3):e70.

Campbell, S. G., P. Croskerry, and W. F. Bond. 2007. Profiles in patient safety: A "perfect storm" in the emergency department. *Academic Emergency Medicine* 14(8):743–749.

Carayon, P., T. B. Wetterneck, A. S. Hundt, S. Rough, and M. Schroeder. 2008. Continuous technology implementation in health care: The case of advanced IV infusion pump technology. In K. Zink (ed.), *Corporate sustainability As a challenge for comprehensive management* (pp. 139–151). New York: Springer.

Carayon, P., B.-T. Karsh, and R. S. Cartmill. 2010. *Incorporating health information technology into workflow redesign: Summary report.* AHRQ Publication No. 10-0098-EF. Rockville, MD: Agency for Healthcare Research and Quality.

Carayon, P., H. Faye, A. S. Hundt, B.-T. Karsh, and T. Wetterneck, T. 2011. Patient safety and proactive risk assessment. In Y. Yuehwern (ed.), *Handbook of Healthcare Delivery Systems* (pp. 12-1–12-15). Boca Raton, FL: Taylor & Francis.

Carayon, P., T. B. Wetterneck, B. Alyousef, R. L. Brown, R. S. Cartmill, K. McGuire, P. L. Hoonakker, J. Slagle, K. S. Van Roy, J. M. Walker, M. B. Weinger, A. Xie, and K. E. Wood. 2015. Impact of electronic health record technology on the work and workflow of physicians in the intensive care unit. *International Journal of Medical Informatics* 84(8):578–594.

Carranza, N., V. Ramos, F. G. Lizana, J. Garcia, A. del Pozo, and J. L. Monteagudo. 2010. A literature review of transmission effectiveness and electromagnetic compatibility in home telemedicine environments to evaluate safety and security. *Telemedicine Journal and E Health* 16(7):818–826.

Castaneda, C., K. Nalley, C. Mannion, P. Bhattacharyya, P. Blake, A. Pecora, A. Goy, and K. S. Suh. 2015. Clinical decision support systems for improving diagnostic accuracy and achieving precision medicine. *Journal of Clinical Bioinformatics* 5(1):4.

CDC (Centers for Disease Control and Prevention). 2014. The Essential Role of Laboratory Professionals: Ensuring the Safety and Effectiveness of Laboratory Data in Electronic Health Record Systems. www.cdc.gov/labhit/paper/Laboratory_Data_in_EHRs_2014.pdf (accessed July 27, 2015).

CDC. 2015. 2014 Ebola outbreak in West Africa. www.cdc.gov/vhf/ebola/outbreaks/2014-west-africa (accessed May 4, 2015).

CHCF (California HealthCare Foundation). 2014. Ten years in: Charting the progress of health information exchange in the U.S. www.chcf.org/~/media/MEDIA%20LIBRARY%20Files/PDF/T/PDF%20TenYearsProgressHIE.pdf (accessed February 9, 2015).

Chomutare, T., L. Fernandez-Luque, E. Arsand, and G. Hartvigsen. 2011. Features of mobile diabetes applications: Review of the literature and analysis of current applications compared against evidence-based guidelines. *Journal of Medical Internet Research* 13(3):e65.

CLIAC (Clinical Laboratory Improvement Advisory Committee). 2012. Letter to HHS Secretary. wwwn.cdc.gov/CLIAC/pdf/2012_Oct_CLIAC_%20to_Secretary_re_EHR.pdf (accessed August 11, 2015).

Cortez, N. G., I. G. Cohen, and A. S. Kesselheim. 2014. FDA regulation of mobile health technologies. *New England Journal of Medicine* 371(4):372–379.

CQPI (Center for Quality and Productivity Improvement). 2015. Usability tools. www.cqpi.wisc.edu/usability-tools.htm (accessed May 3, 2015).

Dallas Morning News. 2014. Full transcript: Dr. Joseph Howard Meier's responses to questions from The Dallas Morning News. www.dallasnews.com/ebola/headlines/20141206-full-transcript-dr.-joseph-howard-meier-s-responses-to-questions-from-the-dallas-morning-news.ece (accessed March 30, 2015).

de la Cruz, J. E., J. C. Shabosky, M. Albrecht, T. R. Clark, J. C. Milbrandt, S. J. Markwell, and J. A. Kegg. 2014. Typed versus voice recognition for data entry in electronic health records: Emergency physician time use and interruptions. *Western Journal of Emergency Medicine* 15(4):541–547.

Del Fiol, G., P. J. Haug, J. J. Cimino, S. P. Narus, C. Norlin, and J. A. Mitchell. 2008. Effectiveness of topic-specific infobuttons: A randomized controlled trial. *Journal of the American Medical Informatics Association* 15(6):752–759.

Divall, P., J. Camosso-Stefinovic, and R. Baker. 2013. The use of personal digital assistants in clinical decision making by health care professionals: A systematic review. *Health Informatics Journal* 19(1):16–28.

Dunklin, R., and S. Thompson. 2014. ER doctor discusses role in Ebola patient's initial misdiagnosis. *Dallas Morning News*, December 6. www.dallasnews.com/ebola/headlines/20141206-er-doctor-discusses-role-in-ebola-patients-initial-misdiagnosis.ece (accessed August 11, 2015).

Dunn, B. E., H. Choi, D. L. Recla, S. E. Kerr, and B. L. Wagenman. 2009. Robotic surgical telepathology between the Iron Mountain and Milwaukee Department of Veterans Affairs Medical Centers: A twelve year experience. *Seminars in Diagnostic Pathology* 26(4):187–193.

Dwoskin, E., and J. Walker. 2014. Can data from your fitbit transform medicine? *The Wall Street Journal,* June 23. www.wsj.com/articles/health-data-at-hand-with-trackers-1403561237 (accessed July 30, 2015).

El-Kareh, R., O. Hasan, and G. Schiff. 2013. Use of health information technology to reduce diagnostic error. *BMJ Quality and Safety* 22(Suppl 2):ii40–ii51.

Energy & Commerce Committee. 2014. Examining the U.S. public health response to the Ebola outbreak. Hearing. U.S. House of Representatives, Committee on Energy and Commerce, Subcommittee on Oversight and Investigations. October 16. http://energycommerce.house.gov/hearing/examining-us-public-health-response-ebola-outbreak (accessed June 6, 2015).

Epner, P. 2015. Input submitted to the Committee on Diagnostic Error in Health Care. January 13, 2015, Washington, DC.

Fratzke, J., S. Tucker, H. Shedenhelm, J. Arnold, T. Belda, and M. Petera. 2014. Enhancing nursing practice by utilizing voice recognition for direct documentation. *Journal of Nursing Administration* 44(2):79–86.

Friedman, A., J. C. Crosson, J. Howard, E. C. Clark, M. Pellerano, B. T. Karsh, B. Crabtree, C. R. Jaen, and D. J. Cohen. 2014. A typology of electronic health record workarounds in small-to-medium size primary care practices. *Journal of the American Medical Informatics Association* 21(e1):e78–e83.

Friedman, C. P., A. S. Elstein, F. M. Wolf, G. C. Murphy, T. M. Franz, P. S. Heckerling, P. L. Fine, T. M. Miller, and V. Abraham. 1999. Enhancement of clinicians' diagnostic reasoning by computer-based consultation: A multisite study of 2 systems. *JAMA* 282:1851–1856.

Furukawa, M. F., J. King, V. Patel, C. J. Hsiao, J. Adler–Milstein, and A. K. Jha. 2014. Despite substantial progress in EHR adoption, health information exchange and patient engagement remain low in office settings. *Health Affairs (Millwood)* 33(9):1672–1679.

Gandhi, T. K., D. F. Sittig, M. Franklin, A. J. Sussman, D. G. Fairchild, and D. W. Bates. 2000. Communication breakdown in the outpatient referral process. *Journal of General Internal Medicine* 15(9):626–631.

Gasson, S. 2003. Human-centered vs. user-centered approaches to information system design. *Journal of Information Technology Theory and Application* 5(2):29–46.

Gawande, A. 2002. *Complications: A surgeon's notes on an imperfect science.* New York: Picador.

Goddard, K., A. Roudsari, and J. C. Wyatt. 2012. Automation bias: A systematic review of frequency, effect mediators, and mitigators. *Journal of the American Medical Informatics Association* 19(1):121–127.

Goodman, K. W., E. S. Berner, M. A. Dente, B. Kaplan, R. Koppel, D. Rucker, D. Z. Sands, P. Winkelstein, and AMIA Board of Directors. 2011. Challenges in ethics, safety, best practices, and oversight regarding HIT vendors, their customers, and patients: A report of an AMIA special task force. *Journal of the American Medical Informatics Association* 18(1):77–81.

Graber, M. 2013. The incidence of diagnostic error in medicine. *BMJ Quality and Safety* 22(Suppl 2):ii21–ii27.

Graber, M. L., and A. Mathew. 2008. Performance of a web-based clinical diagnosis support system for internists. *Journal of General Internal Medicine* 23(Suppl 1):37–40.

Graham, A. R., A. K. Bhattacharyya, K. M. Scott, F. Lian, L. L. Grasso, L. C. Richter, J. B. Carpenter, S. Chiang, J. T. Henderson, A. M. Lopez, G. P. Barker, and R. S. Weinstein. 2009. Virtual slide telepathology for an academic teaching hospital surgical pathology quality assurance program. *Human Pathology* 40(8):1129–1136.

Greenhalgh, T., S. Hinder, K. Stramer, T. Bratan, and J. Russell. 2010. Adoption, non-adoption, and abandonment of a personal electronic health record: case study of HealthSpace. *BMJ* 341:c5814.

Harrington, L., D. Kennerly, and C. Johnson. 2011. Safety issues related to the electronic medical record (EMR): Synthesis of the literature from the last decade, 2000–2009. *Journal of Healthcare Management* 56(1):31–43; discussion 43–44.

Hartung, D. M., J. Hunt, J. Siemienczuk, H. Miller, and D. R. Touchette. 2005. Clinical implications of an accurate problem list on heart failure treatment. *Journal of General Internal Medicine* 20(2):143–147.

Hawkins, C. M., C. G. Anton, W. M. Bankes, A. D. Leach, M. J. Zeno, R. M. Pryor, and D. B. Larson. 2014. Improving the availability of clinical history accompanying radiographic examinations in a large pediatric radiology department. *American Journal of Roentgenology* 202(4):790–796.

HealthIT.gov. 2013. Clinical decision support (CDS). www.healthit.gov/policy-researchers-implementers/clinical-decision-support-cds (accessed June 6, 2015).

Hill, R. G., Jr., L. M. Sears, and S. W. Melanson. 2013. 4000 clicks: A productivity analysis of electronic medical records in a community hospital ED. *American Journal of Emergency Medicine* 31(11):1591–1594.

HIMSS (Healthcare Information and Management Systems Society). 2009. *Defining and testing EMR usability: Principles and proposed methods of EMR usability evaluation and rating.* Chicago, IL: HIMSS.

HIMSS. 2014. What is interoperability? www.himss.org/library/interoperability-standards/what-is-interoperability (accessed February 9, 2015).

Holmes, C., M. Brown, D. St. Hilaire, and A. Wright. 2012. Healthcare provider attitudes towards the problem list in an electronic health record: A mixed-methods qualitative study. *BMC Medical Informatics and Decision Making* 12(1):127.

Houston, J. D., and F. W. Rupp. 2000. Experience with implementation of a radiology speech recognition system. *Journal of Digital Imaging* 13(3):124–128.

Howard, J., E. C. Clark, A. Friedman, J. C. Crosson, M. Pellerano, B. F. Crabtree, B. T. Karsh, C. R. Jaen, D. S. Bell, and D. J. Cohen. 2013. Electronic health record impact on work burden in small, unaffiliated, community-based primary care practices. *Journal of General Internal Medicine* 28(1):107–113.

Hoyt, R., and A. Yoshihashi. 2010. Lessons learned from implementation of voice recognition for documentation in the military electronic health record system. Perspectives in health information management/AHIMA, *American Health Information Management Association* 7(Winter).

Hripcsak, G., and D. K. Vawdrey. 2013. Innovations in clinical documentation. Paper presented at HIT Policy Meaningful Use and Certification /Adoption Workgroups Clinical Documentation Hearing. Arlington, Virginia, February 13, 2013.

Hripcsak, G., D. K. Vawdrey, M. R. Fred, and S. B. Bostwick. 2011. Use of electronic clinical documentation: Time spent and team interactions. *Journal of the American Medical Informatics Association* 18(2):112–117.

Huff, C. 2014. Virtual visits pose real issues for physicians. www.acpinternist.org/archives/2014/11/virtual-visit.htm (accessed May 24, 2015).

IEA (International Ergonomics Assocation). 2000. The discipline of ergonomics. www.iea.cc/whats/index.html (accessed April 10, 2015).

IOM (Institute of Medicine). 2012a. *Health IT and patient safety: Building safer systems for better care.* Washington, DC: The National Academies Press.

IOM. 2012b. *The role of telehealth in an evolving health care environment.* Washington, DC: The National Academies Press.

ISO (International Organization for Standardization). 1998. Ergonomic requirements for office work with visual display terminals (VDTs)—Part 11: Guidance on usability. www.iso.org/obp/ui/#iso:std:iso:9241:-11:ed-1:v1:en (accessed February 25, 2015).

Jacobs, L. 2009. Interview with Lawrence Weed, MD—The father of the problem-oriented medical record looks ahead. *The Permanente Journal* 13(3):84–89.

Johnson, M., S. Lapkin, V. Long, P. Sanchez, H. Suominen, J. Basilakis, and L. Dawson. 2014. A systematic review of speech recognition technology in health care. *BMC Medical Informatics and Decision Making* 14(94).

Johnson, P. T., S. L. Zimmerman, D. Heath, J. Eng, K. M. Horton, W. W. Scott, and E. K. Fishman. 2012. The iPad as a mobile device for CT display and interpretation: Diagnostic accuracy for identification of pulmonary embolism. *Emergency Radiology* 19(4):323–327.

The Joint Commission. 2015a. Preventing copy-and-paste errors in the EHR. www.jointcommission.org/issues/article.aspx?Article=bj%2B%2F2w37MuZrouWveszI1we WZ7ufX%2FP4tLrLI85oCi0%3D (accessed March 27, 2015).

The Joint Commission. 2015b. Sentinel event alert. www.jointcommission.org/assets/1/18/SEA_54.pdf (accessed April 30, 2015).

Jutel, A., and D. Lupton. 2015. Digitizing diagnosis: A review of mobile applications in the diagnostic process. *Diagnosis* 2(2):89–96.

Kayser, K., M. Beyer, S. Blum, and G. Kayser. 2000. Recent developments and present status of telepathology. *Analytical Cellular Pathology* 21(3–4):101–106.

Koppel, R., T. Wetterneck, J. L. Telles, and B. T. Karsh. 2008. Workarounds to barcode medication administration systems: Their occurrences, causes, and threats to patient safety. *Journal of the American Medical Informatics Association* 15(4):408–423.

Kostopoulou, O., A. Rosen, T. Round, E. Wright, A. Douiri, and B. Delaney. 2015. Early diagnostic suggestions improve accuracy of GPs: A randomised controlled trial using computer-simulated patients. *British Journal of General Practice* 65(630):e49–e54.

Krupinski, E. A. 2014. Teleradiology: Current perspectives. *Reports in Medical Imaging* 2014(7):5–14.

Kuhn, T., P. Basch, M. Barr, and T. Yackel. 2015. Clinical documentation in the 21st century: Executive summary of a policy position paper from the American College of Physicians. *Annals of Internal Medicine* 162(4):301–303.

Kuperman, G., and S. T. Rosenbloom. 2013. Paper presented at HIT Policy Meaningful Use and Certification/Adoption Workgroups Clinical Documentation Hearing. Arlington, Virginia, February 13, 2013.

Laksanasopin, T., T. W. Guo, S. Nayak, A. A. Sridhara, S. Xie, O. O. Olowookere, P. Cadinu, F. Meng, N. H. Chee, J. Kim, C. D. Chin, E. Munyazesa, P. Mugwaneza, A. J. Rai, V. Mugisha, A. R. Castro, D. Steinmiller, V. Linder, J. E. Justman, S. Nsanzimana, and S. K. Sia. 2015. A smartphone dongle for diagnosis of infectious diseases at the point of care. *Science Translational Medicine* 7(273):273re1.

Lau, J. K., N. Lowres, L. Neubeck, D. B. Brieger, R. W. Sy, C. D. Galloway, D. E. Albert, and S. B. Freedman. 2013. iPhone ECG application for community screening to detect silent atrial fibrillation: A novel technology to prevent stroke. *International Journal of Cardiology* 165(1):193–194.

Lobach, D. F., and W. E. Hammond. 1997. Computerized decision support based on a clinical practice guideline improves compliance with care standards. *American Journal of Medicine* 102(1):89–98.

Low, J. 2013. Telepathology: Guidance from The Royal College of Pathologists. www.rcpath.org/Resources/RCPath/Migrated%20Resources/Documents/G/G026_Telepathology_Oct13.pdf (accessed May 24, 2015).

Makam, A. N., H. J. Lanham, K. Batchelor, L. Samal, B. Moran, T. Howell-Stampley, L. Kirk, M. Cherukuri, N. Santini, L. K. Leykum, and E. A. Halm. 2013. Use and satisfaction with key functions of a common commercial electronic health record: A survey of primary care providers. *BMC Medical Informatics and Decision Making* 13:86.

Mangalmurti, S. S., L. Murtagh, and M. M. Mello. 2010. Medical malpractice liability in the age of electronic health records. *New England Journal of Medicine* 363(21):2060–2067.

Marceglia, S., P. Fontelo, and M. J. Ackerman. 2015. Transforming consumer health informatics: Connecting CHI applications to the health-IT ecosystem. *Journal of the American Medical Informatics Association* 22(e1):e210–e212.

Massone, C., H. P. Soyer, G. P. Lozzi, A. Di Stefani, B. Leinweber, G. Gabler, M. Asgari, R. Boldrini, L. Bugatti, V. Canzonieri, G. Ferrara, K. Kodama, D. Mehregan, F. Rongioletti, S. A. Janjua, V. Mashayekhi, I. Vassilaki, B. Zelger, B. Zgavec, L. Cerroni, and H. Kerl. 2007. Feasibility and diagnostic agreement in teledermatopathology using a virtual slide system. *Human Pathology* 38(4):546–554.

McLaughlin, P., S. O. Neill, N. Fanning, A. M. Mc Garrigle, O. J. Connor, G. Wyse, and M. M. Maher. 2012. Emergency CT brain: Preliminary interpretation with a tablet device: Image quality and diagnostic performance of the Apple iPad. *Emergency Radiology* 19(2):127–133.

Meeks, D. W., M. W. Smith, L. Taylor, D. F. Sittig, J. M. Scott, and H. Singh. 2014. An analysis of electronic health record-related patient safety concerns. *Journal of the American Medical Informatics Association* 21(6):1053–1059.

Meigs, J. B., E. Cagliero, A. Dubey, P. Murphy-Sheehy, C. Gildesgame, H. Chueh, M. J. Barry, D. E. Singer, and D. M. Nathan. 2003. A controlled trial of web-based diabetes disease management: The MGH diabetes primary care improvement project. *Diabetes Care* 26(3):750–757.

Middleton, B., M. Bloomrosen, M. A. Dente, B. Hashmat, R. Koppel, J. M. Overhage, T. H. Payne, S. T. Rosenbloom, C. Weaver, J. Zhang, and American Medical Informatics Association. 2013. Enhancing patient safety and quality of care by improving the usability of electronic health record systems: Recommendations from AMIA. *Journal of the American Medical Informatics Association* 20(e1):e2–e8.

Moacdieh, N., and N. B. Sarter. 2015. Display clutter: A review of definitions and measurement techniques. *Human Factors* 57(1):61–100.

Mosa, A. S., I. Yoo, and L. Sheets. 2012. A systematic review of healthcare applications for smartphones. *BMC Medical Informatics and Decision Making* 12:67.

NIST (National Institute of Standards and Technology). 2015. Usability. www.nist.gov/healthcare/usability (accessed April 6, 2015).

Obara, P., M. Sevenster, A. Travis, Y. Qian, C. Westin, and P. J. Chang. 2015. Evaluating the referring physician's clinical history and indication as a means for communicating chronic conditions that are pertinent at the point of radiologic interpretation. *Journal of Digital Imaging* 28(3):272–282.

Ober, K. P. 2015. The electronic health record: Are we the tools of our tools? *The Pharos* 78(1):8–14.

O'Malley, A. S., K. Draper, R. Gourevitch, D. A. Cross, and S. H. Scholle. 2015. Electronic health records and support for primary care teamwork. *Journal of the American Medical Informatics Association* 22(2):426–434.

ONC (Office of the National Coordinator for Health Information Technology). 2014a. *Connecting health and care for the nation: A 10-year vision to achieve an interoperable health IT infrastructure.* Washington, DC: The Office of the National Coordinator for Health Information Technology. www.healthit.gov/sites/default/files/ONC10year InteroperabilityConceptPaper.pdf (accessed February 9, 2015).

ONC. 2014b. *Health information technology adverse event reporting: Analysis of two databases.* Washington, DC: Office of the National Coordinator for Health Information Technology.

ONC. 2015. *Report on health information blocking.* Washington, DC: Office of the National Coordinator for Health Information Technology. http://healthit.gov/sites/default/files/reports/info_blocking_040915.pdf (accessed April 10, 2015).

Otte-Trojel, T., A. de Bont, J. van de Klundert, and T. G. Rundall. 2014. Characteristics of patient portals developed in the context of health information exchanges: Early policy effects of incentives in the meaningful use program in the United States. *Journal of Medical Internet Research* 16(11):e258.

Park, J. B., H. J. Choi, J. H. Lee, and B. S. Kang. 2013. An assessment of the iPad 2 as a CT teleradiology tool using brain CT with subtle intracranial hemorrhage under conventional illumination. *Journal of Digital Imaging* 26(4):683–690.

Parkash, V., A. Domfeh, P. Cohen, N. Fischbach, M. Pronovost, G. K. Haines 3rd, and P. Gershkovich. 2014. Are amended surgical pathology reports getting to the correct responsible care provider? *American Journal of Clinical Pathology* 142(1):58–63.

Peterson, M. C., J. H. Holbrook, D. Von Hales, N. L. Smith, and L. V. Staker. 1992. Contributions of the history, physical examination, and laboratory investigation in making medical diagnoses. *Western Journal of Medicine* 156(2):163–165.

Poon, E. G., J. S. Haas, A. Louise Puopolo, T. K. Gandhi, E. Burdick, D. W. Bates, and T. A. Brennan. 2004. Communication factors in the follow-up of abnormal mammograms. *Journal of General Internal Medicine* 19(4):316–323.

Powell, A. C., A. B. Landman, and D. W. Bates. 2014. In search of a few good apps. *JAMA* 311(18):1851–1852.

Prevedello, L. M., S. Ledbetter, C. Farkas, and R. Khorasani. 2014. Implementation of speech recognition in a community-based radiology practice: Effect on report turnaround times. *Journal of the American College of Radiology* 11(4):402–406.

Quint, L. E., D. J. Quint, and J. D. Myles. 2008. Frequency and spectrum of errors in final radiology reports generated with automatic speech recognition technology. *Journal of the American College of Radiology* 5(12):1196–1199.

Ramirez, E. 2012. Talking data with your doc: The doctors. http://quantifiedself.com/2012/04/talking-data-with-your-doc-the-doctors (accessed July 30, 2015).

Ramnarayan, P., R. R. Kapoor, J. Coren, V. Nanduri, A. Tomlinson, P. M. Taylor, J. C. Wyatt, and J. Britto. 2003. Measuring the impact of diagnostic decision support on the quality of clinical decision making: Development of a reliable and valid composite score. *Journal of the American Medical Informatics Association* 10:563–572.

Ramnarayan, P., G. C. Roberts, M. Coren, V. Nanduri, A. Tomlinson, P. M. Taylor, J. C. Wyatt, and J. F. Britto. 2006. Assessment of the potential impact of a reminder system on the reduction of diagnostic errors: A quasi-experimental study. *BMC Medical Informatics and Decision Making* 6:22.

Ramnarayan, P., N. Cronje, R. Brown, R. Negus, B. Coode, P. Moss, T. Hassan, W. Hamer, and J. Britto. 2007. Validation of a diagnostic reminder system in emergency medicine: A multi-centre study. *Emergency Medicine Journal* 24(9):619–624.

Rao, V. M., D. C. Levin, L. Parker, B. Cavanaugh, A. J. Frangos, and J. H. Sunshine. 2010. How widely is computer-aided detection used in screening and diagnostic mammography? *Journal of the American College of Radiology* 7(10):802–805.

Reiner, B., E. Siegel, Z. Protopapas, F. Hooper, H. Ghebrekidan, and M. Scanlon. 1999. Impact of filmless radiology on frequency of clinician consultations with radiologists. *American Journal of Roentgenology* 173(5):1169–1172.

Robison, J. 2014. Two major insurers recognize telemedicine. *Las Vegas Review-Journal*, October 5. www.reviewjournal.com/business/two-major-insurers-recognize-telemedicine (accessed May 24, 2015).

Rosenbloom, S. T., J. C. Denny, H. Xu, N. Lorenzi, W. W. Stead, and K. B. Johnson. 2011. Data from clinical notes: A perspective on the tension between structure and flexible documentation. *Journal of the American Medical Informatics Association* 18(2):181–186.

Roshanov, P. S., J. J. You, J. Dhaliwal, D. Koff, J. A. Mackay, L. Weise-Kelly, T. Navarro, N. L. Wilczynski, and R. B. Haynes. 2011. Can computerized clinical decision support systems improve practitioners' diagnostic test ordering behavior? A decision-maker-researcher partnership systematic review. *Implementation Science* 6:88.

RTI International. 2014. RTI International to develop road map for health IT safety center. www.rti.org/newsroom/news.cfm?obj=FCC8767E-C2DA-EB8B-AD7E2F778E6CB91A (accessed March 27, 2015).

Rubin, M. N., and B. M. Demaerschalk. 2014. The use of telemedicine in the management of acute stroke. *Neurosurgery Focus* 36(1):E4.

Schiff, G. D. 2005. Introduction: Communicating critical test results. *Joint Commission Journal of Quality and Patient Safety* 31(2):63–65.

Schiff, G., and D. W. Bates. 2010. Can electronic clinical documentation help prevent diagnostic errors? *New England Journal of Medicine* 362(12):1066–1069.

Semigran, H.L., J.A. Linder, C. Gidengil, and A. Mehrotra. 2015. Evaluation of symptom checkers for self diagnosis and triage: Audit study. *BMJ* 351:h3480.

Sequist, T. D., T. K. Gandhi, A. S. Karson, J. M. Fiskio, D. Bugbee, M. Sperling, E. F. Cook, E. J. Orav, D. G. Fairchild, and D. W. Bates. 2005. A randomized trial of electronic clinical reminders to improve quality of care for diabetes and coronary artery disease. *Journal of the American Medical Informatics Association* 12(4):431–437.

Shenvi, E., and R. El-Kareh. 2014. Clinical criteria to screen for inpatient diagnostic errors: A scoping review. *Diagnosis* 2:3–19.

Silva, G. S., S. Farrell, E. Shandra, A. Viswanathan, and L. H. Schwamm. 2012. The Status of telestroke in the United States: A survey of currently active stroke telemedicine programs. *Stroke* 43:2078–2085.

Simborg, D. W., B. H. Starfield, S. D. Horn, and S. A. Yourtee. 1976. Information factors affecting problem follow-up in ambulatory care. *Medical Care* 14(10):848–856.

Singh, H., H. S. Arora, M. S. Vij, R. Rao, M. M. Khan, and L. A. Petersen. 2007a. Communication outcomes of critical imaging results in a computerized notification system. *Journal of the American Medical Informatics Association* 14(4):459–466.

Singh, H., E. J. Thomas, M. M. Khan, and L. A. Petersen. 2007b. Identifying diagnostic errors in primary care using an electronic screening algorithm. *Archives of Internal Medicine* 167(3):302–308.

Singh, H., A. D. Naik, R. Rao, and L. A. Petersen. 2008. Reducing diagnostic errors through effective communication: Harnessing the power of information technology. *Journal of General Internal Medicine* 23(4):489–494.

Singh, H., T. Giardina, S. Forjuoh, M. Reis, S. Kosmach, M. Khan, and E. Thomas. 2012. Electronic health record-based surveillance of diagnostic errors in primary care. *BMJ Quality and Safety* 21:93–100.

Singh, H., C. Spitzmueller, N. J. Petersen, M. K. Sawhney, and D. F. Sittig. 2013. Information overload and missed test results in electronic health record-based settings. *JAMA Internal Medicine* 173(8):702–704.

Singh, M., and T. R. Pal. 2011. Voice recognition technology implementation in surgical pathology: Advantages and limitations. *Archives of Pathology & Laboratory Medicine* 135(11):1476–1481.

Sittig, D., and H. Singh. 2010. A new sociotechnical model for studying health information technology in complex adaptive healthcare systems. *Quality and Safety in Health Care* 19:i68–i74.

Sittig, D. F., and H. Singh. 2012. Electronic health records and national patient-safety goals. *New England Journal of Medicine* 367(19):1854–1860.

Sittig, D. F., D. C. Classen, and H. Singh. 2014a. Patient safety goals for the proposed Federal Health Information Technology Safety Center. *Journal of the American Medical Informatics Association.*

Sittig, D. F., J. S. Ash, and H. Singh. 2014b. The SAFER guides: Empowering organizations to improve the safety and effectiveness of electronic health records. *American Journal of Managed Care* 20(5):418–423.

Sittig, D. F., D. R. Murphy, M. W. Smith, E. Russo, A. Wright, and H. Singh. 2015. Graphical display of diagnostic test results in electronic health records: A comparison of 8 systems. *Journal of the American Medical Informatics Association,* March 18 [Epub ahead of print]. jamia.oxfordjournals.org/content/jaminfo/early/2015/03/18/jamia.ocv013. full.pdf (accessed December 8, 2015).

Tsai, T. C., and A. K. Jha. 2014. Hospital consolidation, competition, and quality: Is bigger necessarily better? *JAMA* 312(1):29–30.

Upadhyay, D. K., D. F. Sittig, and H. Singh. 2014. Ebola US Patient Zero: Lessons on misdiagnosis and effective use of electronic health records. *Diagnosis* October 23 [Epub ahead of print]. www.degruyter.com/dg/viewarticle.fullcontentlink:pdfeventlink/$002fj $002fdx.ahead-of-print$002fdx-2014-0064$002fdx-2014-0064.pdf?t:ac=j$002fdx.ahead-of-print$002fdx-2014-0064$002fdx-2014-0064.xml (accessed December 8, 2015).

Uzuner, O., I. Goldstein, Y. Luo, and I. Kohane. 2008. Identifying patient smoking status from medical discharge records. *Journal of the American Medical Informatics Association* 15(1):14–24.

Vargas, B. B., D. D. Channer, D. W. Dodick, and B. M. Demaerschalk. 2012. Teleconcussion: An innovative approach to screening, diagnosis, and management of mild traumatic brain injury. *Telemedicine and E Health* 18(10):803–806.

Verghese, A. 2008. Culture shock—patient as icon, icon as patient. *New England Journal of Medicine* 359(26):2748–2751.

Wachter, R. M. 2015. *The digital doctor.* New York: McGraw-Hill.

Walker, J. M., P. Carayon, N. Leveson, R. A. Paulus, J. Tooker, H. Chin, A. Bothe, Jr., and W. F. Stewart. 2008. EHR safety: The way forward to safe and effective systems. *Journal of the American Medical Informatics Association* 15(3):272–277.

Watson, W. 2014. Texas Health Presbyterian Hospital Dallas implements changes after Ebola event. www.texashealth.org/news/ebola-update-changes-implemented-after-ebola-event (accessed April 7, 2015).

Weed, L. L. 1968. Medical Records That Guide and Teach. *New England Journal of Medicine* 278(11):593–600.

Weed, L. L., and L. Weed. 2011. *Medicine in denial.* USA: Createspace.

Weed, L. L., and L. Weed. 2014. Diagnosing diagnostic failure. *Diagnosis* 1(1):13–17.

Weed, L. L., and N. J. Zimny. 1989. The problem-oriented system, problem-knowledge coupling, and clinical decision making. *Physical Therapy* 69(7):565–568.

Westat. 2013. EHR contracts: Key contract terms for users to understand. www.healthit. gov/.../ehr_contracting_terms_final_508_compliant.pdf (accessed May 25, 2015).

XPRIZE. 2015. The prize: Empowering personal healthcare. http://tricorder.xprize.org/about/overview (accessed May 24, 2015).

Zakim, D., N. Braun, P. Fritz, and M. D. Alscher. 2008. Underutilization of information and knowledge in everyday medical practice: Evaluation of a computer-based solution. *BMC Medical Informatics and Decision Making* 8:50.

6

Organizational Characteristics, the Physical Environment, and the Diagnostic Process: Improving Learning, Culture, and the Work System

This chapter focuses on the actions that health care organizations can take to design a work system that supports the diagnostic process and reduces diagnostic errors (see Figure 6-1). The term "health care organization" is meant to encompass all settings of care in which the diagnostic process occurs, such as integrated care delivery settings, hospitals, clinician practices, retail clinics, and long-term care settings, such as nursing and rehabilitation centers. To improve diagnostic performance, health care organizations need to engage in organizational change and participate in continuous learning. The committee recognizes that health care organizations may differ in the challenges they face related to diagnosis and in their capacity to improve diagnostic performance. They will need to tailor the committee's recommendations to their resources and challenges with diagnosis.

The first section of this chapter describes how organizational learning principles can improve the diagnostic process by providing feedback to health care professionals about their diagnostic performance and by better characterizing the occurrence of and response to diagnostic errors. The second section highlights organizational characteristics—in particular, culture and leadership—that enable organizational change to improve the work system in which the diagnostic process occurs. The third section discusses actions that health care organizations can take to improve the work system and support the diagnostic process. For example, the physical environment (i.e., the design, layout, and ambient conditions) can affect diagnosis and is often under the control of health care organizations.

The Work System

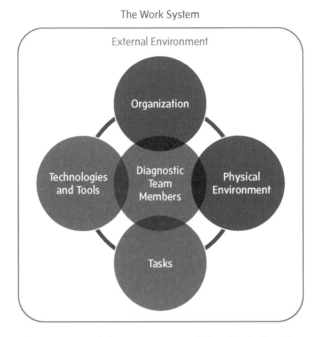

FIGURE 6-1 Organizational characteristics and the physical environment are two elements of the work system in which the diagnostic process occurs.

ORGANIZATIONAL LEARNING TO IMPROVE DIAGNOSIS

In any health care organization, prioritizing continuous learning is key to improving clinical practice (Davies and Nutley, 2000; IOM, 2013; WHO, 2006). The Institute of Medicine (IOM) report *Best Care at Lower Cost* concluded that health care organizations focused on continuous learning are able to more "consistently deliver reliable performance, and constantly improve, systematically and seamlessly, with each care experience and transition" than systems that do not practice continuing learning (IOM, 2013, p. 1). These learning health care organizations ensure that individual health care professionals and health care teams learn from their successes and mistakes and also use this information to support improved performance and patient outcomes (Davies and Nutley, 2000). Box 6-1 describes the characteristics of a continuously learning health care organization.

A focus on continuous learning in the diagnostic process has the potential to improve diagnosis and reduce diagnostic errors (Dixon-Woods et al., 2011; Gandhi, 2014; Grumbach et al., 2014; IOM, 2013; Trowbridge, 2014). To support continuous learning in the diagnostic process, health care organizations need to establish approaches to identify diagnostic errors and near misses and to implement feedback mechanisms on diagnostic performance. The challenges related to identifying and learning from diagnostic errors and near misses, as well as actions health care

---

BOX 6-1
Characteristics of a Continuously Learning
Health Care Organization

Science and Informatics

Real-time access to knowledge—A learning health care organization continuously and reliably captures, curates, and delivers the best available evidence to guide, support, tailor, and improve clinical decision making and the safety and quality of care.

Digital capture of the care experience—A learning health care organization captures the care experience on digital platforms for the real-time generation and application of knowledge for care improvement.

Patient–Clinician Partnerships

Engaged, empowered patients—A learning health care organization is anchored on patient needs and perspectives and promotes the inclusion of patients, families, and other caregivers as vital members of the continuously learning care team.

Incentives

Incentives aligned for value—In a learning health care organization, incentives are actively aligned to encourage continuous improvement, identify and reduce waste, and reward high-value care.

Full transparency—A learning health care organization systematically monitors the safety, quality, processes, prices, costs, and outcomes of care and makes information available for care improvement and informed choices and decision making by clinicians, patients, and their families.

Culture

Leadership-instilled culture of learning—A learning health care organization is stewarded by leadership committed to a culture of teamwork, collaboration, and adaptability in support of continuous learning as a core aim.

Supportive system competencies—In a learning health care organization, complex care operations and processes are constantly refined through ongoing team training and skill building, systems analysis and information development, and the creation of feedback loops for continuous learning and system improvement.

SOURCE: IOM, 2013.

organizations and health care professional societies can take to achieve this goal, are discussed below.

Identifying, Learning from, and Reducing Diagnostic Errors and Near Misses

Diagnostic errors have long been an understudied and underappreciated quality challenge in health care organizations (Graber, 2005; Shenvi and El-Kareh, 2015; Wachter, 2010). In a presentation to the committee, Paul Epner reported that the Society to Improve Diagnosis in Medicine "know[s] of no effort initiated in any health system to routinely and effectively assess diagnostic performance" (2014; see also Graber et al., 2014). The paucity of attention on diagnostic errors in clinical practice has been attributed to a number of factors. Two major contributors are the lack of effective measurement of diagnostic error and the difficulty in detecting these errors in clinical practice (Berenson et al., 2014; Graber et al., 2012b; Singh and Sittig, 2015). Additional factors may include a health care organization's competing priorities in patient safety and quality improvement, the perception that diagnostic errors are inevitable or that they are too difficult to address, and the need for financial resources to address this problem (Croskerry, 2003, 2012; Graber et al., 2005; Schiff et al., 2005; Singh and Sittig, 2015). These challenges make it difficult to identify, analyze, and learn from diagnostic errors in clinical practice (Graber, 2005; Graber et al., 2014; Henriksen, 2014; Singh and Sittig, 2015).

Compared to diagnostic errors, other types of medical errors—including medication errors, surgical errors, and health care–acquired infections—have historically received more attention within health care organizations (Graber et al., 2014; Kanter, 2014; Singh, 2014; Trowbridge, 2014). This is partly attributable to the lack of focus on diagnostic errors within national patient safety and quality improvement efforts. For example, the Agency for Healthcare Research and Quality's (AHRQ's) Patient Safety Indicators and The Joint Commission's list of specific sentinel events do not focus on diagnostic errors (AHRQ, 2015b; The Joint Commission, 2015a; Schiff et al., 2005). The National Quality Forum's Serious Reportable Events list includes only one event closely tied to diagnostic error, which is "patient death or serious injury resulting from a failure to follow up or communicate laboratory, pathology, or radiology test results" (NQF, 2011). The neglect of diagnostic performance measures for accountability purposes means that hospitals today could meet standards for high-quality care and be rewarded through public reporting and pay-for-performance initiatives even if they have major challenges with diagnostic accuracy (Wachter, 2010).

While current research estimates indicate that diagnostic errors are a common occurrence, health care organizations "do not have the tools and strategies to measure diagnostic safety and most have not integrated diagnostic error into their existing patient safety programmes" (Singh and Sittig, 2015, p. 103). Identifying diagnostic errors within clinical practice is critical to improving diagnosis for patients, but measurement has become an "unavoidable obstacle to progress" (Singh, 2013, p. 789). The lack of comprehensive information on diagnostic errors within clinical practice perpetuates the belief that these errors are uncommon or unavoidable and impedes progress on reducing diagnostic errors. Improving diagnosis will likely require a concerted effort among all health care organizations and across all settings of care to better identify diagnostic errors and near misses, learn from them, and, ultimately, take steps to improve the diagnostic process. **Thus, the committee recommends that health care organizations monitor the diagnostic process and identify, learn from, and reduce diagnostic errors and near misses as a component of their research, quality improvement, and patient safety programs.** In addition to identifying near misses and errors, health care organizations can also benefit from evaluating factors that are contributing to improved diagnostic performance.

Given the nascent field of measurement of the diagnostic process, the committee concluded that bottom-up experimentation will be necessary to develop approaches for monitoring the diagnostic process and identifying diagnostic errors and near misses. It is unlikely that one specific method will be successful at identifying all diagnostic errors and near misses; some approaches may be more appropriate than others for specific organizational settings, types of diagnostic errors, or for identifying specific causes. It may be necessary for health care organizations to use a variety of methods in order to have a better sense of their diagnostic performance (Shojania, 2010). As further information is collected regarding the validity and feasibility of specific methods for monitoring the diagnostic process and identifying diagnostic errors and near misses, this information will need to be disseminated in order to inform efforts within other health care organizations. The dissemination of this information will be especially important for health care organizations that do not have the financial and human resources available to pilot-test some of the potential methods for the identification of diagnostic errors and near misses. In some cases, small group practices may find it useful to pool their resources as they explore alternative approaches to identify errors and near misses and monitor the diagnostic process.

As discussed in Chapter 3, there are a number of methods being employed by researchers to describe the incidence and nature of diagnostic errors, including postmortem examinations, medical record reviews, health insurance claims analysis, medical malpractice claims analysis, second reviews of diagnostic testing, and surveys of patients and clinicians. Some of these methods may be better suited than others for identifying diagnostic errors and near misses in clinical practice. Medical record reviews, medical malpractice claims analysis, health insurance claims analysis, and second reviews in diagnostic testing may be more pragmatic approaches for health care organizations because they leverage readily available data sources. Patient surveys may also be an important mechanism for health care organizations to consider. It is important to note that many of the methods described below are just beginning to be applied to diagnostic error detection in clinical practice; very few are validated or available for widespread use in clinical practice (Bhise and Singh, 2015; Graber, 2013; Singh and Sittig, 2015).

Medical record reviews can be a useful method to identify diagnostic errors and near misses because health care organizations can leverage their electronic health records (EHRs) for these analyses. The committee's recommendation on health information technology (health IT) highlights the need for EHRs to include user-friendly platforms that enable health care organizations to measure diagnostic errors (see Chapter 5). Trigger tools, or algorithms that scan EHRs for potential diagnostic errors, can be used to identify patients who have a higher likelihood of experiencing a diagnostic error. For example, they can identify patients who return for inpatient hospitalization within 2 weeks of a primary care visit or patients who require follow-up after abnormal diagnostic testing results. Review of their EHRs can evaluate whether a diagnostic error occurred, using explicit or implicit criteria. For diagnostic errors, these tools have been piloted primarily in outpatient settings, but they are also being considered in the inpatient setting (Murphy et al., 2014; Shenvi and El-Kareh, 2015; Singh et al., 2012a). EHR surveillance, such as Kaiser Permanente's SureNet System,[1] is another opportunity to detect patients at risk of experiencing a diagnostic error (Danforth et al., 2014; Graber et al., 2014; HIMSS Analytics, 2015; Kanter, 2014). The SureNet System identifies patients who may have inadvertent lapses in care (such as a patient with iron deficiency anemia who has not had a colonoscopy to rule out colon cancer) and ensures that follow-up occurs by proactively reaching out to affected patients and members of their care team.

Medical malpractice claims analysis is another approach to identifying diagnostic errors and near misses in clinical practice. Chapter 7 discusses the importance of leveraging the expertise of professional liability insurers in efforts to improve diagnosis and reduce diagnostic errors and near misses. Health care professionals and organizations can collaborate with professional liability insurers in efforts to identify diagnostic errors

---

[1] Kaiser Permanente's SureNet System was previously known as the SafetyNet System.

and near misses in clinical practice; because of the richness of the data source, this method could also be helpful in identifying the reasons why diagnostic errors occur. However, there are limitations with malpractice claims data because these claims may not be representative; few people who experience adverse events file claims, and the ones who do are more likely to have experienced serious harm.

Although there are few examples of using health insurance claims data to identify diagnostic errors and near misses, this may be a useful method, especially if it is combined with other approaches (e.g., if it is linked to medical records or diagnostic testing results). One of the advantages of this data source is that it makes it possible to assess the downstream clinical consequences and costs of errors. It also enables comparisons across different settings, types of clinicians, and days of the week (which can be important because there may be some days when staffing is low and the volume of patients unexpectedly high).

Second reviews of diagnostic testing results could also help health care organizations identify diagnostic errors and near misses related to the interpretive aspect of the diagnostic testing processes. A recent guideline recommended that health care organizations use second reviews in anatomic pathology to identify disagreements and potential interpretive errors (Nakhleh et al., 2015). The guideline notes that organizations will likely need to tailor the second review process that they employ and the number of reviews they conduct to their specific needs and resources (Nakhleh et al., 2015). Some organizations include anatomic pathology second reviews as part of their quality assurance and improvement efforts. The Veterans Health Administration requires that "[a]t least 10 percent of the cytotechnologist's gynecologic cases that have been interpreted to be negative are routinely rescreened, and are diagnosed and documented as being negative by a qualified pathologist" (VHA, 2008, p. 32). Though the infrastructure for peer review in radiology is still evolving, there are now frameworks specific to radiology for identifying and learning from diagnostic errors (Allen and Thorwarth, 2014; Lee et al., 2013; Provenzale and Kranz, 2011). In addition to the use of peer review in identifying errors, there is an increasing emphasis on using peer review tools to promote peer learning and improve practice quality (Allen and Thorwarth, 2014; Brook et al., 2015; Fotenos and Nagy, 2012; Iyer et al., 2013; Kruskal et al., 2008). Organizations can participate in the American College of Radiology's RADPEER™ program, which includes a second review process that can help identify diagnostic performance issues related to medical image interpretation (ACR, 2015).

Patient surveys represent another opportunity. The use of such surveys is in line with the committee's recommendation to create environments in which patients and their families feel comfortable sharing their feedback and concerns about diagnostic errors and near misses (see Chapter 4). Eliciting this information via surveys may be helpful in identifying errors and near misses, and it can also provide useful feedback to the organization and health care professionals (see section below on feedback). For example, a recent patient-initiated voluntary survey of adverse events found that harm was commonly associated with reported diagnostic errors and the survey identified actions that patients believed could improve care (Southwick et al., 2015).

In addition to identifying diagnostic errors that have already occurred, some methods used to monitor the diagnostic process and identify diagnostic errors can be used for error recovery. Error recovery is the process of identifying failures early in the diagnostic process so that actions can be taken to reduce or avert negative effects resulting from the failure (IOM, 2000). Methods that identify failures in the diagnostic process or catch diagnostic errors before significant harm is incurred could make it possible to avoid diagnostic errors or to intervene early enough to avert significant harm. By scanning medical records to identify lapses in care, the SureNet system supports error recovery by identifying patients at risk of experiencing a diagnostic error (Danforth et al., 2014; HIMSS Analytics, 2015; Kanter, 2014) (see also section on a supportive work system).

Beyond identifying diagnostic errors and near misses, organizational learning aimed at improving diagnostic performance and reducing diagnostic errors will also require a focus on understanding where in the diagnostic process the failures occur, the work system factors that contribute to their occurrence, what the outcomes were, and how these failures may be prevented or mitigated (see Chapter 3). For example, the committee's conceptual model of the diagnostic process describes the steps within the process that are vulnerable to failure: engagement, information gathering, integration, interpretation, establishing a diagnosis, and communication of the diagnosis. If a health care organization is evaluating where in the diagnostic testing process a failure occurs, the brain-to-brain loop model may be helpful in conducting these analyses, in particular by articulating the five phases of testing: pre-pre-analytical, pre-analytical, analytical, post-analytical, and post-post-analytical (Plebani and Lippi, 2011; Plebani et al., 2011).

It is also important to determine the work system factors that contribute to diagnostic errors and near misses. Some of the data sources and methods mentioned above, such as malpractice claims analyses and medical record reviews, can provide valuable insights into the causes and outcomes of diagnostic errors. Health care organizations can also employ formal error analysis and other risk assessment methods to understand the work system factors that contribute to diagnostic errors and near misses. Relevant analytical methods include root cause analysis, cognitive autopsies, and morbidity and mortality (M&M) conferences (Gandhi, 2014; Graber et al., 2014; Reilly et al., 2014). Root cause analysis is a problem-solving method that attempts to identify the factors that contributed to an error; these analyses take a systems approach by trying to identify all of the underlying factors rather than focusing exclusively on the health care professionals involved (AHRQ, 2014b). Maine Medical Center recently conducted a demonstration program to inform clinicians about the root causes of diagnostic errors. They created a novel fishbone root cause analysis procedure, which visually represents the multiple cause and effect relationships responsible for an error (Trowbridge, 2014). Organizations and individuals can also take advantage of continuing education opportunities focused on using root cause analysis to study diagnostic errors in order to improve their ability to identify and under-stand diagnostic errors (Reilly et al., 2015). The cognitive autopsy is a variation of a root cause analysis that involves a clinician reflecting on the reasoning process that led to the error in order to identify causally relevant shortcomings in reasoning or decision making (Croskerry, 2005). M&M conferences bring a diverse group of health care professionals to-gether to learn from errors (AHRQ, 2008). These can be useful, especially if they are framed from a patient safety perspective rather than focusing on attributing blame. Other analytical methods used in human factors and ergonomics research could also be applied in health care organizational settings to further elucidate the work system components that contribute to diagnostic errors (see Chapter 3) (Bisantz and Roth, 2007; Carayon et al., 2014; Kirwan and Ainsworth, 1992; Rogers et al., 2012; Roth, 2008; Salas et al., 1995).

As health care organizations develop a better understanding of diag-nostic errors within their organizations, they can begin to implement and evaluate interventions to prevent or mitigate these errors as part of their patient safety, research, and quality improvement efforts. To date, there have been relatively few studies that have evaluated the impact of inter-ventions on improving diagnosis and reducing diagnostic errors and near misses; three recent systematic reviews summarized current interventions (Graber et al., 2012a; McDonald et al., 2013; Singh et al., 2012b). These reviews found that the measures used to evaluate the interventions were quite heterogeneous, and there were concerns about the generalizability of some of the findings to clinical practice. Health care organizations can take into consideration some of the methodological challenges identified in these reviews in order to ensure that their evaluations generate much-needed evidence to identify successful interventions.

The Medicare conditions of participation and accreditation organi-zations can be leveraged to ensure that health care organizations have appropriate programs in place to identify diagnostic errors and near misses, learn from them, and improve the diagnostic process. The Medicare conditions of participation are requirements that health care organizations must meet in order to receive payment (CMS, 2015a). State survey agencies and accreditation organizations (such as The Joint Commission, the Healthcare Facilities Accreditation Program, the Accreditation Commission for Health Care, the College of American Pathologists, and Det NorskeVeritas-Germanischer Lloyd) determine whether organizations are in compliance with the Medicare conditions of participation through surveys and site visits. Some of these organizations accredit the broad range of health care organizations, while others confine their scope to a single type of health care organization. Other accreditation bodies, such as the National Committee for Quality Assurance (NCQA), provide administrative and clinical accreditation and certification of health plans and provider organizations. For example, NCQA offers accountable care organization (ACO) accreditation, which evaluates an organization's capacity to provide the coordinated, high-quality care and performance-reporting that is required of ACOs (NCQA, 2013). Accreditation processes, federal oversight, and quality improvement efforts specific to diagnostic testing can also be used to ensure quality in the diagnostic process (see Chapter 2). By leveraging the Medicare conditions of participation requirements and accreditation processes, it may be possible to use the existing oversight programs that health care organizations have in place to monitor the diagnostic process and to ensure that the organizations are identifying diagnostic errors and near misses, learning from them, and making timely efforts to improve diagnosis. **Thus, the committee recommends that accreditation organizations and the Medicare conditions of participation should require that health care organizations have programs in place to monitor the diagnostic process and identify, learn from, and reduce diagnostic errors and near misses in a timely fashion. As more is learned about successful program approaches, accreditation organizations and the Medicare conditions of participation should incorporate these proven approaches into updates of these requirements.**

Postmortem Examinations

The committee recognized that many approaches to identifying diagnostic errors are important, but the committee thought that the postmortem examination (also referred to as an autopsy) warranted additional committee focus because of its role in understanding the epidemiology of diagnostic error. Postmortem examinations are typically performed to determine cause of death and can reveal discrepancies between premortem and postmortem clinical findings (see Chapter 3). However, the number of postmortem examinations performed in the United States has declined substantially since the 1960s (Hill and Anderson, 1988; Lundberg, 1998; MedPAC, 1999). One of the contributors to the decline is that in 1971 The Joint Commission eliminated the requirement that hospitals conduct these examinations on a certain percentage of deaths in their facility—20 percent in community hospitals and 25 percent in teaching facilities—in order to receive accreditation (Allen, 2011; CDC, 2001). Cost is another factor; according to a survey of medical institutions in eight states, researchers in 2006 estimated that the mean cost of performing a postmortem examination was $1,275 (Nemetz et al., 2006). Insurers do not directly pay for postmortem examinations, as they typically limit payment to procedures for living patients. Medicare bundles payment for postmortem examinations into its payment for quality improvement activities, which may also disincentivize their performance (Allen, 2011).

Given the steep decline in postmortem examinations, there is interest in increasing their use. For example, Hill and Anderson (1988) recommended that half of all deaths in hospitals, nursing homes, and other accredited medical facilities receive a postmortem examination. Lundberg (1998) recommended reinstating the mandate that a percentage of hospital deaths undergo postmortem examination, either to meet Medicare conditions of participation or accreditation standards. The Medicare Payment Advisory Commission proposed a number of recommendations designed to increase the postmortem examination rate and evaluate their potential for use in "quality improvement and error reduction initiatives" (MedPAC, 1999, p. xviii).

The committee concluded that a new approach to increasing the use of postmortem examinations is warranted. The committee weighed the relative merits of increasing the number of postmortem examinations conducted throughout the United States versus a more targeted approach. The requirements for postmortem examinations in the current Medicare conditions of participation state that postmortem examinations should be performed when there is an unusual death; in particular, these requirements state that "medical staff should attempt to secure an autopsy [postmortem examination] in all cases of unusual death and of medical–legal and educational interest" (CMS, 2015b, p. 210). In these circumstances, the committee concluded that health care organizations should continue to perform these postmortem examinations. In addition, the committee concluded that it is appropriate to have a limited number of highly qualified health care systems participate in conducting routine postmortem exams that produce research-quality information about the incidence and nature of diagnostic errors. **Thus, the committee recommends that the Department of Health and Human Services (HHS) should provide funding for a designated subset of health care systems to conduct routine postmortem examinations on a representative sample of patient deaths.** To accomplish this, these health care systems need to reflect a broad array of different settings of care and could receive funding to perform routine postmortem examinations in a representative sample of patient deaths. A competitive grant process could be used to identify these systems.

In recognition that not all patients' next of kin will consent to the performance of a postmortem examination, these systems can characterize the frequency with which the request for a postmortem examination is refused and thus better describe the risk of response bias in results. This approach will likely provide better epidemiologic data and it represents an advance over current selection methods for performing postmortem examinations, because clinicians do not seem to be able to predict cases in which diagnostic errors will be found (Shojania et al., 2002, 2003). The data collected from health care systems that are highly qualified to conduct routine postmortem examinations may not be representative of all systems of care. However, the committee concluded that this is a more feasible approach, given the financial and workforce demands of conducting postmortem examinations.

Findings from the health care systems that perform routine postmortem examinations can then be disseminated to the broader health care community. Participating health care systems could be required to produce annual reports on the epidemiology of diagnostic errors found by postmortem exams, the value of postmortem examinations as a tool for identifying and reducing such errors, and, if relevant, the role and value of postmortem examinations in quality improvement efforts.

These health care systems could also investigate how new, minimally invasive postmortem approaches compare with traditional full body postmortem examinations. Less invasive approaches include the use of medical imaging, laparoscopy, biopsy, histology, and cytology. Given the advances in molecular diagnostics and advanced imaging techniques, these new approaches could provide useful insights into the incidence of diagnostic error and may be more acceptable options for patients' next of kin. For example, instead of conducting a full body postmortem exam, pathologists could biopsy tissue samples from an organ where disease is suspected and conduct molecular analysis (van der Linden et al., 2014). Some studies suggest that minimally invasive postmortem examinations (including a combination of medical imaging with other minimally invasive postmortem investigations) have been found to have accuracy similar to that of conventional postmortem examinations in fetuses, newborns, and infants (Lavanya et al., 2008; Pichereau et al., 2015; Ruegger et al., 2014; Thayyil et al., 2013; Weustink et al., 2009). Postmortem imaging in adults has shown less promise for replacing postmortem exams, but these techniques continue to be actively explored (O'Donnell and Woodford, 2008; Roberts et al., 2012). A concern with minimally invasive postmortem imaging is that it may be subject to similar limitations that affect imaging in living patients, and may not detect premortem and postmortem discrepancies. Further understanding the benefits and limitations of minimally invasive approaches may provide critical information moving forward. If successful approaches to minimally invasive postmortem examinations are found, they could play a role in reestablishing the practice of routine postmortem investigation in medicine (Saldiva, 2014).

Improving Feedback

Feedback is a critical mechanism that health care organizations can use to support continuous learning in the diagnostic process. The *Best Care at Lower Cost* report called for the creation of feedback loops that support continuous learning and system improvement (IOM, 2013). As it relates to diagnosis, feedback entails informing an individual, team, or organization about its diagnostic performance, including its successes, near misses, and diagnostic errors (Black, 2011; Croskerry, 2000; Gandhi, 2014; Gandhi et al., 2005; Schiff, 2008, 2014; Trowbridge, 2014). The committee received substantial input indicating that there are limited opportunities for feedback on diagnostic performance (Dhaliwal, 2014; Henriksen, 2014; Schiff, 2014; Singh, 2014; Trowbridge, 2014). There are often not systems in place to provide clinicians with input on whether they made an accurate, timely diagnosis or if their patients experienced a diagnostic error. The failure to follow up with patients about their diagnosis and treatment—in both the near term and the long term—is a major gap in improving diagnosis.

The committee concluded that improving diagnostic performance requires feedback at all levels of health care. Feedback can help clinicians assess how well they are performing in the diagnostic process, correct overconfidence, identify when remediation efforts are needed, and reduce the likelihood of repeated mistakes (Berner and Graber, 2008; Croskerry and Norman, 2008). Feedback on diagnostic performance can also provide opportunities for health care organizational learning and improvements to the work system (Plaza et al., 2011). **To improve the opportunities for feedback, the committee recommends that health care organizations should implement procedures and practices to provide systematic feedback on diagnostic performance to individual health care professionals, care teams, and clinical and organizational leaders.**

Box 6-2 identifies some characteristics for effective feedback interventions (Hysong et al., 2006; Ivers et al., 2014). Feedback interventions in high-performing organizations have been found to share a number of characteristics, including being actionable, timely, individualized, and nonpunitive; a nonpunitive culture helps foster an environment in which

---

BOX 6-2
Characteristics of Effective Feedback Interventions

Feedback
- Is nonpunitive
- Is actionable
- Is timely
- Is individualized
- Comes from the appropriate individual (i.e., a trusted source)
- Targets behavior that can be affected by feedback
- Is provided to recipients who are responsible for improvement
- Includes a description of the desired performance/behavior

SOURCES: Hysong et al., 2006; Ivers et al., 2014.

---

mistakes can be viewed as opportunities for growth and improvement (Hysong et al., 2006). Other studies have found that feedback is likely to have the largest effect when baseline performance is low and feedback occurs regularly (Ivers et al., 2012; Lopez-Campos et al., 2014). Tailoring the feedback approach to the individual recipient and choosing an appropriate source of feedback (e.g., supervisor versus a peer as the provider of feedback) are important variables in determining how well recipients will respond (Ilgen et al., 1979).

Health care organizations need to be aware of the factors that can impede the provision of feedback, such as the fragmentation of the health care system, resistance to critical feedback from clinicians, and the lack of time for follow-up (Schiff, 2008). In addition, improving feedback will likely require health care organizations to invest additional time and resources for developing systematic feedback mechanisms.

There are many opportunities to provide feedback in clinical practice. Methods to monitor the diagnostic process and identify diagnostic errors and near misses can be leveraged as mechanisms to provide feedback. Feedback opportunities include disseminating postmortem examination results to clinicians who were involved in the patient's care; sharing the results of patient surveys, medical record reviews, or information gained through follow-up with the health care professionals; using patient-actors or simulated care scenarios to assess and inform health care professionals' diagnostic performance; and others (Schwartz and Weiner, 2014; Schwartz et al., 2012; Southwick et al., 2015; Weiner et al., 2010). As discussed in Chapter 4, patients and their families have unique insights into the diagnostic process and the occurrence of diagnostic error; therefore, following up with patients and their families about their experiences and outcomes will be an important source of feedback (Schiff, 2008). AHRQ recently proposed recommendations for the development of consumer and patient safety reporting systems, which organizations can use for feedback and learning purposes (AHRQ, 2011). M&M conferences, root cause analyses, departmental meetings, and leadership WalkRounds[2] provide additional opportunities to provide feedback to health care professionals, care teams, and leadership about diagnostic performance.

Peer review processes, including second reviews of anatomic pathology specimens and medical images, can also be utilized for feedback, and there is an increasing emphasis on using peer-review tools to promote peer learning and improve practice quality (Allen and Thorwarth, 2014; Brook et al., 2015; Fotenos and Nagy, 2012; Iyer et al., 2013; Kruskal et al., 2008). For example, RADPEER™ allows anonymous peer review of previous image interpretations by integrating previous images into current workflow to allow for a nondisruptive peer review process. Summary statistics of image reviews are made available to participating groups and clinicians to improve performance (ACR, 2015). As of 2013, 16,450 clinicians in 1,127 groups were enrolled in the RADPEER™ program; 1,218 clinicians had used or were using the program as part of the American Board of Radiology's Practice Quality Improvement project for maintenance of certification (ACR, 2013). Performance monitoring programs designed to satisfy the requirements of the Mammography Quality Standards Act have been used to improve feedback on diagnostic performance on mammography to radiologists and medical imaging facilities (Allen and Thorwarth, 2014).

Leveraging Health Care Professional Societies' Efforts to Improve Diagnosis

Health care organizations can leverage external input from health care professional societies to inform the organizations' efforts to monitor and improve the diagnostic process. For example, health care professional societies and their members can help develop and prioritize approaches to improve diagnosis specific to their specialties. By engaging health care professional societies, efforts to improve diagnosis can build on professionalism and intrinsic motivation. **Thus, the committee recommends**

---

[2] Leadership WalkRounds are a tool to connect leadership with frontline clinicians and health care professionals. They consist of leadership (senior executives, vice presidents, etc.) making announced or unannounced visits to different areas of the organization to engage with frontline employees (IHI, 2004).

that health care professional societies should identify opportunities to improve accurate and timely diagnoses and reduce diagnostic errors in their specialties.

Such an effort could be modeled on the Choosing Wisely initiative, which was initiated by the American Board of Internal Medicine Foundation to encourage patient and health care professional communication as a way to ensure high-quality, high-value care. The initiative invited health care professional societies to each develop a list of five services (i.e., tests, treatments, and procedures) that are commonly used in practice but may be unnecessary or not supported by the evidence as improving patient care. These lists were made publicly available as a way of encouraging discussions about appropriate care between patients and health care professionals. Choosing Wisely received national media attention and engaged more than 50 health care professional societies (Choosing Wisely, 2015). A major lesson from the Choosing Wisely initiative is the importance of beginning with a small group of founding organizations and then expanding membership. Engaging consumer groups as the program progressed was also an important component of the initiative. Another factor in the initiative's success was that it allowed flexibility within limits; participating health care professional societies and boards were given flexibility in identifying their "Top 5" lists, but items on each list had to be evidence-based and within the purview of that particular society.

Early efforts on prioritization could focus on identifying the most common diagnostic errors and "don't miss" health conditions, such as those that present the greatest likelihood for diagnostic errors and harm (Newman-Toker et al., 2013). For example, stroke, acute myocardial infarction, or pulmonary embolism may be important areas of focus in the emergency department setting while cancer is a frequently missed diagnosis in the ambulatory care setting (CRICO, 2014; Gandhi et al., 2006; Newman-Toker et al., 2013; Schiff et al., 2013). Efforts to improve diagnosis can include a focus on the quality and safety of diagnosis as well as increasing efficiency and value, such as identifying inappropriate diagnostic testing. Another approach may be for societies to identify "low-hanging fruit," or targets that are easily remediable, as a high priority. Doing this may increase the likelihood of having early successes that can contribute to the long-term success of the effort (Kotter, 1995). Some groups may identify particular actions, tools, or approaches to reduce errors associated with a particular diagnosis within their specialties (such as checklists, second reviews, or decision support tools).

Each society could identify five high-priority areas to improve diagnosis. The groups would need to be given latitude in the identification of their targets, and, as was the case in Choosing Wisely, a primary constraint could be that there must be evidence indicating that adopting the recommendation would result in improving diagnosis or reducing diagnostic error. This could also be an opportunity for health care professional societies to collaborate, especially in cases of diagnoses that may be missed because of the inappropriate isolation of symptoms among specialties. For example, urologists, primary care clinicians, and neurologists could collaborate to make the diagnosis of normal pressure hydrocephalus (symptoms include frequent urination, a type of balance problem, and some memory loss) a "not to be missed" diagnosis (McDonald, 2014).

ORGANIZATIONAL CHARACTERISTICS FOR LEARNING AND IMPROVED DIAGNOSIS

Health care organizations influence the work system in which diagnosis occurs and also play a vital role in implementing changes to improve diagnosis and prevent diagnostic errors. The committee identified organizational culture and organizational leadership and management as key characteristics for ensuring continuous learning from and improvements to the diagnostic process. Health care organizations are responsible for developing a culture that promotes a safe place for all health care professionals to identify and learn from diagnostic errors. Organizational leaders and managers can facilitate this culture and set the priorities to achieve progress in improving diagnostic performance and reducing diagnostic errors. The committee drew on the broader quality and patient safety literature to inform this discussion; making connections to previous efforts to improve quality and safety is particularly important, given the limited focus on improving diagnosis in the patient safety and quality improvement literature. The committee concluded that many of the findings from the broader fields of quality improvement and patient safety have the potential to reduce diagnostic errors and improve diagnosis. However, this also represents a research need—further studies need to evaluate the generalizability of these findings to diagnosis (see Chapter 8).

Promoting a Culture for Improved Diagnosis

As discussed in Chapter 1, health care organizations can leverage four major cultural movements in health care—patient safety, professionalism, patient engagement, and collaboration—to create a local environment that supports continuous learning and improvement in diagnosis. Organizational culture refers to an organization's norms of behavior and the shared basic assumptions and values that sustain those norms (Kotter, 2012; Schein, 2004). Though the cultures in most health care organizations exhibit common elements, they can differ considerably due to varying missions, values, and histories. Another factor that makes culture in health care organizations more complicated is the presence of subcultures (multiple distinct sets of norms and beliefs within a single organization) (Schein, 2004). Subcultures can reflect the individual attitudes of a nurse manager on a specific hospital floor or interprofessional differences that spring from the long history and social concerns of each health care profession (Hall, 2005). The existence of multiple cultures within a single health care organization may make it difficult to promote the shared values, goals, and approaches necessary for improving diagnosis.

Some aspects of culture may promote diagnostic accuracy, such as the intrinsic motivation of health care professionals to deliver high-quality care and the dedicated focus on quality and safety found in some health care organizations. Other aspects of culture may be detrimental to efforts to improve diagnosis, including the persistence of punitive, fault-based cultures; cultural taboos on providing peer feedback; hierarchical attitudes that are misaligned with team-based practice; and the acceptance of the inevitability of errors. Punitive cultures that emphasize discipline and punishment for those who make mistakes are not conducive to improved diagnostic performance; this type of culture thwarts the learning process because health care professionals fear the consequences of reporting errors (Hoffman and Kanzaria, 2014; Khatri et al., 2009; Larson, 2002; Schiff, 1994). Clinicians within these settings may also feel uneasy about providing feedback to colleagues about their diagnostic performance or the occurrence of diagnostic errors (Gallagher et al., 2013; Tucker and Edmondson, 2003).

There have been multiple calls for health care organizations to create nonpunitive cultures that encourage communication and learning (IOM, 2000, 2004, 2013). Despite these efforts, a punitive culture persists within some health care organizations (Chassin, 2013; Chassin and Loeb, 2013). For example, a recent survey found that less than half (44 percent) of health care professionals perceived that their organizations had a nonpunitive response to error (AHRQ, 2014a). The fault-based medical liability system and, in rare cases, clinicians who exhibit unprofessional or intimidating behavior also contribute to the persistence of punitive cultures (Chassin, 2013; Chassin and Loeb, 2013).

Cultures that continue to view diagnosis as a solitary clinician activity discount the important roles of teamwork and collaboration. A culture that validates the perspective that diagnostic errors are inevitable may also pose problems. When these cultural attitudes are pervasive within health care organizations, attempts to improve diagnosis are challenging (Berner and Graber, 2008).

Changing an organization's culture is often difficult, and there are many opportunities throughout the change process where failure can occur (Kotter, 1995). Health care organizations may be hesitant to attempt culture change because of system inertia, concern that benefits due to the present culture could be lost, or because there is uncertainty regarding which approaches to improving culture work best in a given organizational setting (Chassin, 2013; Coiera, 2011; Parmelli et al., 2011). Organizations may attempt to implement multiple change processes simultaneously, and this can lead to change fatigue, where employees experience burnout[3] and apathy (Perlman, 2011). Other factors may include: the failure to convey the urgent need for change; poor communication of the successes that have resulted from change; the inadequate identification, preparation, or removal of barriers to change; and insufficient involvement of leadership and management in the change initiative (Chassin, 2013; Hines et al., 2008; IOM, 2013; Kotter, 1995, 2012). Although the challenges to cultural change can be significant, the committee concluded that addressing organizational culture is central to improving diagnosis (Gandhi, 2014; Kanter, 2014; Thomas, 2014). **Thus, the committee recommends that health care organizations should adopt policies and practices that promote a nonpunitive culture that values open discussion and feedback on diagnostic performance.**

There are a variety of approaches that can be employed to improve culture (Davies et al., 2000; Etchegaray et al., 2012; Schein, 2004; Schiff, 2014; Williams et al., 2007). The measurement of an organization's culture is often a first step in the improvement process because it facilitates the identification of cultural challenges and the evaluation of interventions (IOM, 2013). A number of measurement tools are available, including surveys to identify health care professionals' perception of their organization's culture (AHRQ, 2014c; Farley et al., 2009; Modak et al., 2007; Sexton et al., 2006; Watts et al., 2010).

Organizations can create a culture that supports learning and continual improvement by implementing a just culture, also referred to as a culture of safety (IOM, 2004; Kanter, 2014; Khatri et al., 2009; Larson, 2002; Marx, 2001; Milstead, 2005). A just culture balances competing priorities—learning from error and personal accountability—by understanding that health care is a complex activity involving imperfect individuals who will make mistakes, while not tolerating reckless behavior (AHRQ, 2015a). The just culture approach distinguishes between "human error" (an inadvertent act by a clinician, such as a slip or lapse), "at-risk behavior" (taking shortcuts, violating a safety rule without perceiving it as likely to cause harm), and "reckless behavior" (conscious choices by clinicians to

---

[3] The term "burnout" is defined as occupational stress resulting from demanding and emotional relationships between health care professionals and patients that is marked by emotional exhaustion, a negative attitude toward one's patients, and the belief that one is no longer effective at work with patients (Bakker et al., 2005).

engage in behavior they know poses a significant risk, such as ignoring required safety steps). The just culture model recommends "consoling the clinician" involved in human error, "coaching the clinician" who engages in at-risk behavior, and reserving discipline only for clinicians whose behavior is truly reckless. Further refinements to this approach employ a "substitution test" (i.e., would three other clinicians with similar skills and knowledge do the same in similar circumstances?) to identify situations in which system flaws have developed that create predisposing conditions for the error in question to occur. Finally, whether or not the clinician has a history of repeatedly making the same or similar mistakes is considered in formulating an appropriate response to error.

Health care organizations can also look to high reliability organizations (HROs), which operate in high-stakes conditions but maintain high safety levels (such as those found in the nuclear power and aviation industries). Health care organizations can benefit from adapting the traits of HRO cultures, such as rejecting complacency and focusing on error reduction (Chassin and Loeb, 2011; Singh, 2014; Thomas, 2014; Weick and Sutcliffe, 2011). The involvement of supportive and committed leadership is another component of successful attempts to improve culture and is a key component of HRO success (Chassin, 2013; Hines et al., 2008; IOM, 2013; Kotter, 1995, 2012).

Health care organizations can espouse cultural values that support the open discussion of diagnostic performance and improvement (Davies and Nutley, 2000) (see Box 6-3). The culture needs to promote the discussion of error and offer psychological safety (Jeffe et al., 2004; Kachalia, 2013). Successes need to be celebrated, and mistakes need to be treated as opportunities to learn and improve. Complacency with regard to current diagnostic performance needs to be replaced with an enduring desire for continuing improvement. An emphasis on teamwork is critical, and it can be facilitated by a culture that values the development of trusting, mutually respectful relationships among health care professionals, patients and their family members, and organizational leadership.

Despite the difficulties one faces in implementing culture change, health care organizations have begun to make changes that can improve patient safety (Chassin and Loeb, 2013). For instance, changing culture was a critical factor in sustaining the reduction in intensive care unit–acquired central line bloodstream infections in Michigan state hospitals (Pronovost et al., 2006, 2008, 2010). Cincinnati Children's Hospital has focused on better process design that leverages human factors expertise and on building a culture of reliability (Cincinnati Children's Hospital, 2014). A number of health care organizations have undertaken the process of instituting a just culture by prioritizing learning and fairness and creating an atmosphere of transparency and psychological safety (Marx,

BOX 6-3
Important Cultural Values for Continuously
Learning Health Care Systems

- Celebration of success. If excellence is to be pursued with vigor and commitment, its attainment needs to be valued within the organizational culture.
- Absence of complacency. Learning organizations value innovation and change—they are searching constantly for new ways to improve their outcomes.
- Recognition of mistakes as opportunities to learn. Learning from failure is a prerequisite for achieving improvement. This requires a culture that accepts the positive spin-offs from errors, rather than seeking to blame. This does not imply a tolerance of routinely poor or mediocre performance from which no lessons are learned or of reckless disregard for safe practices.
- Belief in human potential. It is people who drive success in organizations—using their creativity, energy, and innovation. Therefore, the culture within a learning organization values people and fosters their professional and personal development.
- Recognition of tacit knowledge. Learning organizations recognize that those individuals closest to processes have the best and most intimate knowledge of their potential and flaws. Therefore, the learning culture values tacit knowledge and shows a belief in empowerment (the systematic enlargement of discretion, responsibility, and competence).
- Openness. Because learning organizations try to foster a systems view, sharing knowledge throughout the organization is one key to developing learning capacity. "Knowledge mobility" emphasizes informal channels and personal contacts over written reporting procedures. Cross disciplinary and multifunction teams, staff rotations, on-site inspections, and experiential learning are essential components of this informal exchange.
- Trust. For individuals to give their best, take risks, and develop their competencies, they must trust that such activities will be appreciated and valued by colleagues and managers. In particular, they must be confident that should they err, they will be supported, not castigated. In turn, managers must be able to trust that subordinates will use wisely the time, space, and resources given to them through empowerment programs—and not indulge in opportunistic behavior. Without trust, learning is a faltering process.
- Outward looking. Learning organizations are engaged with the world outside as a rich source of learning opportunities. They look to their competitors for insights into their own operations and are attuned to the experiences of other stakeholders, such as their suppliers. In particular, they are focused on obtaining a deep understanding of clients' needs.

SOURCE: Davies and Nutley, 2000. Adapted by permission from BMJ Publishing Group Limited. Developing learning organizations in the new NHS, H. T. O. Davies and S. N. Nutley, *BMJ* 320, 998–1001, 2000.

2001; Wyatt, 2013). For example, after two high-profile medical mistakes, the Dana-Farber Cancer Institute implemented a plan to develop a just culture in order to improve learning from error and care performance (Connor et al., 2007). Its plan centered on incorporating a set of principles into practice that promoted learning, the open discussion of error, individual accountability, and program evaluation; this plan was endorsed and supported by organizational leadership (Connor et al., 2007). Organizations can explore the strategies that are best suited to their needs and aims (e.g., specific strategies for small practices to improve culture) (Gandhi and Lee, 2010; Shostek, 2007).

Leadership and Management

Organizational leaders are responsible for setting the priorities and expectations that guide a health care organization and for determining the rules and policies necessary to achieve the organization's goals. Organizational leaders can include the health care organization's governing body, the chief executive officer and other senior managers, and clinical leaders; collaboration among these leaders is critical to achieving the organization's quality goals. According to The Joint Commission (2009, p. 3), only "the leaders of a health care organization have the resources, influence, and control" to ensure that an organization has the right elements in place to meet quality and safety priorities, including a nonpunitive culture, the availability of appropriate resources (including human, financial, physical, and informational), a sufficient number of competent staff, and an ongoing evaluation of the quality and safety of care. In particular, health care organization governing boards have an obligation to ensure the quality and safety of care within their organizations (Arnwine, 2002; Callender et al., 2007; The Joint Commission, 2009).[4] As a part of their oversight function, governing boards routinely identify emerging quality of care trends and can help prioritize efforts to address these issues within an organization.

The involvement of organizational leaders and managers is crucial for successful change initiatives (Dixon-Woods et al., 2011; Firth-Cozens, 2004; Gandhi, 2014; Kotter, 1995; Larson, 2002; Moran and Brightman, 2000; Silow-Carroll et al., 2007). In many health care organizations, organizational leaders have not focused significant attention on improving diagnosis and reducing diagnostic errors (Gandhi, 2014; Graber, 2005; Graber et al., 2014; Henriksen, 2014; Wachter, 2010; Zwaan et al., 2013). However, facilitating change will require the support and involvement of these

---

[4] 42 C.F.R. § 482.12(a)(5); Caremark International Inc. Derivative Litigation, 698 A. 2d 959 (Del. Ch. 1996).

leaders. To start, health care governing boards can prioritize diagnosis and can support senior managers in implementing policies and practices that support continued learning and improved diagnostic performance. For example, potential policies and practices could focus on team-based care in diagnosis, the adoption of a continuously learning culture, opportunities to provide feedback to clinicians, and approaches to monitor the diagnostic process and identify diagnostic errors and near misses. All organizational leaders can raise awareness of the quality and safety challenges related to diagnostic error as well as dispelling the myth that diagnostic errors are inevitable (Leape, 2010; Wachter, 2010). Importantly, organizational leaders can appeal to the intrinsic motivation of health care professionals to drive improvements in diagnosis.

Focusing on improving diagnosis and reducing diagnostic error is necessary to improve the quality and safety of care; in addition, it has the potential to reduce organizational costs (IOM, 2013). For example, a recent study identified a link between inpatient harm and negative financial consequences for hospitals (Adler et al., 2015). The downstream effects associated with diagnostic error, including patient harm, malpractice claims, and inappropriate use of resources, suggest that organizations that focus on improving diagnosis could extend benefits beyond patient outcomes to include reducing costs. Research that evaluates the economic impact of diagnostic errors may be helpful in building the business case for prioritizing diagnosis within health care organizations (see Chapter 8).

There are a variety of strategies that can be drawn upon as leaders chart a course toward improved diagnostic performance, including Six Sigma and lean management principles (Chassin and Loeb, 2013; James and Savitz, 2011; Jimmerson et al., 2005; Pronovost et al., 2006; Todnem By, 2005; Varkey et al., 2007; Vest and Gamm, 2009). Involving leadership in WalkRounds, M&M conferences, and departmental meetings can help increase leadership visibility as diagnostic performance improvements are implemented (Frankel et al., 2003, 2005; Thomas et al., 2005). It may also be beneficial for leaders to pursue improvement efforts that are person-centered and community-driven, contribute to shaping the desired culture, and leverage interdisciplinary relationships (Swensen et al., 2013). Insights from HROs and just culture may also be useful as leaders consider the opportunities to improve diagnosis (Pronovost et al., 2006). In addition, leaders could adapt the IOM's CEO Checklist for High Value Health Care for improving diagnosis (see Box 6-4) (IOM, 2012). Because a majority of change initiatives fail, leaders need to be aware of the reasons for failure and take precautions to ensure that efforts to improve diagnosis are feasible and sustainable (Coiera, 2011; Etheridge et al., 2013; Henriksen and Dayton, 2006; Kotter, 1995). Ongoing evaluation of the change effort is also warranted.

BOX 6-4
A CEO Checklist for High-Value Health Care

Foundational Elements

- Governance priority—visible and determined leadership by chief executive officer (CEO) and board
- Culture of continuous improvement—commitment to ongoing, real-time learning

Infrastructure Fundamentals

- Information technology (IT) best practices—automated, reliable information to and from the point of care
- Evidence protocols—effective, efficient, and consistent care
- Resource utilization—optimized use of personnel, physical space, and other resources

Care Delivery Priorities

- Integrated care—right care, right setting, right clinicians, right teamwork
- Shared decision making—patient–clinician collaboration on care plans
- Targeted services—tailored community and clinic interventions for resource-intensive patients

Reliability and Feedback

- Embedded safeguards—supports and prompts to reduce injury and infection
- Internal transparency—visible progress in performance, outcomes, and costs

SOURCE: Adapted from IOM, 2012.

A SUPPORTIVE WORK SYSTEM TO FACILITATE DIAGNOSIS

Many components of the work system are under the purview of health care organizations. Thus, organizations can implement changes that ensure a work system that supports the diagnostic process. **The committee recommends that health care organizations should design the work system in which the diagnostic process occurs to support the work and activities of patients, their families, and health care professionals and to facilitate accurate and timely diagnoses.** The previous section described how health care organizations can use organizational culture, leadership, and management to facilitate organizational change. This section considers additional actions that organizations can take, including a focus on error recovery, on results reporting and communication, and on ensuring that additional work system elements (i.e., diagnostic team members and their tasks, the tools and technologies they employ, and the physical and external environment) support the diagnostic process.

Error Recovery

One principle that health care organizations can apply to the design of the work system is error recovery (IOM, 2000). There are a variety of opportunities for health care organizations to improve error recovery and resiliency in the diagnostic process. For example, improved patient access to clinical notes and diagnostic testing results is a form of error recovery; this gives patients the opportunity to identify and correct errors in their medical records that could lead to diagnostic errors, potentially before any harm results (Bell et al., 2014) (see Chapter 4). Informal, real-time collaboration among professionals, including face-to-face and virtual communication, presents another opportunity for error detection and recovery. Wachter (2015) noted that before the computerization of medical imaging, treating health care professionals often collaborated with radiologists in reading rooms while reviewing films together, whereas today communication is primarily facilitated electronically, through the radiology report. Health care organizations can consider how to promote these types of opportunities for clinicians to discuss cases and to facilitate more collaborative working relationships during the diagnostic process. For example, some organizations are now situating medical imaging reading stations in clinical areas, such as the emergency department and the intensive care unit (Wachter, 2015). The thoughtful use of redundancies, such as second reviews of anatomic pathology specimens and medical images, consultations, and second opinions in challenging cases or complex care environments, are also a form of error recovery that health care organizations can consider (Durning, 2014; Nakhleh et al., 2015). For example, the tele-intensive care unit is a telemedicine process that helps support clinicians' care for acutely ill patients by using off-site clinicians and software systems to provide a "second set of eyes" to remotely monitor intensive care unit patients (Berenson et al., 2009; Khunlertkit and Carayon, 2013).

Results Reporting and Communication

The Joint Commission has identified improved communication of critical test results as a key safety issue and urges organizations to "[r]eport critical results of tests and diagnostic procedures on a timely basis" (The Joint Commission, 2015b, p. 2). Input to the committee echoed this call and emphasized the importance of improving communication between treating health care professionals, pathologists, radiologists, and other diagnostic testing clinicians (Allen and Thorwarth, 2014; Epner, 2015; Gandhi, 2014; Myers, 2014). **To facilitate the timely collaboration among health care professionals in the diagnostic process, the committee recommends that health care organizations should develop and implement processes to ensure effective and timely communication between diagnostic testing health care professionals and treating health care professionals across all health care delivery settings.** For example, closed loop reporting systems for diagnostic testing and referral can be implemented to ensure that test results or specialist findings are reported back to the treating health care professional in a timely manner (Gandhi, 2014; Gandhi et al., 2005; Myers, 2014; SHIEP, 2012). These systems can also help to ensure that relevant information is being communicated among the appropriate health care professionals. Recent efforts to improve closed loop reporting include the American Medical Association's Closing the Referral Loop Project and the Office of the National Coordinator for Health Information Technology's 360X Project, which aim to develop guidelines for closed loop referral system implementation (AMA, 2015; Williams, 2012). Early lessons from the 360X Project include the importance of seamless workflow integration, tailoring the amount of information transmitted between clinicians and specialists, and the importance of national standards for system interoperability (SHIEP, 2012). A task force comprised of pathologists, radiologists, other clinicians, risk managers, patient safety specialists, and IT specialists recommended four actions to improve communication and follow-up related to clinically significant test results: (1) standardize policies and definitions across networked organizations, (2) identify the patient's care team, (3) results management and tracking, and (4) develop shared quality and reporting metrics (Roy et al., 2013).

Health care organizations can leverage health IT resources to improve communication and collaboration among pathologists, radiologists, and treating health care professionals (Allen and Thorwarth, 2014; Gandhi, 2014; Kroft, 2014; Schiff et al., 2003). HHS's Tests Results Reporting and Follow-Up SAFER Guide offers insight on how to use EHRs to safely facilitate communication and the reporting of results (HHS, 2015). Some closed loop reporting systems include an alert notification mechanism designed to inform ordering clinicians when critical diagnostic testing results are available (Lacson et al., 2014a,b; Singh et al., 2010). Dalal and colleagues (2014) identified an automated e-mail notification system as a "promising strategy for managing" the results of tests that were pending when the patient was discharged. There is some evidence that the use of alert notification mechanisms improves timely communication of results reports (Lacson et al., 2014a,b). However, closed loop reporting systems need to be carefully designed to support clinician cognition and workflow in the diagnostic process; if there is a high volume of alerts, a clinician may experience cognitive overload, which can limit the effectiveness of such alerts (Singh et al., 2009, 2010).

The use of standard formats may also improve the communication of test results. Studies have shown that structured radiology reports are more complete, have more relevant content, and have greater clarity than free-form reports (Marcovici and Taylor, 2014; Schwartz et al., 2011). Similar to a checklist, structured reports have a template with standardized headings and often use standardized language. Input to the committee suggests that similar standardized formats for anatomic and clinical pathology results reports are likely to improve communication (Gandhi, 2014; Myers, 2014). Encouraging the use of simpler and more transparent language in results reports may also improve communication between health care professionals.

Additional Work System Elements

In addition to improving error recovery and results reporting and communication, health care organizations can focus more broadly on improving the work system in which the diagnostic process occurs. To ensure that their work systems are designed to support the diagnostic process, health care organizations need to consider all of the elements of the work system and recognize that these elements are interrelated and dynamically interact. For example, a new EHR system (tools and technology) will be most beneficial when an organization ensures that its health care professionals are trained on how to use the system (team members and tasks), when the system meets usability standards (external environment), and when the tool is located in the appropriate location (physical environment). The following sections highlight some of the ways in which health care organizations can improve the design of work systems for improved diagnostic performance. The actions discussed are not meant to be exhaustive; rather, they are offered as examples of steps organizations can take. Discussions in Chapters 4, 5, and 7 further augment these discussions.

In addition to improving a specific work system, health care organizations need to recognize that patients may cross organizational boundaries when seeking a diagnosis. This fragmentation has the potential to contribute to diagnostic errors and the failures to learn from them. Though health care organizations are not solely responsible for this problem, they have a responsibility to ensure, to the best of their abilities, that the health care system as a whole supports the diagnostic process. Teamwork and health IT interoperability will help, but to meet this responsibility, organizations will need to take steps to improve communication with other organizations. One mechanism, discussed earlier, focuses on improving the communication of diagnostic testing results and referrals. Implementing systematic feedback mechanisms that track patient outcomes over time could also identify diagnostic errors that transcend health care organization boundaries. In addition, payment and care delivery reforms that incentivize accountability and collaboration may alleviate some of the challenges that the fragmented nature of the health care system presents for diagnosis (see Chapter 7).

Physical Environment

The design and characteristics of the physical environment can influence human performance and the quality and safety of health care (Carayon, 2012; Hogarth, 2010; Reiling et al., 2008). Elements of the physical environment include the layout and ambient conditions such as distractions, noise, temperature, and lighting. Researchers have focused primarily on the design of hospital environments and how these environments may influence patient safety, patient outcomes, and task performance. For example, a review of 600 articles on the impact of physical design found three studies that linked medication errors with factors in the hospital environment, including lighting, distractions, and interruptions (Ulrich et al., 2004). Another study found that operational failures occurring in two large hospitals were the result of insufficient workspace (29 percent), poor process design (23 percent), and a lack of integration in the internal supply chains (23 percent); only 14 percent of the failures could be attributed to training and human error (Tucker et al., 2013).

Although the impact of the physical environment on diagnostic error has not been well studied, there are indications that it may be an important contributor to diagnostic performance. For example, the emergency department has been described as a challenging environment in which to make diagnoses because of the presence of high-acuity illness, incomplete information, time constraints, and frequent interruptions and distractions (Croskerry and Sinclair, 2001). Cognitive performance is vulnerable to distractions and interruptions, which influence the likelihood of error (Chisholm et al., 2000). Other physical environment factors that could influence the diagnostic process include the location of health technologies designed to support the diagnostic process, adequate space for team members to complete their tasks related to the diagnostic process, and ambient conditions that can affect cognition, such as noise, lighting, odor, and temperature (Chellappa et al., 2011; Johnson, 2011; Mehta et al., 2012; Parsons, 2000; Ward, 2013). Poorly designed systems that require health care professionals to traverse long distances to perform their tasks may increase fatigue and reduce face-to-face time with patients (Ulrich et al., 2004).

To address the challenges associated with the physical environment, health care organizations can design workplaces that align with work patterns and support workflow, can locate health technology near the point of care, and can reduce ambient noise (Durning, 2014; Reiling et al., 2008; Ulrich et al., 2004). Other possible actions include using the appropriate lighting, providing adequate ventilation, and maintaining an appropriate temperature to ensure that the ambient conditions do not negatively affect diagnostic performance. Studies suggest that such changes may improve both patient outcomes and patient and family satisfaction with care provision (Reiling et al., 2008; Ulrich et al., 2004).

Diagnostic Team Members and Their Tasks

Health care organizations need to ensure that their clinicians have the needed competencies and support to perform their tasks in the diagnostic process. Health care professional certification and accreditation standards can be leveraged to ensure that health care professionals within an organization are well prepared to fulfill their roles in the diagnostic process. Health care organizations can also offer more opportunities for team-based training in diagnosis and can expand the use of integrated practice units, treatment planning conferences, and diagnostic management teams (see Chapter 4). Ensuring adequate supervision and support of health care professionals—especially the many health care professional trainees involved in the diagnostic process—is another way for health care organizations to improve the work system (ACGME, 2011; IOM, 2009). For example, many health care organizations have adopted policies to address patient safety risks caused by fatigue (including decision fatigue), sleep deprivation, and sleep debt for medical residents (Croskerry and Musson, 2009; IOM, 2009; Zwaan et al., 2009). Health care professionals who work in high-stress environments may also experience mental health difficulties and burnout, which can increase the chance of error (AHRQ, 2005; Bakker et al., 2005; Dyrbye and Shanafelt, 2011). Several studies have identified certain characteristics of the workplace and high patient care demands as a cause of this stress and have suggested workforce and culture changes as potential solutions (AHRQ, 2005; Bakker et al., 2005; Dyrbye and Shanafelt, 2011). For example, work scheduling practices can ensure that a health care organization has the appropriate clinicians for facilitating the diagnostic process (both amount of clinicians and appropriate areas of expertise).

Health care organizations can also make improvements to the work system to better involve patients and their families in the diagnostic process and in efforts to improve diagnosis (Kelly et al., 2013). For example, health care organizations can improve patient access to their EHRs, incorporate patient and family advisory groups, and involve patients and their families in processes to learn about errors when appropriate. In addition, these organizations can offer patients and their families more opportunities to provide feedback on their experiences with diagnosis (see Chapter 4).

Tools and Technologies

Health care organizations will need to consider how the tools and technologies they provide for the delivery of health care affect the diagnostic process. For example, Chapter 5 highlights the need for health IT tools to incorporate human-centered design principles, fit within clinical workflow, integrate measurement capability, provide decision support, and facilitate the timely flow of information. Health care organizations can consider these issues when choosing health IT tools to incorporate, considering implementation issues, and ensuring that use is safe and aligned with clinical workflow. Some organizations may need to consider workflow redesign when adopting new health IT. Resources are available to guide health care organizations as they integrate new health IT or redesign their workflow (HealthIT.gov, 2013).

External Environment

External environmental factors can influence the work system in which diagnosis occurs, and although they are typically not under the control of health care organizations, they need to be taken into account as efforts to improve the work system are implemented at the level of health care organizations (see Chapter 7).

RECOMMENDATIONS

Goal 4: Develop and deploy approaches to identify, learn from, and reduce diagnostic errors and near misses in clinical practice

Recommendation 4a: Accreditation organizations and the Medicare conditions of participation should require that health care organizations have programs in place to monitor the diagnostic process and identify, learn from, and reduce diagnostic errors and near misses in a timely fashion. Proven approaches should be incorporated into updates of these requirements.

Recommendation 4b: Health care organizations should:
- Monitor the diagnostic process and identify, learn from, and reduce diagnostic errors and near misses as a component of their research, quality improvement, and patient safety programs.
- Implement procedures and practices to provide systematic feedback on diagnostic performance to individual health care professionals, care teams, and clinical and organizational leaders.

Recommendation 4c: The Department of Health and Human Services should provide funding for a designated subset of health care systems to conduct routine postmortem examinations on a representative sample of patient deaths.

Recommendation 4d: Health care professional societies should identify opportunities to improve accurate and timely diagnoses and reduce diagnostic errors in their specialties.

Goal 5: Establish a work system and culture that supports the diagnostic process and improvements in diagnostic performance

Recommendation 5: Health care organizations should:
- Adopt policies and practices that promote a nonpunitive culture that values open discussion and feedback on diagnostic performance.
- Design the work system in which the diagnostic process occurs to support the work and activities of patients, their families, and health care professionals and to facilitate accurate and timely diagnoses.
- Develop and implement processes to ensure effective and timely communication between diagnostic testing health care professionals and treating health care professionals across all health care delivery settings.

REFERENCES

ACGME (Accreditation Council for Graduate Medical Education). 2011. *The ACGME 2011 duty hour standards: enhancing quality of care, supervision, and resident professional development*. Chicago, IL: Accreditation Council for Graduate Medical Education.

ACR (American College of Radiology). 2013. RADPEER™ marks a decade of service. www.acr.org/Quality-Safety/eNews/Issue-01-March-2013/RADPEER (accessed July 15, 2015).

ACR. 2015. RADPEER. www.acr.org/Quality-Safety/RADPEER (accessed June 7, 2015).

Adler, L., D. Yi, M. Li, B. McBroom, L. Hauck, C. Sammer, C. Jones, T. Shaw, and D. Classen. 2015. Impact of inpatient harms on hospital finances and patient clinical outcomes. *Journal of Patient Safety*, March 23 [Epub ahead of print].

AHRQ (Agency for Healthcare Research and Quality). 2005. Organizational climate, stress, and error in primary care: the MEMO Study. In K. Henriksen, J. B. Battles, E. S. Marks, and D. I. Lewin (eds.), *Advances in patient safety: From research to implementation (Vol. 1: Research findings)* (pp. 65–77). AHRQ Publication No. 05-0021-1. Rockville, MD: Agency for Healthcare Research and Quality.

AHRQ. 2008. Transforming the morbidity and mortality conference into an instrument for systemwide improvement. In K. Henriksen, J. B. Battles, M. A. Keyes, and M. L. Grady (eds.), *Advances in patient safety: New directions and alternative approaches (Vol. 2: Culture and redesign)* (pp. 357-363). AHRQ Publication No. 08-0034-2. Rockville, MD: Agency for Healthcare Research and Quality. www.ahrq.gov/professionals/quality-patient-safety/patient-safety-resources/resources/advances-in-patient-safety-2/vol2/advances-deis_82.pdf (accessed June 7, 2015).

AHRQ. 2011. *Designing consumer reporting systems for patient safety events.* AHRQ Publication No. 11-0060-EF. Rockville, MD: Agency for Healthcare Research and Quality. www.ahrq.gov/professionals/quality-patient-safety/patient-safety-resources/resources/consumer-experience/reporting/11-0060-EF.pdf

AHRQ. 2014a. *Hospital survey on patient safety culture: 2014 user comparative database report.* AHRQ Publication No. 14-0019-EF. Rockville, MD: Agency for Healthcare Research and Quality. www.ahrq.gov/professionals/quality-patient-safety/patientsafety culture/hospital/2014/hsops14pt1.pdf (accessed February 25, 2014).

AHRQ. 2014b. Patient safety primers: Root cause analysis. www.psnet.ahrq.gov/primer. aspx?primerID=10 (accessed May 25, 2015).

AHRQ. 2014c. Surveys on patient safety culture. www.ahrq.gov/professionals/quality-patient-safety/patientsafetyculture (accessed April 28, 2015).

AHRQ. 2015a. Glossary entry: Just culture. http://psnet.ahrq.gov/popup_glossary. aspx?name=justculture (accessed June 7, 2015).

AHRQ. 2015b. Patient safety indicators overview. www.qualityindicators.ahrq.gov/modules/psi_resources.aspx (accessed April 6, 2015).

Allen, B., and W. T. Thorwarth. 2014. Comments from the American College of Radiology. Input submitted to the Committee on Diagnostic Error in Health Care, November 5 and December 29, 2014, Washington, DC.

Allen, M. 2011. Without autopsies, hospitals bury their mistakes. *ProPublica*, December 15. www.propublica.org/article/without-autopsies-hospitals-bury-their-mistakes (accessed May 4, 2015).

AMA (American Medical Association). 2015. Closing the Referral Loop project. www. ama-assn.org/ama/pub/physician-resources/physician-consortium-performance-improvement/about-pcpi/focus-on-quality/quality-improvement/closing-referral-loop.page? (accessed March 27, 2015).

Arnwine, D. L. 2002. Effective governance: The roles and responsibilities of board members. *Proceedings (Baylor University. Medical Center)* 15(1):19–22.

Bakker, A. B., P. M. Le Blanc, and W. B. Schaufeli. 2005. Burnout contagion among intensive care nurses. *Journal of Advanced Nursing* 51(3):276–287.

Bell, S., M. Anselmo, J. Walker, and T. Delbanco. 2014. OpenNotes. Input submitted to the Committee on Diagnostic Error in Health Care, December 2, 2014, Washington, DC.

Berenson, R. A., J. M. Grossman, and E. A. November. 2009. Does telemonitoring of patients—the eICU—improve intensive care? *Health Affairs* 28(5):w937–w947.

Berenson, R. A., D. Upadhyay, and D. R. Kaye. 2014. *Placing diagnosis errors on the policy agenda*. Washington, DC: Urban Institute. www.urban.org/research/publication/placing-diagnosis-errors-policy-agenda (accessed June 7, 2015).

Berner, E. S., and M. L. Graber. 2008. Overconfidence as a cause of diagnostic error in medicine. *American Journal of Medicine* 121(5 Suppl):S2–S23.

Bhise, V., and H. Singh. 2015. Measuring diagnostic safety of inpatients: Time to set sail in uncharted waters. *Diagnosis* 2(1):1–2.

Bisantz, A., and E. Roth. 2007. Analysis of cognitive work. *Reviews of Human Factors and Ergonomics* 3(1):1–43.

Black, L. M. 2011. Tragedy into policy: A quantitative study of nurses' attitudes toward patient advocacy activities. *American Journal of Nursing* 111(6):26–35; quiz 36–37.

Brook, O. R., J. Romero, A. Brook, J. B. Kruskal, C. S. Yam, and D. Levine. 2015. The complementary nature of peer review and quality assurance data collection. *Radiology* 274(1):221–229.

Callender, A. N., D. Hastings, M. Hemsley, L. Morris, and M. Peregrine. 2007. *Corporate responsibility and health care quality: A resource for health care boards of directors.* Washington, DC: Department of Health and Human Services Office of the Inspector General and American Health Lawyers Association.

Carayon, P. 2012. The physical environment in health care. In C. J. Alvarado (ed.), *Handbook of human factors and ergonomics in health care and patient safety* (pp. 215–234). Boca Raton, FL: Taylor & Francis Group.

Carayon, P., Y. Li, M. M. Kelly, L. L. DuBenske, A. Xie, B. McCabe, J. Orne, and E. D. Cox. 2014. Stimulated recall methodology for assessing work system barriers and facilitators in family-centered rounds in a pediatric hospital. *Applied Ergonomics* 45(6):1540–1546.

CDC (Centers for Disease Control and Prevention). 2001. *The autopsy, medicine, and mortality statistics. Vital Health Statistics* 3(32). Hyattsville, MD: Centers for Disease Control and Prevention.

Chassin, M. R. 2013. Improving the quality of health care: What's taking so long? *Health Affairs* 32(10):1761–1765.

Chassin, M. R., and J. M. Loeb. 2011. The ongoing quality improvement journey: Next stop, high reliability. *Health Affairs* 30(4):559–568.

Chassin, M. R., and J. M. Loeb. 2013. High-reliability health care: Getting there from here. *Milbank Quarterly* 91(3):459–490.

Chellappa, S. L., M. Gordijn, and C. Cajochen. 2011. Can light make us bright? Effects of light on cognition and sleep. *Progress in Brain Research* 190:119–133.

Chisholm, C. D., E. K. Collison, D. R. Nelson, and W. H. Cordell. 2000. Emergency department workplace interruptions: Are emergency physicians "interrupt-driven" and "multi-tasking"? *Academic Emergency Medicine* 7(11):1239–1243.

Choosing Wisely. 2015. Choosing Wisely: An initiative of the ABIM Foundation. www.choosingwisely.org (accessed March 3, 2015).

Cincinnati Children's Hospital. 2014. Becoming a high reliability organization. www.cincinnatichildrens.org/service/j/anderson-center/safety/methodology/high-reliability (accessed March 9, 2015).

CMS (Centers for Medicare & Medicaid Services). 2015a. Conditions for coverage (CfCs) & Conditions of Participations (CoPs). www.cms.gov/Regulations-and-Guidance/Legislation/CFCsAndCoPs/index.html?redirect=/cfcsandcops/16_asc.asp (accessed March 26, 2015).

CMS. 2015b. State Operations Manual, Appendix A - Survey Protocol, Regulations and Interpretive Guidelines for Hospitals. www.cms.gov/Regulations-and-Guidance/Guidance/Manuals/Downloads/som107ap_a_hospitals.pdf (accessed June 30, 2015).

Coiera, E. 2011. Why system inertia makes health reform so difficult. *BMJ* 342:d3693.

Connor, M., D. Duncombe, E. Barclay, S. Bartel, C. Borden, E. Gross, C. Miller, and P. R. Ponte. 2007. Creating a fair and just culture: One institution's path toward organizational change. *Joint Commission Journal on Quality and Patient Safety* 33(10):617–624.

CRICO. 2014. *Annual benchmarking report: Malpractice risks in the diagnostic process.* Cambridge, MA: CRICO. www.rmfstrategies.com/benchmarking (accessed June 4, 2015).

Croskerry, P. 2000. The feedback sanction. *Academic Emergency Medicine* 7(11):1232–1238.

Croskerry, P. 2003. The importance of cognitive errors in diagnosis and strategies to minimize them. *Academic Medicine* 78(8):775–780.

Croskerry, P. 2005. Diagnostic failure: A cognitive and affective approach. In *Advances in patient safety: From research to implementation, Vol. 2* (pp. 241–254). AHRQ Publication No. 050021. Rockville, MD: Agency for Healthcare Research and Quality.

Croskerry, P. 2012. Perspectives on diagnostic failure and patient safety. *Healthcare Quarterly* 15(Special Issue):50–56.

Croskerry, P., and D. Musson. 2009. Individual Factors in Patient Safety. In P. Croskerry, K. S. Cosby, S. M. Schenkel, and R. L. Wears (eds.), *Patient Safety in Emergency Medicine* (pp. 269–276). Philadelphia, PA: Lippincott Williams and Wilkins.

Croskerry, P., and G. Norman. 2008. Overconfidence in clinical decision making. *American Journal of Medicine* 121(5 Suppl):S24–S29.

Croskerry, P., and D. Sinclair. 2001. Emergency medicine: A practice prone to error. *Canadian Journal of Emergency Medicine* 3(4):271–276.

Dalal, A. K., C. L. Roy, E. G. Poon, D. H. Williams, N. Nolido, C. Yoon, J. Budris, T. Gandhi, D. W. Bates, and J. L. Schnipper. 2014. Impact of an automated email notification system for results of tests pending at discharge: a cluster-randomized controlled trial. *Journal of the American Medical Informatics Association* 21(3):473–480.

Davies, H. T. O., and S. M. Nutley. 2000. Developing learning organisations in the new NHS. *BMJ* 320(7240):998–1001.

Davies, H. T. O., S. M. Nutley, and R. Mannion. 2000. Organisational culture and quality of health care. *Quality in Health Care* 9(2):111–119.

Dhaliwal, G. 2014. Blueprint for diagnostic excellence. Presentation to the Committee on Diagnostic Error in Health Care, November 21, 2014, Washington, DC.

Dixon-Woods, M., C. Bosk, E. Aveling, C. Goeschel, and P. Pronovost. 2011. Explaining Michigan: Developing an ex-post theory of a quality improvement program. *Milbank Quarterly* 89(2):167–205.

Durning, S. J. 2014. Submitted input. Input submitted to the Committee on Diagnostic Error in Health Care, October 24, 2014, Washington, DC.

Dyrbye, L. N., and T. D. Shanafelt. 2011. Physician burnout: A potential threat to successful health care reform. *JAMA* 305(19):2009–2010.

Epner, P. 2014. An Overview of Diagnostic Error in Medicine. Presentation to the Committee on Diagnostic Error in Health Care, April 28, 2014, Washington, DC.

Epner, P. 2015. Submitted input. Input submitted to the Committee on Diagnostic Error in Health Care, January 13, 2015, Washington, DC.

Etchegaray, J. M., T. H. Gallagher, S. K. Bell, B. Dunlap, and E. J. Thomas. 2012. Error disclosure: A new domain for safety culture assessment. *BMJ Quality & Safety* 21(7):594–599.

Etheridge, F., Y. Couturier, J.-L. Denis, L. Tremblay, and C. Tannenbaum. 2013. Explaining the success or failure of quality improvement initiatives in long-term care organizations from a dynamic perspective. *Journal of Applied Gerontology* 33(6):672–689.

Farley, D. O., M. S. Ridgely, P. Mendel, S. S. Teleki, and C. L. Damberg. 2009. *Assessing patient safety practices and outcomes in the US health care system.* Santa Monica, CA: RAND Corporation.

Firth-Cozens, J. 2004. Organisational trust: The keystone to patient safety. *Quality and Safety in Health Care* 13(1):56–61.

Fotenos, A., and P. Nagy. 2012. What are your goals for peer review? A framework for understanding differing methods. *Journal of the American College of Radiology* 9(12):929–930.

Frankel, A., E. Graydon-Baker, C. Neppl, T. Simmonds, M. Gustafson, and T. K. Gandhi. 2003. Patient safety leadership WalkRounds. *Joint Commission Journal on Quality and Patient Safety* 29(1):16–26.

Frankel, A., S. P. Grillo, E. G. Baker, C. N. Huber, S. Abookire, M. Grenham, P. Console, M. O'Quinn, G. Thibault, and T. K. Gandhi. 2005. Patient safety leadership WalkRounds at Partners HealthCare: Learning from implementation. *Joint Commission Journal on Quality and Patient Safety* 31(8):423–437.

Gallagher, T. H., M. M. Mello, W. Levinson, M. K. Wynia, A. K. Sachdeva, L. Snyder Sulmasy, R. D. Truog, J. Conway, K. Mazor, A. Lembitz, S. K. Bell, L. Sokol-Hessner, J. Shapiro, A. L. Puopolo, and R. Arnold. 2013. Talking with patients about other clinicians' errors. *New England Journal of Medicine* 369(18):1752–1757.

Gandhi, T. K. 2014. Focus on diagnostic errors: Understanding and prevention. Presentation to the Committee on Diagnostic Error in Health Care, August 7, 2014, Washington, DC.

Gandhi, T. K., and T. H. Lee. 2010. Patient safety beyond the hospital. *New England Journal of Medicine* 363(11):1001–1003.

Gandhi, T. K., E. Graydon-Baker, C. Neppl Huber, A. D. Whittemore, and M. Gustafson. 2005. Closing the loop: Follow-up and feedback in a patient safety program. *Joint Commission Journal on Quality and Patient Safety* 31(11):614–621.

Gandhi, T. K., A. Kachalia, E. J. Thomas, A. L. Puopolo, C. Yoon, T. A. Brennan, and D. M. Studdert. 2006. Missed and delayed diagnoses in the ambulatory setting: A study of closed malpractice claims. *Annals of Internal Medicine* 145(7):488–496.

Graber, M. L. 2005. Diagnostic errors in medicine: A case of neglect. *Joint Commission Journal on Quality and Patient Safety* 31(2):106–113.

Graber, M. L. 2013. The incidence of diagnostic error in medicine. *BMJ Quality & Safety* 22(Suppl 2):ii21–ii27.

Graber, M. L., N. Franklin, and R. Gordon. 2005. Diagnostic error in internal medicine. *Archives of Internal Medicine* 165(13):1493–1499.

Graber, M. L., S. Kissam, V. L. Payne, A. N. D. Meyer, A. Sorensen, N. Lenfestey, E. Tant, K. Henriksen, K. LaBresh, and H. Singh. 2012a. Cognitive interventions to reduce diagnostic error: A narrative review. *BMJ Quality & Safety* 21(7):535–557.

Graber, M. L., R. M. Wachter, and C. K. Cassel. 2012b. Bringing diagnosis into the quality and safety equations. *JAMA* 308(12):1211–1212.

Graber, M. L., R. Trowbridge, J. S. Myers, C. A. Umscheid, W. Strull, and M. H. Kanter. 2014. The next organizational challenge: Finding and addressing diagnostic error. *Joint Commission Journal on Quality and Patient Safety* 40(3):102–110.

Grumbach, K., C. R. Lucey, and S. C. Johnston. 2014. Transforming from centers of learning to learning health systems: The challenge for academic health centers. *JAMA* 311(11):1109–1110.

Hall, P. 2005. Interprofessional teamwork: Professional cultures as barriers. *Journal of Interprofessional Care* 19(Suppl 1):188–196.

HealthIT.gov. 2013. What is workflow redesign? Why is it important? www.healthit.gov/providers-professionals/faqs/ehr-workflow-redesign (accessed May 1, 2015).

Henriksen, K. 2014. Improving diagnostic performance: Some unrecognized obstacles. *Diagnosis* 1(1):35–38.

Henriksen, K., and E. Dayton. 2006. Organizational silence and hidden threats to patient safety. *Health Services Research* 41(4p2):1539–1554.

HHS (Department of Health and Human Services). 2015. Test results reporting and follow-up. www.healthit.gov/safer/guide/sg008 (accessed April 9, 2015).

Hill, R. B., and R. E. Anderson. 1988. *The autopsy—Medical practice and public policy*. Boston: Butterworths.

HIMSS (Healthcare Information and Management Systems Society) Analytics. 2015. HIMSS analytics stage 7 Case study: Kaiser Permanente. http://himssanalytics.org/case-study/kaiser-permanente-stage-7-case-study (accessed May 10, 2015).

Hines, S., K. Luna, J. Lofthus, M. Marquardt, and D. Stelmokas. 2008. *Becoming a high reliability organization: Operational advice for hospital leaders*. Rockville, MD: Agency for Healthcare Research and Quality.

Hoffman, J. R., and H. K. Kanzaria. 2014. Intolerance of error and culture of blame drive medical excess. *BMJ* 349:g5702.

Hogarth, R. 2010. On the learning of intuition. In H. Plessner, C. Betsch, and T. Betsch (eds.), *Intuition in judgment and decision making* (pp. 91–105). New York: Taylor & Francis.

Hysong, S. J., R. G. Best, and J. A. Pugh. 2006. Audit and feedback and clinical practice guideline adherence: Making feedback actionable. *Implementation Science* 1(9).

IHI (Institute for Healthcare Improvement). 2004. Patient safety leadership WalkRounds. www.ihi.org/resources/Pages/Tools/PatientSafetyLeadershipWalkRounds.aspx (accessed June 7, 2015).

Ilgen, D. R., C. D. Fisher, and M. S. Taylor. 1979. Consequences of individual feedback on behavior in organizations. *Journal of Applied Psychology* 64(4):349–371.

IOM (Institute of Medicine). 2000. *To err is human: Building a safer health system*. Washington, DC: National Academy Press.

IOM. 2004. *Patient safety: Achieving a new standard for care*. Washington, DC: The National Academies Press.

IOM. 2009. *Resident duty hours: Enhancing sleep, supervision, and safety*. Washington, DC: The National Academies Press.

IOM. 2012. *A CEO checklist for high-value health care: Discussion paper*. Washington, DC: The National Academies. http://nam.edu/wp-content/uploads/2015/06/CEOHigh ValueChecklist.pdf (accessed July 25, 2015).

IOM. 2013. *Best care at lower cost: The path to continuously learning health care in America*. Washington, DC: The National Academies Press.

Ivers, N., G. Jamtvedt, S. Flottorp, J. M. Young, J. Odgaard-Jensen, S. D. French, M. A. O'Brien, M. Johansen, J. Grimshaw, and A. D. Oxman. 2012. Audit and feedback: Effects on professional practice and healthcare outcomes. *Cochrane Database Systematic Reviews* Issue 6:Cd000259.

Ivers, N., A. Sales, H. Colquhoun, S. Michie, R. Foy, J. Francis, and J. Grimshaw. 2014. No more "business as usual" with audit and feedback interventions: Towards an agenda for a reinvigorated intervention. *Implementation Science* 9(1):14.

Iyer, R. S., J. O. Swanson, R. K. Otto, and E. Weinberger. 2013. Peer review comments augment diagnostic error characterization and departmental quality assurance: 1-year experience from a children's hospital. *American Journal of Roentgenology* 200(1):132–137.

James, B. C., and L. A. Savitz. 2011. How Intermountain trimmed health care costs through robust quality improvement efforts. *Health Affairs (Millwood)* 30(6):1185–1191.

Jeffe, D. B., W. C. Dunagan, J. Garbutt, T. E. Burroughs, T. H. Gallagher, P. R. Hill, C. B. Harris, K. Bommarito, and V. J. Fraser. 2004. Using focus groups to understand physicians' and nurses' perspectives on error reporting in hospitals. *Joint Commission Journal on Quality and Patient Safety* 30(9):471–479.

Jimmerson, C., D. Weber, and D. K. Sobek. 2005. Reducing waste and errors: Piloting lean principles at Intermountain Healthcare. *Joint Commission Journal on Quality and Patient Safety* 31(5):249–257.

Johnson, A. J. 2011. Cognitive facilitation following intentional odor exposure. *Sensors* 11(5):5469–5488.

The Joint Commission. 2009. Leadership in healthcare organizations: A guide to joint commission leadership standards. www.jointcommission.org/Leadership_in_Healthcare_Organizations (accessed May 1, 2015).

The Joint Commission. 2015a. Sentinel Event Policy and Procedures. www.jointcommission.org/Sentinel_Event_Policy_and_Procedures (accessed March 26, 2015).

The Joint Commission. 2015b. National Patient Safety Goals Effective January 1, 2015. www.jointcommission.org/assets/1/6/2015_NPSG_HAP.pdf (accessed November 30, 2015).

Kachalia, A. 2013. Improving patient safety through transparency. Presentation to the Committee on Diagnostic Error in Health Care, August 7, 2014, Washington, DC.

Kanter, M. H. 2014. Diagnostic errors—Patient safety. Presentation to the Committee on Diagnostic Error in Health Care, August 7, 2014, Washington, DC.

Kelly, M. M., A. Xie, P. Carayon, L. L. DuBenske, M. L. Ehlenbach, and E. D. Cox. 2013. Strategies for improving family engagement during family-centered rounds. *Journal of Hospital Medicine* 8(4):201–207.

Khatri, N., G. D. Brown, and L. L. Hicks. 2009. From a blame culture to a just culture in health care. *Health Care Management Review* 34(4):312–322.

Khunlertkit, A., and P. Carayon. 2013. Contributions of tele-intensive care unit (Tele-ICU) technology to quality of care and patient safety. *Journal of Critical Care* 28(3):315. e311–312.

Kirwan, B., and L. K. Ainsworth (eds.). 1992. *A guide to task analysis: The task analysis working group*. Boca Raton, FL: CRC Press.

Kotter, J. P. 1995. Leading change: Why transformation efforts fail. *Harvard Business Review.* January 2007. https://hbr.org/2007/01/leading-change-why-transformation-efforts-fail (accessed June 29, 2015).

Kotter, J. P. 2012. The key to changing organizational culture. *Forbes*, September 27. www.forbes.com/sites/johnkotter/2012/09/27/the-key-to-changing-organizational-culture (accessed March 9, 2015).

Kroft, S. 2014. American Society for Clinical Pathology. Input submitted to the Committee on Diagnostic Error in Health Care, April 28, 2014, Washington, DC.

Kruskal, J. B., B. Siewert, S. W. Anderson, R. L. Eisenberg, and J. Sosna. 2008. Managing an acute adverse event in a radiology department. *RadioGraphics* 28(5):1237–1250.

Lacson, R., S. D. O'Connor, K. P. Andriole, L. M. Prevedello, and R. Khorasani. 2014a. Automated critical test result notification system: Architecture, design, and assessment of provider satisfaction. *American Journal of Roentgenology* 203(5):W491–W496.

Lacson, R., L. M. Prevedello, K. P. Andriole, S. D. O'Connor, C. Roy, T. Gandhi, A. K. Dalal, L. Sato, and R. Khorasani. 2014b. Four-year impact of an alert notification system on closed-loop communication of critical test results. *American Journal of Roentgenololgy* 203(5):933–938.

Larson, E. B. 2002. Measuring, monitoring, and reducing medical harm from a systems perspective: A medical director's personal reflections. *Academic Medicine* 77(10):993–1000.

Lavanya, T., M. Cohen, S. V. Gandhi, T. Farrell, and E. H. Whitby. 2008. A case of a Dandy-Walker variant: The importance of a multidisciplinary team approach using complementary techniques to obtain accurate diagnostic information. *British Journal of Radiology* 81(970):e242–e245.

Leape. L. 2010. Q&A with Lucian Leape, M.D., adjunct professor of health policy, Harvard University. www.commonwealthfund.org/publications/newsletters/states-in-action/2010/jan/january-february-2010/ask-the-expert/ask-the-expert (accessed September 23, 2014).

Lee, C. S., P. G. Nagy, S. J. Weaver, and D. E. Newman-Toker. 2013. Cognitive and system factors contributing to diagnostic errors in radiology. *American Journal of Roentgenology* 201(3):611–617.

Lopez-Campos, J. L., M. I. Asensio-Cruz, A. Castro-Acosta, C. Calero, and F. Pozo-Rodriguez. 2014. Results from an audit feedback strategy for chronic obstructive pulmonary disease in hospital care: A joint analysis from the AUDIPOC and European COPD Audit Studies. *PLoS ONE* 9(10):e110394.

Lundberg, G. D. 1998. Low-tech autopsies in the era of high-tech medicine: Continued value for quality assurance and patient safety. *JAMA* 280(14):1273–1274.

Marcovici, P. A., and G. A. Taylor. 2014. Structured radiology reports are more complete and more effective than unstructured reports. *American Journal of Roentgenology* 203(6): 1265–1271.

Marx, D. A. 2001. Patient safety and the "just culture": A primer for health care executives. Medical Event Reporting System–Transfusion Medicine. www.safer.healthcare.ucla. edu/safer/archive/ahrq/FinalPrimerDoc.pdf (accessed June 7, 2015).

McDonald, K. M. 2014. The diagnostic field's players and interactions: From the inside out. *Diagnosis* 1(1):55–58.

McDonald, K. M., B. Matesic, D. G. Contopoulos–Ioannidis, J. Lonhart, E. Schmidt, N. Pineda, and J. P. A. Ioannidis. 2013. Patient safety strategies targeted at diagnostic errors: A systematic review. *Annals of Internal Medicine* 158(5 Part 2):381–389.

MedPAC (Medicare Payment Advisory Commission). 1999. *Report to the Congress: Selected Medicare issues.* Washington, DC: MedPAC. http://medpac.gov/documents/reports/Jun99Entirereport.pdf?sfvrsn=0 (accessed June 7, 2015).

Mehta, R., R. Zhu, and A. Cheema. 2012. Is noise always bad? Exploring the effects of ambient noise on creative cognition. *Journal of Consumer Research* 39(4):784–799.

Milstead, J. A. 2005. The culture of safety. *Policy, Politics, & Nursing Practice* 6(1):51–54.

Modak, I., J. B. Sexton, T. Lux, R. Helmreich, and E. Thomas. 2007. Measuring safety culture in the ambulatory setting: The Safety Attitudes Questionnaire—Ambulatory Version. *Journal of General Internal Medicine* 22(1):1–5.

Moran, J. W., and B. K. Brightman. 2000. Leading organizational change. *Journal of Workplace Learning* 12(2):66–74.

Murphy, D. R., A. Laxmisan, B. A. Reis, E. J. Thomas, A. Esquivel, S. N. Forjuoh, R. Parikh, M. M. Khan, and H. Singh. 2014. Electronic health record-based triggers to detect potential delays in cancer diagnosis. *BMJ Quality & Safety* 23(1):8–16.

Myers, J. 2014. Diagnostic errors in (. . . and around) pathology. Presentation to the Committee on Diagnostic Error in Health Care, August 7, 2014, Washington, DC.

Nakhleh, R. E., V. Nose, C. Colasacco, L. A. Fatheree, T. J. Lillemoe, D. C. McCrory, F. A. Meier, C. N. Otis, S. R. Owens, S. S. Raab, R. R. Turner, C. B. Ventura, and A. A. Renshaw. 2015. Interpretive diagnostic error reduction in surgical pathology and cytology: Guideline from the College of American Pathologists Pathology and Laboratory Quality Center and the Association of Directors of Anatomic and Surgical Pathology. *Archives of Pathology and Laboratory Medicine*, May 12 [Epub ahead of print].

NCQA (National Committee for Quality Assurance). 2013. Accountable care organization accreditation. www.ncqa.org/Programs/Accreditation/AccountableCareOrganization ACO.aspx (accessed May 1, 2015).

Nemetz, P. N., E. Tangalos, L. P. Sands, W. P. Fisher Jr, W. P. Newman III, and E. C. Burton. 2006. Attitudes toward the autopsy—An 8-state survey. *Medscape General Medicine* 8(3):80.

Newman-Toker, D. E., K. M. McDonald, and D. O. Meltzer. 2013. How much diagnostic safety can we afford, and how should we decide? A health economics perspective. *BMJ Quality & Safety* 22(Suppl 2):ii11–ii20.

NQF (National Quality Forum). 2011. *Serious reportable events in healthcare—2011 update: A consensus report.* Washington, DC: National Quality Forum.

O'Donnell, C., and N. Woodford. 2008. Post-mortem radiology—A new sub-speciality? *Clinical Radiology* 63(11):1189–1194.

Parmelli, E., G. Flodgren, F. Beyer, N. Baillie, M. Schaafsma, and M. Eccles. 2011. The effectiveness of strategies to change organisational culture to improve healthcare performance: A systematic review. *Implementation Science* 6(1):33.

Parsons, K. C. 2000. Environmental ergonomics: A review of principles, methods and models. *Applied Ergonomics* 31(6):581–594.

Perlman, K. 2011. Change fatigue: Taking its toll on your employees? *Forbes*, September 15. www.forbes.com/sites/johnkotter/2011/09/15/can-i-use-this-method-for-change-in-my-organization (accessed April 29, 2011).

Pichereau, C., E. Maury, L. Monnier-Cholley, S. Bourcier, G. Lejour, M. Alves, J.-L. Baudel, H. Ait Oufella, B. Guidet, and L. Arrivé. 2015. Post-mortem CT scan with contrast injection and chest compression to diagnose pulmonary embolism. *Intensive Care Medicine* 41(1):167–168.

Plaza, C., L. Beard, A. D. Fonzo, M. D. Tommaso, Y. Mujawaz, M. Serra-Julia, and D. Morra. 2011. Innovation in healthcare team feedback. *Healthcare Quarterly* 14(2):61–68.

Plebani, M., and G. Lippi. 2011. Closing the brain-to-brain loop in laboratory testing. *Clinical Chemistry and Laboratory Medicine* 49(7):1131–1133.

Plebani, M., M. Laposata, and G. D. Lundberg. 2011. The brain-to-brain loop concept for laboratory testing 40 years after its introduction. *American Journal of Clinical Pathology* 136(6):829–833.

Pronovost, P. J., S. M. Berenholtz, C. A. Goeschel, D. M. Needham, J. B. Sexton, D. A. Thompson, L. H. Lubomski, J. A. Marsteller, M. A. Makary, and E. Hunt. 2006. Creating high reliability in health care organizations. *Health Services Research* 41(4p2):1599–1617.

Pronovost, P. J., S. M. Berenholtz, and D. M. Needham. 2008. Translating evidence into practice: a model for large scale knowledge translation. *BMJ* 337:a1714.

Pronovost, P. J., C. A. Goeschel, E. Colantuoni, S. Watson, L. H. Lubomski, S. M. Berenholtz, D. A. Thompson, D. J. Sinopoli, S. Cosgrove, J. B. Sexton, J. A. Marsteller, R. C. Hyzy, R. Welsh, P. Posa, K. Schumacher, and D. Needham. 2010. Sustaining reductions in catheter related bloodstream infections in Michigan intensive care units: Observational study. *BMJ* 340:c309.

Provenzale, J., and P. Kranz. 2011. Understanding errors in diagnostic radiology: Proposal of a classification scheme and application to emergency radiology. *Emergency Radiology* 18(5):403–408.

Reiling, J., G. Hughes, and M. Murphy. 2008. Chapter 28: The impact of facility design on patient safety. In R. G. Hughes (ed.), *Patient safety and quality: An evidence-based handbook for nurses* (pp. 700–725). Rockville, MD: Agency for Healthcare Research and Quality.

Reilly, J. B., J. S. Myers, D. Salvador, and R. L. Trowbridge. 2014. Use of a novel, modified fishbone diagram to analyze diagnostic errors. *Diagnosis* 1(2):167–171.

Reilly, J. B., M. L. Graber, and R. L. Trowbridge. 2015. How to do a root cause analysis of diagnostic error. http://c.ymcdn.com/sites/www.npsf.org/resource/collection/A81D4178-F1E9-4F87-8A85-CA89DEBB953F/How_to_Do_a_Root_Cause_Analysis_of_Diagnostic_Error_Handout_Slides.pdf (accessed March 2, 2015).

Roberts, I. S. D., R. E. Benamore, E. W. Benbow, S. H. Lee, J. N. Harris, A. Jackson, S. Mallett, T. Patankar, C. Peebles, C. Roobottom, and Z. C. Traill. 2012. Post-mortem imaging as an alternative to autopsy in the diagnosis of adult deaths: A validation study. *Lancet* 379(9811):136–142.

Rogers, M. L., E. S. Patterson, and M. L. Render. 2012. Cognitive work analysis in health care. In P. Carayon (ed.), *Handbook of human factors and ergonomics in health care and patient safety* (pp. 465–474). Boca Raton, FL: Taylor & Francis Group.

Roth, E. M. 2008. Uncovering the requirements of cognitive work. *Human Factors: The Journal of the Human Factors and Ergonomics Society* 50(3):475–480.

Roy, C. L., J. M. Rothschild, A. S. Dighe, G. D. Schiff, E. Graydon-Baker, J. Lenoci-Edwards, C. Dwyer, R. Khorasani, and T. K. Gandhi. 2013. An initiative to improve the management of clinically significant test results in a large health care network. *Joint Commission Journal on Quality and Patient Safety* 39(11):517–527.

Ruegger, C., C. Bartsch, R. Martinez, S. Ross, S. Bolliger, B. Koller, L. Held, E. Bruder, P. Bode, R. Caduff, B. Frey, L. Schaffer, and H. Bucher. 2014. Minimally invasive, imaging guided virtual autopsy compared to conventional autopsy in foetal, newborn and infant cases: Study protocol for the paediatric virtual autopsy trial. *BMC Pediatrics* 14(1):15.

Salas, E., C. Prince, D. P. Baker, and L. Shrestha. 1995. Situation awareness in team performance: Implications for measurement and training. *Human Factors: The Journal of the Human Factors and Ergonomics Society* 37(1):123–136.

Saldiva, P. H. N. 2014. Minimally invasive autopsies: A promise to revive the procedure. *Autopsy and Case Reports* 4(3).

Schein, E. H. 2004. *Organizational culture and leadership*, 3rd ed. San Francisco, CA: John Wiley & Sons.

Schiff, G. D. 1994. Commentary: Diagnosis tracking and health reform. *American Journal of Medical Quality* 9(4):149–152.

Schiff, G. D. 2008. Minimizing diagnostic error: The importance of follow-up and feedback. *American Journal of Medicine* 121(5):S38–S42.

Schiff, G. D. 2014. Presentation. Presentation to the Committee on Diagnostic Error in Health Care, August 7, 2014, Washington, DC.

Schiff, G. D., D. Klass, J. Peterson, G. Shah, and D. W. Bates. 2003. Linking laboratory and pharmacy: Opportunities for reducing errors and improving care. *Archives of Internal Medicine* 163(8):893–900.

Schiff, G. D., S. Kim, R. Abrams, K. Cosby, A. S. Elstein, S. Hasler, N. Krosnjar, R. Odwanzy, M. F. Wisniewsky, and R. A. McNutt. 2005. Diagnosing diagnosis errors: Lessons from a multi-institutional collaborative project for the diagnostic error evaluation and research project investigators. In K. Henrikson, J. B. Battles, E. S. Marks, and D. I. Lewin (eds.), *Advances in Patient Safety: From Research to Implemenation* (*Volume 2: Concepts and methodology*) (pp. 255–278). Rockville, MD: Agency for Healthcare Research and Quality.

Schiff, G. D., A. L. Puopolo, A. Huben-Kearney, W. Yu, C. Keohane, P. McDonough, B. R. Ellis, D. W. Bates, and M. Biondolillo. 2013. Primary care closed claims experience of Massachusetts malpractice insurers. *JAMA Internal Medicine* 173(22): 2063-2068.

Schwartz, A., and S. J. Weiner. 2014. The value of direct observation and feedback on provider performance in diagnosis. Input submitted to the Committee on Diagnostic Error in Health Care, October 24, 2014, Washington, DC.

Schwartz, A. W., S. J. Weiner, F. Weaver, R. Yudkowsky, G. Sharma, A. Binns-Calvey, B. Preyss, and N. Jordan. 2012. Uncharted territory: Measuring costs of diagnostic errors outside the medical record. *BMJ Quality & Safety* 21(11):918–924.

Schwartz, L. H., D. M. Panicek, A. R. Berk, Y. Li, and H. Hricak. 2011. Improving communication of diagnostic radiology findings through structured reporting. *Radiology* 260(1):174–181.

Sexton, J., R. Helmreich, T. Neilands, K. Rowan, K. Vella, J. Boyden, P. Roberts, and E. Thomas. 2006. The Safety Attitudes Questionnaire: Psychometric properties, benchmarking data, and emerging research. *BMC Health Services Research* 6(1):1–10.

Shenvi, E. C., and R. El-Kareh. 2015. Clinical criteria to screen for inpatient diagnostic errors: A scoping review. *Diagnosis* 2(1):3–19.

SHIEP (State Health Information Exchange Program). 2012. Getting to impact: Harnessing health information technology to support improved care coordination. http://healthit. gov/sites/default/files/bright-spots-synthesis_care-coordination-part-i_final_012813. pdf (accessed June 8, 2015).

Shojania, K. G. 2010. The elephant of patient safety: What you see depends on how you look. *Joint Commission Journal of Quality and Patient Safety* 36(9):399–401.

Shojania, K., E. Burton, K. McDonald, and L. Goldman. 2002. *The autopsy as an outcome and performance measure.* AHRQ Publication No. 03-E002. Rockville, MD: Agency for Healthcare Research and Quality.

Shojania, K. G., E. C. Burton, K. M. McDonald, and L. Goldman. 2003. Changes in rates of autopsy-detected diagnostic errors over time: A systematic review. *JAMA* 289(21): 2849–2856.

Shostek, K. 2007. Developing a culture of safety in ambulatory care settings. *Journal of Ambulatory Care Management* 30(2):105–113.

Silow-Carroll, S., T. Alteras, and J. A. Meyer. 2007. *Hospital quality improvement: Strategies and lessons from U.S. hospitals.* www.commonwealthfund.org/publications/ fund-reports/2007/apr/hospital-quality-improvement--strategies-and-lessons-from- u-s--hospitals (accessed June 7, 2015).

Singh, H. 2013. Diagnostic errors: Moving beyond "no respect" and getting ready for prime time. *BMJ Quality & Safety* 22(10):789–792.

Singh, H. 2014. Building a robust conceptual foundation for defining and measuring diagnostic errors. Presentation to the Committee on Diagnostic Error in Health Care, August 7, 2014, Washington, DC.

Singh, H., and D. F. Sittig. 2015. Advancing the science of measurement of diagnostic errors in healthcare: The Safer Dx framework. *BMJ Quality & Safety* 24:103–110.

Singh, H., E. J. Thomas, S. Mani, D. Sittig, H. Arora, D. Espadas, M. M. Khan, and L. A. Petersen. 2009. Timely follow-up of abnormal diagnostic imaging test results in an outpatient setting: Are electronic medical records achieving their potential? *Archives of Internal Medicine* 169(17):1578–1586.

Singh, H., E. J. Thomas, D. F. Sittig, L. Wilson, D. Espadas, M. M. Khan, and L. A. Petersen. 2010. Notification of abnormal lab test results in an electronic medical record: Do any safety concerns remain? *American Journal of Medicine* 123(3):238–244.

Singh, H., T. D. Giardina, S. N. Forjuoh, M. D. Reis, S. Kosmach, M. M. Khan, and E. J. Thomas. 2012a. Electronic health record-based surveillance of diagnostic errors in primary care. *BMJ Quality and Safety* 21(2):93–100.

Singh, H., M. L. Graber, S. M. Kissam, A. V. Sorensen, N. F. Lenfestey, E. M. Tant, K. Henriksen, and K. A. LaBresh. 2012b. System-related interventions to reduce diagnostic errors: A narrative review. *BMJ Quality and Safety* 21(2):160–170.

Southwick, F. S., N. M. Cranley, and J. A. Hallisy. 2015. A patient-initiated voluntary online survey of adverse medical events: The perspective of 696 injured patients and families. *BMJ Quality & Safety* 24:620–629.

Thayyil, S., N. J. Sebire, L. S. Chitty, A. Wade, W. K. Chong, O. Olsen, R. S. Gunny, A. C. Offiah, C. M. Owens, D. E. Saunders, R. J. Scott, R. Jones, W. Norman, S. Addison, A. Bainbridge, E. B. Cady, E. D. Vita, N. J. Robertson, and A. M. Taylor. 2013. Post-mortem MRI versus conventional autopsy in fetuses and children: a prospective validation study. *Lancet* 382(9888):223–233.

Thomas, E. J. 2014. Safety culture and diagnostic error: A rising tide lifts all boats. Presentation to the Committee on Diagnostic Error in Health Care, November 5, 2014, Washington, DC.

Thomas, E. J., J. B. Sexton, T. B. Neilands, A. Frankel, and R. L. Helmreich. 2005. The effect of executive walk rounds on nurse safety climate attitudes: A randomized trial of clinical units. *BMC Health Services Research* 5(1):28.

Todnem By, R. 2005. Organisational change management: A critical review. *Journal of Change Management* 5(4):369–380.

Trowbridge, R. 2014. Diagnostic performance: Measurement and feedback. Presentation to the Committee on Diagnostic Error in Health Care, August 7, 2014, Washington, DC.

Tucker, A., and A. C. Edmondson. 2003. Why hospitals don't learn from failures. *California Management Review* 45(2):55–72.

Tucker, A., W. S. Heisler, and L. D. Janisse. 2013. Organizational factors that contribute to operational failures in hospitals. Harvard Business School Working Paper. http://hbswk.hbs.edu/item/7352.html (accessed June 29, 2015).

Ulrich, R., X. Quan, C. Zimring, A. Joseph, and R. Choudhary. 2004. The role of the physical environment in the hospital of the 21st century: A once-in-a-lifetime opportunity. Designing the 21st Century Hospital Project. www.healthdesign.org/sites/default/files/Role%20Physical%20Environ%20in%20the%2021st%20Century%20Hospital_0.pdf (accessed June 7, 2015).

van der Linden, A., B. M. Blokker, M. Kap, A. C. Weustink, P. H. J. Riegman, and J. W. Oosterhuis. 2014. Post-Mortem tissue biopsies obtained at minimally invasive autopsy: An RNA-quality analysis. *PLoS ONE* 9(12):e115675.

Varkey, P., M. K. Reller, and R. K. Resar. 2007. Basics of quality improvement in health care. *Mayo Clinic Proceedings* 82(6):735–739.

Vest, J., and L. Gamm. 2009. A critical review of the research literature on Six Sigma, Lean and StuderGroup's Hardwiring Excellence in the United States: The need to demonstrate and communicate the effectiveness of transformation strategies in healthcare. *Implementation Science* 4(35):1–9.

VHA (Veterans Health Administration). 2008. *Pathology and laboratory medicine service procedures.* Washington, DC: Department of Veterans Affairs, Veterans Health Administration.

Wachter, R. M. 2010. Why diagnostic errors don't get any respect—and what can be done about them. *Health Affairs* 29(9):1605–1610.

Wachter, R. M. 2015. *The digital doctor: Hope, hype, and harm at the dawn of medicine's computer age.* New York: McGraw-Hill.

Ward, A. F. 2013. Winter wakes up your mind—and warm weather makes it harder to think straight. *Scientific American,* February 12. www.scientificamerican.com/article/warm-weather-makes-it-hard-think-straight (accessed June 7, 2015).

Watts, B. V., K. Percarpio, P. West, and P. D. Mills. 2010. Use of the Safety Attitudes Questionnaire as a measure in patient safety improvement. *Journal of Patient Safety* 6(4):206–209.

Weick, K. E., and K. M. Sutcliffe. 2011. Business organizations must learn to operate "mindfully" to ensure high performance. www.bus.umich.edu/FacultyResearch/Research/ManagingUnexpected.htm (accessed May 26, 2015).

Weiner, S. J., A. Schwartz, F. Weaver, J. Goldberg, R. Yudkowsky, G. Sharma, A. Binns-Calvey, B. Preyss, M. M. Schapira, and S. D. Persell. 2010. Contextual errors and failures in individualizing patient care: A multicenter study. *Annals of Internal Medicine* 153(2):69–75.

Weustink, A. C., M. G. M. Hunink, C. F. v. Dijke, N. S. Renken, G. P. Krestin, and J. W. Oosterhuis. 2009. Minimally invasive autopsy: An alternative to conventional autopsy? *Radiology* 250(3):897–904.

WHO (World Health Organization). 2006. *The world health report 2006: Working together for health.* Geneva: World Health Organization.

Williams, C. 2012. Health information exchange: It should just work. www.healthit.gov/buzz-blog/state-hie/health-information-exchange-work (accessed March 27, 2015).

Williams, E. S., L. B. Manwell, T. R. Konrad, and M. Linzer. 2007. The relationship of organizational culture, stress, satisfaction, and burnout with physician-reported error and suboptimal patient care: Results from the MEMO study. *Health Care Management Review* 32(3):203–212.

Wyatt, R. M. 2013. Blameless or blameworthy errors—Does your organization make a distinction? *Joint Commission Physician Blog*, December 18. www.jointcommission.org/jc_physician_blog/blameless_or_blameworthy_errors (accessed June 7, 2015).

Zwaan, L., A. Thijs, C. Wagner, G. van der Wal, and D. R. Timmermans. 2009. Design of a study on suboptimal cognitive acts in the diagnostic process, the effect on patient outcomes and the influence of workload, fatigue and experience of physician. *BMC Health Services Research* 9:65.

Zwaan, L., G. D. Schiff, and H. Singh. 2013. Advancing the research agenda for diagnostic error reduction. *BMJ Quality & Safety* 22(Suppl 2):ii52–ii57.

7

The External Environment
Influencing Diagnosis: Reporting,
Medical Liability, and Payment

This chapter focuses on the external environment and how it contributes to the diagnostic process and the occurrence of diagnostic errors (see Figure 7-1). The category of external environmental factors is quite broad and may include: error reporting, medical liability and risk management, payment and care delivery, and oversight processes (such as accreditation, certification, and regulatory requirements). While the committee does consider oversight processes to be external environmental factors, they are discussed in the sections on health care professional education and competency in Chapter 4 and in the section on the oversight of health care organizations in Chapter 6.

In this chapter the committee emphasizes the need for safe environments for voluntary error reporting, without the threat of legal discovery or disciplinary action, where health care organizations can analyze and learn from diagnostic errors in order to improve diagnosis. The role of medical liability reform is also described as an opportunity to increase the disclosure of diagnostic errors as well as to promote improved reporting, analysis, and learning from diagnostic errors. The committee highlights the potential for payment models—both current and new—to incentivize improved diagnostic performance. Importantly, this chapter reflects the committee's commitment to consider recommendations from both a pragmatic and an aspirational perspective. The committee's recommendations balance the urgent need to improve diagnosis by identifying immediate opportunities for improvement while also considering more fundamental changes that are likely to take significant effort and time to achieve. As noted elsewhere in the report, the committee's recommenda-

The Work System

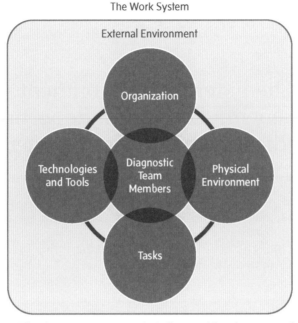

FIGURE 7-1 The diagnostic process is influenced by the external environment, including factors such as payment, reporting, medical liability, and oversight processes.

tions to improve diagnosis in this chapter may also improve patient safety and health care more generally. For example, the evaluation of the Patient Safety Organization (PSO) program is likely to be informative for error reporting broadly; adoption of communication and resolution programs (CRPs) has the potential to improve disclosure and error analysis for all types of errors in health care; and reforming fee-for-service (FFS) payment and documentation guidelines could also benefit the health care system more broadly.

REPORTING AND LEARNING FROM DIAGNOSTIC ERRORS

The committee concluded that there need to be safe, confidential places for health care organizations and professionals to share and learn from their experiences of diagnostic errors, adverse events, and near misses. Conducting systems-based analyses of these events presents the best opportunity to learn from such experiences and to implement changes to improve the diagnostic process. The Institute of Medicine's (IOM's) *To Err Is Human: Building a Safer Health System* (2000) report recommended that reporting systems be used to collect this information. Various groups, including individual states, The Joint Commission, the Department of Veterans Affairs, and PSOs, have developed a number of reporting systems which collect different types of information for different purposes. Characteristics of successful reporting systems include: reporting is safe for those individuals who report; reporting leads to constructive responses; adequate expertise and resources enable learning from reporting; and the results of reporting can be disseminated (Barach and Small, 2000; WHO, 2005). In contrast, if health care organizations focus on punishing individuals who make mistakes, it will prevent people from reporting because they fear that a report may be used as evidence of fault, could precipitate lawsuits, or could result in disciplinary action by state professional licensing boards and employers (IOM, 2012; WHO, 2005). Thus, there is a need for safe environments in which there is not the threat of legal discovery or disciplinary action, where diagnostic errors, adverse events, and near misses can be analyzed and learned from in order to improve the quality of diagnosis and prevent future diagnostic errors. **In line with the *To Err Is Human* report, the committee recommends that the Agency for Healthcare Research and Quality (AHRQ) or other appropriate agencies or independent entities should encourage and facilitate the voluntary reporting of diagnostic errors and near misses.**

Unfortunately, it is often difficult to create environments where diagnostic errors, adverse events, and near misses can be shared and discussed. Health care organizations and clinicians have been challenged by the limitations of inconsistent and individual state-enacted peer review and quality improvement processes for the protection of information relating to adverse events and medical errors, the external use of such information, and what benefits the health care organizations and clinicians receive from reporting. In response to this challenge, the *To Err Is Human* report recommended that "Congress should pass legislation to extend peer review protections to data related to patient safety and quality improvement that are collected and analyzed by health care organizations for internal use or shared with others solely for purposes of improving safety and quality" (IOM, 2000, p. 10). In 2005 the Patient Safety and Quality Improvement Act (PSQIA) was passed by Congress; the act confers privilege and confidentiality protections to health care organizations that share specific types of patient safety information with federally listed PSOs (HHS, 2015). According to AHRQ, which shares responsibility for implementing PSQIA with the Office for Civil Rights, "The Act promotes increased patient safety event reporting and analysis, as adverse event information reported to a … PSO is protected from disclosure in medical malpractice cases. This legislation supports and stimulates advancement of a culture of safety in health care organizations across the country, leading to provision of safer care to patients" (AHRQ, 2015a, p. 23). The PSO program provides an important national lever to increase voluntary error reporting and analysis which is well aligned with the committee's recommendation. However, progress in implementing the PSO program has been slow (AHRQ, 2015a; GAO, 2010). The committee is concerned that a number of challenges with the current program may limit the extent to which it can facilitate much-needed voluntary reporting, analysis, and learning of diagnostic errors and near misses (see section below on the evaluation of the PSO program).

Due to this concern, the committee's recommendation recognizes that additional federal efforts across the Department of Health and Human Services (HHS), as well as the involvement of other independent entities, need to be considered in order to prioritize voluntary event reporting for diagnostic errors and near misses. Support of this recommendation can be found in the IOM report *Health IT and Patient Safety: Building Safer Systems for Better Care*, which reviewed the existing reporting systems in health care and concluded that despite the various reporting systems and numerous calls for change, adverse event reports are not being collected and analyzed in a comprehensive manner (IOM, 2012). The report concluded that "learning from these systems is limited because a multitude of different data is collected by each system, hampering any attempt to aggregate data between reporting systems" (IOM, 2012, p. 152). After reviewing the opportunities to improve adverse event reporting, the committee that produced the 2012 report made a recommendation for a new entity, akin to the National Transportation Safety Board, that could investigate "patient safety deaths, serious injuries, or potentially unsafe conditions" and report results of these activities (IOM, 2012, p. 11). That committee suggested that this entity's purview could include (1) collecting reports of adverse events; (2) analyzing collected reports to identify patterns; (3) investigating reports of patient deaths or serious injuries related to health IT; (4) investigating trends of reports of unsafe conditions; (5) recommending corrective actions; (6) providing feedback based on these investigations; and (7) disclosing the results of the investigations to the public.

Because efforts to improve voluntary reporting and analysis at the national level have been slow, the current committee also recognized the potential for more localized efforts that could be carried out while national efforts continue to be developed and improved. In the interim, smaller-scale efforts to improve voluntary reporting and learning from diagnostic errors, adverse events, and near misses may be helpful for generating and sharing the lessons learned from such efforts. For instance, at the level of health care organizations, quality and patient safety committees can incorporate the analysis of and learning from diagnostic errors, and these activities may be protected from disclosure by state statutes. In an integrated delivery system in Maine, for example, a surgical quality collaborative was established to review the quality and safety of surgical care, compare results to national and regional data, and provide feedback to participating organizations.[1] Another option that some organizations (including PSOs) are incorporating is the use of "safe tables" forums (WSHA, 2014), which are "members-only, shared learning meeting[s] of healthcare peers to exchange patient safety experiences, discuss best practices and learn in an open, uninhibited and legally protected environment" (MHA PSO, 2015). The limitation to this approach is that the best practices and lessons learned cannot be shared beyond the participants.

Evaluation of the PSO Program

The PSO program enables public or private organizations to be listed as a PSO provided that they meet certain qualifications articulated in the patient safety rule (AHRQ, 2015e). PSO designation indicates that an organization is "authorized to serve providers as independent patient safety experts and to receive data regarding patient safety events that will be considered privileged and confidential" (GAO, 2010, p. 2). PSOs do not receive federal funding, but they can recruit health care organizations and clinicians to join their PSO. When health care organizations or health care professionals join a PSO, they can then voluntarily send patient safety data to the PSO for analysis and feedback on how to improve care. Additionally, PSOs can send de-identified patient safety data to the Network of Patient Safety Databases (NPSD) overseen by AHRQ. The intent of the program is that AHRQ will then analyze the aggregated data and publish reports (GAO, 2010). A provision in the Affordable Care Act will likely increase the number of hospitals who join PSOs; per the HHS 2015 Payment Notice, hospitals with more than 50 beds will be required to join a PSO by January 2017 in order to contract with health plans in insurance exchanges (CFPS, 2015).[2] There is very limited information about the impact that PSOs have on learning and improving the quality and safety of care. The Government Accountability Office concluded in 2010 that it was too early to evaluate the effectiveness of the PSO program (GAO, 2010). AHRQ is still in the process of implementing the NPSD, and to this point aggregated information collected from PSOs has not been analyzed or shared.

Currently there are more than 80 listed PSOs (AHRQ, 2015c), and the

---

[1] The MaineHealth Surgical Quality Collaborative was developed in accordance with the provisions of the Maine Health Security Act, 24 Me.Rev.Stat.Ann. § 2501, *et seq* to maintain the confidentiality of information and data reviewed.

[2] See www.federalregister.gov/articles/2013/12/02/2013-28610/patient-protection-and-affordable-care-act-hhs-notice-of-benefit-and-payment-parameters-for-2015 (accessed December 6, 2015).

PSO network is active in sharing information with their members about strategies to mitigate patient safety events, as evidenced by PSO websites. AHRQ has also developed "Common Formats," or generic- and event-specific forms, to encourage standardized event reporting among PSOs (AHRQ, 2015b). However, use of the Common Formats is voluntary, and some organizations are implementing these variably or using legacy reporting formats (ONC, 2014). To facilitate the aggregation of patient safety data, AHRQ established the PSO Privacy Protection Center (PSO PPC). The PSO PPC receives data from PSOs, facilitates use of the Common Formats, de-identifies data in a standardized manner, validates the quality and accuracy of the data, provides technical assistance to PSOs and other Common Formats users, and transmits non-identifiable information to the NPSD (AHRQ, 2015a).

The PSO PPC works with individual PSOs that wish to submit de-identified patient safety event information. In order to submit reports, PSOs are required to sign a data use agreement with the PSO PPC. By the end of fiscal year (FY) 2014, 20 of 76 listed PSOs had established data use agreements with the PSO PPC (AHRQ, 2015a). AHRQ reports that while these data use agreements "grew in number in FY 2014, and some data were transmitted to the PSO PPC, none have been of sufficient quality and volume to ensure that data transmitted to the NPSD is both accurate and non-identifiable" (AHRQ, 2015a, p. 53). For FY 2015, AHRQ expects the volume of data submission to the PSO PPC and the quality of the data submitted to increase significantly. AHRQ's goal is to gather "sufficient patient safety event reports to transmit to the NPSD," and the FY 2015 target is to transfer 25,000 patient safety event reports to the NPSD (AHRQ, 2015a, p. 53).

There are concerns that the federal privilege protections extended by PSQIA are not shielding organizations from state reporting requirements; a recent ruling by the Kentucky Supreme Court found that the information a hospital is required to generate under state law is not protected by PSQIA, even if it is shared with a PSO.[3] This type of court decision could undermine the creation of safe environments for sharing this information and thus make voluntary submissions to PSOs much less likely.

Given that the PSO program has the potential to improve learning

---

[3] *Tibbs v. Bunnel*, Ky., 2012-SC-000603-MR (August 21, 2014). The Kentucky Supreme Court held that the incident report developed by the University of Kentucky Hospital's patient safety evaluation system (PSES), following the death of a patient, was not protected as patient safety work product (PSWP) under PSQIA. While this case may not set any official precedent in other states, it will be considered persuasive case law. Organizations that have established a PSES for reporting to a PSO need to explore any state-mandated safety and quality regulations to ensure that the collection of such information is conducted in harmony with the PSES to ensure protection as PSWP.

about diagnostic errors and to expedite the implementation of solutions and adoption of best practices, it is important to evaluate whether the program is meeting the statutory objectives of PSQIA—namely, that the PSO program is creating opportunities to examine and learn from medical errors, including diagnostic errors. **Thus, the committee recommends that AHRQ should evaluate the effectiveness of PSOs as a major mechanism for voluntary reporting and learning from these events.** Given the concern over the erosion of PSQIA privilege protections at the state level, the evaluation could also focus on whether these protections are consistent with Congress's intent in enacting the legislation. While the evaluation of the PSO program is ongoing, PSOs can help support voluntary reporting efforts by educating their members about the applicable state peer review protections as well as about the PSQIA privilege protections. Health care organizations participating in PSOs can also take steps to ensure that any information and data shared with PSOs are protected by defining their patient safety evaluations systems broadly and by carefully analyzing the information they intend to submit to a PSO in order to minimize the chance that the PSQIA privilege is abrogated (or invalidated) at the state level.

The evaluation of the PSO program could also explore how the PSO program influences efforts to improve transparency within health care organizations. According to a recent report, "PSOs have the potential to foster transparency through increased reporting of complications and errors, and identification and sharing of learning and best practices; however, it remains to be seen how successfully these groups can balance the need for a protected space to which organizations can voluntarily report errors and the need for open sharing of information outside the organization" (National Patient Safety Foundation's Lucian Leape Institute, 2015, p. 16). The committee recognizes that efforts to improve diagnosis can include both a focus on improving the disclosure of medical errors to patients and their families (see discussion on CRPs) and efforts to improve voluntary reporting and learning.

In addition, AHRQ's evaluation needs to focus on how AHRQ and PSOs can improve the voluntary reporting of diagnostic errors and learning from those errors, which have not been a major focus within PSOs to date. **The committee recommends that AHRQ should modify the PSO Common Formats for reporting of patient safety events to include diagnostic errors and near misses.** To implement Common Formats specific to diagnostic error, AHRQ could begin with high-priority areas (such as the most frequent diagnostic errors or "don't miss" health conditions that may result in significant patient harm, such as stroke, acute myocardial infarction, and pulmonary embolism). AHRQ could also consider whether other PSO activities, such as discussions during annual PSO meetings, could focus attention on diagnostic errors.

MEDICAL LIABILITY

The two core functions of the medical liability system are to compensate negligently injured patients and to promote quality by encouraging clinicians and organizations to avoid medical errors. Although the medical liability system may act as a generalized deterrent to medical errors, it is not well aligned with the promotion of high-quality safe care (Mello et al., 2014b). Concerns about medical liability prevent clinicians from disclosing medical errors to patients and their families, despite calls from numerous groups that full disclosure is an ethical necessity (Hendrich et al., 2014; Sage et al., 2014) and despite the fact that such disclosures are a requirement for The Joint Commission accreditation. Clinicians often struggle to fulfill this responsibility: There is limited guidance for clinicians about how to disclose this information effectively, and a number of factors, including embarrassment, inexperience, lack of confidence, and mixed messages from risk managers and health care organizations' senior leadership, can thwart disclosures to patients and their families (Gallagher et al., 2007, 2013; The Joint Commission, 2005; Schiff et al., 2014).

The current tort-based judicial system for resolving medical liability claims creates barriers to improvements in quality and patient safety and stifles continuous learning. Medical malpractice reform could be designed to permit patients and health professionals to become allies in trying to make health care safer by encouraging transparency about errors. Such an approach would allow patients to be promptly and fairly compensated for injuries that were avoidable, while at the same time turning errors into lessons to improve subsequent performance (Berenson, 2005; Mello and Gallagher, 2010; Mello et al., 2014a).

The IOM report *Fostering Rapid Advances in Health Care: Learning from System Demonstrations* concluded that there are numerous challenges to the current medical liability system, including the many instances of negligence that do not result in litigation and, conversely, malpractice claims that are not the result of negligent care, judgments that are inconsistent with the evidence base, and highly variable compensation for similar medical injuries (IOM, 2002). Patients and their families are poorly served by the current system; only a fraction of negligently injured patients receive compensation, typically after a protracted and adversarial litigation process (AHRQ, 2014; Kachalia and Mello, 2011). One analysis found that fewer than 2 percent of patients who experienced adverse events due to medical negligence actually filed malpractice claims (Localio et al., 1991);

another analysis found that the rates of paid medical malpractice claims have steadily declined since the early 2000s (Mello et al., 2014b).

An ongoing medical liability concern is the practice of defensive medicine. Defensive medicine "occurs when doctors order tests, procedures, or visits, or avoid high-risk patients or procedures, primarily (but not necessarily soley) to reduce their exposure to malpractice liability" (OTA, 1994, p. 13). The practice of defensive medicine is a barrier to high-quality care because it can lead to overly aggressive and unnecessary care. For example, clinicians who practice defensive medicine may order more diagnostic tests than are necessary (Hoffman and Kanzaria, 2014; Kessler et al., 2006; Mello et al., 2010). Overtesting in the diagnostic process has the potential to cause patient harm—both from the risk of the diagnostic test itself as well as from the resulting cascade of diagnostic and treatment decisions that stem from the test result (Hoffman and Kanzaria, 2014) (see also Chapter 3).

Diagnostic errors are a leading cause of malpractice claims, and these claims are more likely to be associated with patient deaths than other types of medical errors (Tehrani et al., 2013). Reforming the medical liability system, therefore, has the potential to improve learning from diagnostic errors, to facilitate the disclosure of diagnostic errors to patients and their families, and may produce fairer outcomes in the medical injury resolution processes. **The committee recommends that states, in collaboration with other stakeholders (health care organizations, professional liability insurance carriers, state and federal policy makers, patient advocacy groups, and medical malpractice plaintiff and defense attorneys), should promote a legal environment that facilitates the timely identification, disclosure, and learning from diagnostic errors.**

There have been many calls for changes to the medical liability system. Traditional mechanisms to reform the liability system—such as imposing barriers to bringing lawsuits, limiting compensation, and changing the way that damage awards are paid—have not resulted in improvements in either compensating negligently injured patients or deterring unsafe care (Mello et al., 2014b). Thus, the committee concluded that these stakeholders need to consider alternative approaches to improving the legal environment and promoting learning from diagnostic errors. The *To Err Is Human* report concluded that alternative approaches to the resolution of medical injuries could reduce the incentive to hide medical injuries, and in 2002 the IOM proposed state-level demonstration projects to explore alternative approaches to the current liability system that are patient-centered and focused on patient safety (IOM, 2000, 2002). In 2010, AHRQ allocated approximately $23 million in funding for demonstration and planning grants aimed at finding ways to improve medical injury compensation and patient safety (AHRQ, 2015d; Kachalia and Mello,

2011). Five of the seven demonstration grants (totaling $19.7 million in awarded funds) that were funded by AHRQ focused on CRPs, one on safe harbors for following evidence-based clinical practice guidelines, and one on judge-directed negotiation. The 13 planning grants (totaling $3.5 million) were diverse and included CRPs, safe harbors, and other formats (AHRQ, 2015d). These demonstration and planning grants were somewhat limited, however, because they could not involve approaches that required legislative changes (such as administrative health court demonstrations) (Bovbjerg, 2010). Furthermore, while the Affordable Care Act authorized $50 million to test new approaches to the resolution of medical injury disputes, this funding was never appropriated.

Although enthusiasm for alternative approaches to the current medical liability system is growing, in general the progress toward such approaches has been slow, especially for those that involve more fundamental changes to the medical liability system. Thus, the committee took both a pragmatic and an aspirational approach to considering which changes to medical liability could promote improved disclosure of diagnostic errors and opportunities to learn from these errors. A number of alternative approaches to the current medical liability system were evaluated, and the committee concluded that the most promising approaches included CRPs, the use of clinical practice guidelines as safe harbors, and administrative health courts (see Box 7-1). CRPs represent a more pragmatic approach in that they are more likely to be implemented in the current medical liability climate, and they have a strong focus on improving patient safety as well as on reducing litigation. **Thus, the committee recommends that states, in collaboration with other stakeholders (health care organizations, professional liability insurance carriers, state and federal policy makers, patient advocacy groups, and medical malpractice plaintiff and defense attorneys), should encourage the adoption of CRPs with legal protections for disclosures and apologies under state laws.**

Safe harbors for adherence to clinical practice guidelines may also help facilitate improvements in diagnostic accuracy by encouraging clinicians to follow evidence-based diagnostic approaches; however, most clinical practice guidelines address treatment, not diagnosis. Moreover, implementing safe harbors for adherence to these guidelines will be administratively complex. Administrative health courts offer a fundamental change that would promote a more open environment for identifying, studying, and learning from errors, but their implementation will be a major challenge due to operational complexity and to resistance from stakeholders who are strongly committed to preserving the current tort-based system. **Thus, the committee concluded that these changes are more aspirational, and recommends that states and other stakeholders should conduct demonstration projects of alternative approaches to the**

resolution of medical injuries, including administrative health courts and safe harbors for adherence to evidence-based clinical practice guidelines. The following sections describe the alternative approaches, the challenges influencing their implementation, and the potential benefits for improving diagnosis.

Communication and Resolution Programs

CRPs have recently garnered significant attention as a means of improving the disclosure and resolution of medical injuries and improving patient safety. A number of the AHRQ demonstration projects focused on CRPs, and organizations such as the American College of Physicians and the American College of Surgeons have called for continued experimentation (ACP, 2014; ACS, 2015). At 14 hospitals in 3 health care systems across the country, AHRQ is currently developing and field-testing an educational toolkit on CRPs which teaches about the best practices from the CRP-focused demonstration projects (AHRQ, 2015a). CRPs offer a principled, comprehensive, and systematic approach to responding to patients who have been harmed by their health care. They are an integral component of a larger commitment to quality and patient safety. CRPs seek to meet the needs of the affected patient and his or her family; it is the health care organization's responsibility to address the quality issues and safety gaps that caused the event. While some of the specifics related to CRP implementation may vary based on an organization's circumstances, Box 7-1 describes the essential components of a CRP.

CRPs could improve patient safety generally and reduce diagnostic errors in several ways. CRPs rely on creating transparent health care cultures in which the early reporting of adverse events is the norm and is coupled with systems-based event analysis designed to understand the root causes of the event and to aid in the development of plans for preventing recurrences. Increased transparency surrounding diagnostic errors can help foster an improved culture of reporting, which in turn can promote learning about and identifying interventions to improve the safety and quality of diagnosis (Mello et al., 2014a). CRPs also emphasize remaining transparent about adverse events—including diagnostic errors—with patients and their families.

The disclosure of medical errors also can also improve outcomes for patients, their families, and health care professionals (Delbanco and Bell, 2007; Helmchen et al., 2010; Hendrich et al., 2014; Lopez et al., 2009). In some cases, clinician disclosure of medical errors to patients is associated with higher ratings of quality care by patients (Lopez et al., 2009). When a CRP was implemented at the University of Michigan Health System (UMHS), it was associated with fewer malpractice claims, faster claims

---

BOX 7-1
Description of Alternative Approaches
to the Medical Liability System

- **Communication and resolution programs (CRPs)** are principled comprehensive patient safety programs in which health care professionals and organizations openly discuss adverse outcomes with patients and proactively seek resolution while promoting patient-centeredness, learning, and quality improvement. CRPs typically incorporate the following elements:
  - o Early reporting of adverse events to the health care organization or liability insurer for rapid analysis using human factors[a] and other advanced event analysis techniques
  - o Developing plans for preventing recurrences and communicating these plans to patients and their families
  - o Open communication with patients and their families about unanticipated care outcomes and adverse events
  - o Proactively seeking resolutions, including offering an explanation as to why the event occurred and an acknowledgment of responsibility and/ or an apology
  - o Initiating support services, both emotional and other types of support, for the patient, family, and care team
  - o Where appropriate, offering timely reimbursement for medical expenses not covered by insurance or compensation for economic loss or other remedies
- **Safe harbors for adherence to evidence-based clinical practice guidelines** are laws that provide health care professionals and organizations a defense against a malpractice claim if they can show that they followed a clinical practice guideline in providing care for a patient. Safe harbors:

---

processing times, and reduced liability costs and settlement amounts (Boothman et al., 2009, 2012; Kachalia et al., 2010). Safety culture scores at UMHS also improved with the implementation of the CRP; however, it is difficult to attribute causation to the CRP program (Boothman et al., 2012). CRPs "appear to be effective in improving communication with patients and families. Disclosure reportedly became more routine and robust in implementing hospitals after clinicians were given disclosure training and risk managers began more closely monitoring whether and how disclosures were carried out" (Mello et al., 2014b, pp. 2150–2151).

CRPs continue to expand in the United States. For example, the Massachusetts Alliance for Communication and Resolution following Medical Injury (MACRMI) is committed to spurring adoption of CRPs and sharing lessons learned to improve the dissemination of CRPs throughout Massachusetts (MACRMI, 2015). MACRMI supported enabling legislation

- o May create a rebuttable presumption (i.e., it is introduced as evidence of the standard of care, but is not dispositive) or irrefutable presumption of nonnegligence
- **Administrative health courts** offer a system of administrative compensation for medical injuries which has the following components:
  - o Injury compensation decisions are made outside the regular court system by specially trained judges
  - o Compensation decisions are based on a standard of avoidability of medical injuries rather than a standard of negligence—claimants must show that the injury would not have occurred if best practices had been followed or an optimal system of care had been in place, but they need not show that care fell below the standard expected of a reasonably prudent health care professional
  - o Compensation decisions are guided by previous determinations about the preventability of common medical adverse events; this knowledge, coupled with precedent, is converted to decision aids that allow fast-track compensation decisions for certain types of injury
  - o Previous determinations also inform decisions about the amount of the award for economic and noneconomic damages

---

[a] Human factors (or ergonomics) is: "the scientific discipline concerned with the understanding of interactions among humans and other elements of a system, and the profession that applies theory, principles, data and methods to design in order to optimize human well-being and overall system performance. Practitioners of ergonomics and ergonomists contribute to the design and evaluation of tasks, jobs, products, environments and systems in order to make them compatible with the needs, abilities and limitations of people" (IEA, 2000).

SOURCES: Chow, 2007; Jost, 2006; Mello et al., 2014b; Peters, 2008; Timm, 2010.

that adopted the UMHS CRP model, including a 6-month pre-litigation period and protections for disclosures and apologies (MACRMI, 2015).

Although establishing CRPs does not require legislative changes, CRP adoption could be facilitated by changes to state laws, such as laws protecting disclosures and apologies (Sage et al., 2014). For example, the American College of Physicians has called for "strong, broad legal protections that ensure apologies from physicians and other health care professionals are inadmissible" in a subsequent medical malpractice action (ACP, 2014). Though more than two-thirds of states have apology laws, the majority only protect the clinician's voluntary expression of sympathy from use by a patient in malpractice litigation (Mastroianni et al., 2010). A small number of states also protect explanations of the event or expressions of fault, or both; however, Sage and colleagues concluded that no states protect "the full scope of information that patients report needing when an unexpected outcome arises: a preliminary explanation of what happened; an expression of sympathy; an admission of responsibility; and a final analysis of the causes and consequences of the event, with information about remedial actions taken to prevent such incidents in the future" (Sage et al., 2014, p. 14). Of the nine states that have disclosure laws, a majority require health care organizations to notify patients when an event has caused serious harm: "States vary on whether the disclosure receives protection from subsequent use by a plaintiff in malpractice litigation. For the most part, states provide limited, if any, procedural guidance; some states require written—versus oral—communication or timely communication" (Mastroianni et al., 2010, p. 1614).

The implementation of CRPs face a number of challenges. One challenge is HHS's recent interpretation of the reporting requirements to the National Practitioner Data Bank (NPDB). Federal law requires that medical liability insurers report malpractice payments to the NPDB, which was initially established to prevent clinicians from concealing disciplinary and malpractice histories as they moved across state lines (Sage et al., 2014). An Oregon law attempted to assert that the NPDB reporting was not required if a settlement resulted from a mediation mechanism, such as a CRP (Robeznieks, 2014), but HHS concluded that any payments stemming from written demands (whether part of mediation mechanisms or not) are required to be submitted to the NPDB (HHS, 2014). There are concerns that these reporting requirements will prevent participation in CRPs: "Physicians worry that CRPs will offer compensation when the physician was not at fault, either as a compassionate gesture or because the hospital or insurer deems it prudent to settle, and that, as a result, physicians will be reported to the NPDB more often" (Sage et al., 2014, p. 16). The reporting of settlements arising from mediation mechanisms to the NPDB could have negative effects on clinicians' reputations, credentialing, or disciplinary actions, and at least one medical specialty society, the American College of Physicians, recommends that the reporting requirement be altered to encourage CRP participation (ACP, 2014).

Other considerations will influence the implementation and effectiveness of CRPs, including the presence of organizational champions and a culture that supports the reporting of medical errors; a focus on coaching and support services to help clinicians participate in disclosures and the CRP processes; and buy-in from and coordination with health care organizations and professional liability insurance carriers (Mello et al., 2014a).

Of particular interest is the potential for CRPs to promote widespread learning following adverse events. As growing numbers of health care organizations and professional liability insurers adopt CRPs, close collaboration among these programs and between these programs and PSOs could help ensure that the lessons learned from adverse events are shared widely within and outside the organizations where the events occurred. The establishment of a national collaborative of CRPs could be one way to accelerate the spread of CRPs and to fully realize the quality and safety benefits of these programs.

Safe Harbors for Adherence to Evidence-Based Clinical Practice Guidelines

Safe harbors for following evidence-based clinical guidelines have the potential to raise the quality of health care by creating an incentive—liability protection—for clinicians to follow evidence-based clinical practice guidelines.[4] Safe harbors can create an affirmative defense for health care professionals who adhered to accepted and applicable clinical practice guidelines. Input to the committee suggested that safe harbors, unlike other approaches to improving the medical liability environment, offer direct opportunities to improve diagnosis (Kachalia, 2014). While other approaches to improving medical liability focus on improving learning through improved disclosure, safe harbors focus on aligning clinical care with best practices.

Available evidence suggests that creating national standards of care against which clinicians are judged in malpractice claims can improve quality of care. Providing standardized guidelines for certain diagnostic workups and holding these to be the standard of care has the potential to reduce diagnostic error. Despite calls for safe harbors (ACP, 2014; Mello et al., 2014b), there is limited information about how effective safe harbors are in minimizing medical errors, partly because there have been relatively few pilot programs and those programs have had poor clinician participation (Kachalia et al., 2014; Mello et al., 2014b). A recent simulation analysis evaluated the potential impact of safe harbors and concluded that they constitute a promising approach to driving improvements in the quality of patient care, but their impact on liability costs and patient outcomes is likely to be minimal (Kachalia et al., 2014).

---

[4] Safe harbors for adherence to clinical practice guidelines differ from the current use of clinical practice guidelines in the courts. Typically, malpractice litigation uses expert testimony to determine whether the care provided by a clinician fell below the standard of care (what would be expected of a reasonably prudent clinician). Expert witnesses can introduce clinical practice guidelines as legal evidence, but many states permit defendants to escape liability if they demonstrated customary care, even if it is not considered optimal care (IOM, 2011). This is partly due to variability in how states define the standard of care. Some states employ a national standard (clinicians would be held to the same degree of care and skill that a reasonably competent health care professional in the same field would exercise under similar circumstances). Other states use a local standard of care (clinicians would be held to the degree of knowledge and skill that is generally exercised by the same professionals in the community where they practice).

There are a number of implementation challenges related to safe harbors for adherence to clinical practice guidelines. For example, it requires state endorsement of specific clinical practice guidelines for use in malpractice litigation. Furthermore, safe harbor programs may be administratively complex because they require determining which clinical practice guidelines apply, when they apply, and who makes the determination. Also, given the constantly changing evidence base, ensuring the timely updating of approved guidelines and making clinicians aware of the updates could be challenging (Bovbjerg and Berenson, 2012). Clinician acceptability is another concern. Clinicians may find it burdensome to have to comply with additional clinical practice guidelines for improving diagnostic performance and avoiding liability. Clinicians already encounter multiple guidelines from specialty associations, insurers, health care organizations, hospitals, and others, and these guidelines are likely not all in alignment. Additionally, recent policy changes add to the resistance of using clinical practice guidelines for legal purposes. The legislation that repealed the sustainable growth rate included a provision that prevents the use of guidelines or standards used in federal programs as proof of negligence: The "development, recognition, or implementation of any guideline or other standard" under the Medicare and Medicaid programs and any provision in the Affordable Care Act "shall not be construed to establish the standard of care or duty of care owed by a health care provider to a patient in any medical malpractice or medical product liability action or claim."[5]

Administrative Health Courts

Administrative health courts have been proposed as a way to provide injured patients with expedited compensation decisions for certain types of medical errors and to promote the disclosure of medical errors (such as diagnostic errors). Administrative health courts are a nonjudicial way of handling medical injuries, in which cases are filed through an administrative process. The goal in using these courts is to quickly and equitably compensate patients who have experienced avoidable injuries without requiring them to become plaintiffs within the medical liability system who must prove negligence in an adversarial proceeding (Berenson, 2005).

There are various versions of how such an approach might work. In one version, specially trained judges preside and are assisted by investigations and opinions provided by neutral experts on the matter under consideration. Administrative health courts also take fault—or negligence—terminology out of the determination of liability and sub-

---

[5] Medicare Access and CHIP Reauthorization Act of 2015. P.L. 114-10. (April 16, 2015).

stitute it with the concept of avoidability (IOM, 2002; Mello et al., 2006). "[A] system based on an avoidability standard would award compensation to claimants who could show that their injury would not have occurred in the hands of the best practitioner or system" (Kachalia et al., 2008, p. 388). Proving negligence requires evidence that a clinician failed to meet a standard of care, is very fact-specific, and is more challenging to demonstrate; on the other hand, avoidability represents complications that generally should not occur under competent medical care (Berenson, 2005). Although substituting the negligence standard with an avoidability standard will lower the threshold for making these determinations, claimants will still have to establish cause—that their injuries were the result of their care rather than their underlying illnesses (Kachalia et al., 2008).

The establishment of administrative health courts could help to reduce process inefficiencies and inequities in compensation caused by shortcomings in the current system of tort liability, and adjudicated cases could be used to inform and foster the development of mechanisms to identify and mitigate medical errors (IOM, 2002; Mello et al., 2006). Administrative health courts have been described as holding theoretic appeal because "the model addresses some of the most important problems with the U.S. medical malpractice system, including the difficulty that patients have filing and prevailing in claims, the duration of litigation, the substantial overhead costs, the unpredictability of damages awards, and the punitive effect felt by physicians" (Mello et al., 2014b). Health courts have been used in other countries, including Denmark, New Zealand, and Sweden, and evidence suggests that they provide compensation to a greater number of claimants and are able to reach conclusions more quickly and at lower costs than tort-based mechanisms (ACP, 2006; Bovbjerg and Sloan, 1998; Mello et al., 2011).

Health courts appear to have bipartisan support in the United States: A nationwide poll conducted in 2012 found that 68 percent of Republicans, 67 percent of Democrats, and 61 percent of independents surveyed support the creation of health courts (Howard, 2012). Legislation to experiment with, or create, health courts has been proposed in a number of states—including Georgia, Maryland, New York, Oregon, and Virginia—but none has passed (Peters, 2008). Several organizations and experts have recommended pilot-testing or using health courts in the United States, but very few systems have been implemented or even tested (ACP, 2014; Howard and Maine, 2013; IOM, 2002; Mello et al., 2014b; Peters, 2008). There are only two state systems that implement the principles of health courts, and these uses are confined to cases involving neurological birth injury (Howard and Maine, 2013; Mello et al., 2014b).

There are several challenges associated with health courts, including the need for legislative action, which has been difficult to achieve (Mello et al., 2014b; Peters, 2008). As mentioned earlier, resistance from stakeholders strongly committed to preserving the current tort-based system will be a major challenge to overcome. Another issue that needs to be considered is how a health court should make information on paid claims of avoidable injuries available to state professional licensing boards, state hospital licensing agencies, medical specialty boards, and the NPDB. Such reporting could have a chilling effect on clinician disclosure of diagnostic errors; however, there is a competing concern about limiting the transparency of information on potentially substandard care practices.

RISK MANAGEMENT

Professional liability insurance carriers and health care organizations that participate in captive or other self-insurance arrangements have an inherent interest in improving diagnosis. Many of these organizations are actively exploring opportunities to improve diagnosis and reduce diagnostic errors. According to input the committee received, "[M]edical liability serves as a rich training area for reducing diagnostic error" (Lembitz and Boyle, 2014, p. 1). Given the expertise of professional liability insurance carriers and captive insurers in understanding the contributing factors to diagnostic errors, they can bring an important perspective to efforts to improve diagnosis, both those focused on individual health care professionals and those focused on the work system components that may contribute to diagnostic errors. **Thus, the committee recommends that professional liability insurance carriers and captive insurers should collaborate with health care professionals on opportunities to improve diagnostic performance through education, training, and practice improvement approaches and they should increase participation in such programs.**

One way in which these groups are helping improve diagnosis is by conducting data analyses that characterize the reasons that diagnostic errors occur. PIAA, the industry trade association representing companies in the medical liability insurance field, has a data sharing project that gathers and analyzes data on medical professional liability claims submitted by its members (Parikh, 2014).[6] The project's findings are used to identify opportunities to reduce risk and improve patient safety in health care organizations. Individual carriers can also provide information to help improve the understanding of diagnostic errors that lead to medical

---

[6] As discussed in Chapter 3, one of the limitations of malpractice claims data is that these data are not necessarily representative of diagnostic error in clinical practice; in one analysis, fewer than 2 percent of patients who experienced adverse events due to medical negligence filed malpractice claims (Localio et al., 1991).

liability claims. For example, Physician Reciprocal Insurers (PRI), CRICO, and The Doctors Company have gathered data on submitted and paid malpractice claims that suggest that diagnostic errors are the cause of around 20 percent of all submitted claims and 52 percent of all paid claims (CRICO, 2014; Donohue, 2014; Troxel, 2014). CRICO synthesizes information on important issues in medical injury claims and produces reports on these issues (such as a report on diagnostic errors in ambulatory care settings) (CRICO, 2014). Professional liability insurers often have rich data because they have collected a variety of information (e.g., information from electronic health records [EHRs], statements from various participants in the diagnostic process, and information from court documents) in the course of preparing for medical malpractice lawsuits. This information can lead to important, albeit potentially nonrepresentative, insights about the vulnerabilities in the diagnostic process and about potential areas on which to focus in order to improve care. Improved voluntary participation in malpractice claims databases among all professional liability insurance carriers and captive insurers could be helpful for aggregating information and sharing lessons learned.

Many professional liability insurers offer risk management educational services that are designed to improve diagnostic performance. The associated activities include seminars, workshops, team training, residency training programs, and newsletters (Donohue, 2014; Lembitz and Boyle, 2014). COPIC, a provider of medical liability insurance, reported that it conducts more than 2,000 practice site visits each year, in which specially trained nurses use explicit criteria to identify patient safety and risk issues, including vulnerability to systems errors, communication failures, information transfer, EHR issues, and standardized processes (Lembitz and Boyle, 2014). In some cases, incentives such as discounted insurance premiums are offered to individuals to induce participation (Donohue, 2014; Lembitz and Boyle, 2014). Surveys suggest that clinicians perceive these educational and training approaches as beneficial; for example, PRI reported that 94 percent of the clinicians participating in their case review exercise believe that it will reduce the risk of diagnostic errors occurring in their practice (Donohue, 2014). Unfortunately, because of measurement difficulties, there is little information on the impact of these educational approaches on the occurrence of diagnostic error (Donohue, 2014; Lembitz and Boyle, 2014). However, the committee concluded that the expertise of health professional liability insurance carriers should be leveraged to improve the diagnostic process. Improved collaboration between health professional liability insurance carriers and health care professionals and organizations could help to identify resources, prioritize areas of concern, and devise interventions. Collaboration among health care professional educators and professional liability insurance carriers also could be helpful in developing interventions for trainees. An example of collaborative efforts among medical liability insurers and educators is the recent grant from The Doctors Company Foundation to the Society to Improve Diagnosis in Medicine (SIDM, 2015; TDCF, 2015). This grant will provide funding for diagnostic training, with a focus on clinical reasoning and methods to communicate with patients about diagnostic errors (SIDM, 2015).

PAYMENT AND CARE DELIVERY

FFS payment, the predominant form of payment for health care services in the United States, pays health care professionals for each service they provide. FFS payment has long been recognized for its inability to incentivize well-coordinated, high-quality, and efficient health care (Council of Economic Advisors, 2009; IOM, 2001, 2013a; National Commission on Physician Payment Reform, 2013). There is relatively little information about the impact of payment on the diagnostic process. However, the committee concluded that payment is likely to have an impact on the diagnostic process, and several payment experts who provided input to the committee helped elaborate on some of these consequences (Miller, 2014; Rosenthal, 2014; Wennberg, 2014).

In general, FFS payment may not incentivize a high-quality, efficient diagnostic process because the more services the diagnostic process entails, the more remuneration will result. There is no disincentive for ordering unnecessary diagnostic testing that could lead to false positive results and diagnostic errors (Miller, 2014; Wennberg, 2014). There is also a financial incentive to provide treatment to patients rather than determining that patients do not have health problems; thus, inappropriate diagnoses are better compensated than determining that a patient does not have a health problem. Likewise, accuracy in the diagnostic process is not explicitly rewarded by FFS payment: Clinicians who interpret diagnostic testing or provide a diagnosis during a patient visit receive payment whether or not the work was done adequately to support accurate interpretation and diagnosis and whether or not the interpretations and diagnoses are accurate (Miller, 2014).

Given the importance of team-based care in the diagnostic process, the lack of financial incentives in FFS payment to coordinate care may contribute to challenges in diagnosis and diagnostic errors, particularly delays in diagnosis (Rosenthal, 2014). FFS Medicare and most commercial payers do not pay for time that a clinician spends contacting other clinicians by phone or e-mail to facilitate the diagnostic process: for example, by helping determine the appropriate diagnostic tests for a patient. In addition, clinicians are not reimbursed for proactive outreach to patients to obtain diagnostic testing, to schedule visits with specialists, or to make follow-up appointments (Miller, 2014). **To improve teamwork and care coordination in the diagnostic process, the committee recommends that the Centers for Medicare & Medicaid Services (CMS) and other payers should create current procedural terminology (CPT) codes and provide coverage for additional evaluation and management activities not currently coded or covered, including time spent by pathologists, radiologists, and other clinicians in advising ordering clinicians on the selection, use, and interpretation of diagnostic testing for specific patients.** New CPT codes can help incentivize communication and collaboration among treating clinicians and clinicians who conduct diagnostic testing in order to improve the diagnostic testing process for patients (Allen and Thorwarth, 2014; Kroft, 2014; Miller, 2014). These codes could be modeled on current CPT codes that compensate coordination and planning activities that are recognized for payment by Medicare and some other payers (e.g., CPT codes for radiation therapy planning, post-discharge transitional care coordination, and complex chronic care coordination) (AAFP, 2013; ASTRO, 2014; Bendix, 2013; Blue Cross Blue Shield of North Carolina, 2015; CMS, 2013, 2014b; Edwards and Landon, 2014; Nicoletti, 2005; Texas Medical Association, 2013). The proposed new codes are not meant to capture every discussion among clinicians; rather they are meant to capture discrete work that does not occur routinely in normal interactions to encourage more collaborative activity in the diagnostic process.

The Medicare physician fee schedule sets payment rates based on relative value units that are meant to reflect the level of time, effort, skill, and stress associated with providing each service (MedPAC, 2014). Fee schedule services can include evaluation and management services ("E&M services," such as office, inpatient, or emergency department visits), diagnostic testing, and other procedures. For all medical specialties, there are well-documented fee schedule distortions that result in more generous payments (in relation to the costs of production) being made for procedures and diagnostic testing interpretations than for E&M services (Berenson, 2010; National Commission on Physician Payment Reform, 2013). The existence of these distortions has coincided with a large growth in diagnostic testing in health care (see Figure 7-2); for example, the percent of patients presenting to the emergency department with dizziness who underwent computed tomography (CT) scans rose from 9 percent in 1995 to 40 percent in 2013, but this has not increased diagnoses of stroke or other neurologic diseases (Iglehart, 2009; Newman-Toker et al., 2013).

The lower relative value afforded to E&M services versus procedure-oriented care is problematic for improved diagnostic performance. E&M services reflect the cognitive expertise and skills that all clinicians have

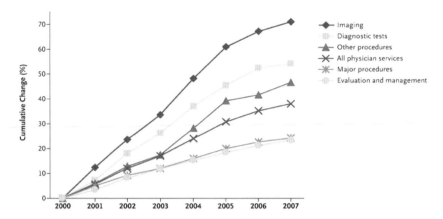

FIGURE 7-2 Rates of use of medical imaging services and diagnostic testing compared with rates of other clinician-ordered services, per Medicare Beneficiary (2000–2007).
SOURCE: J. K. Iglehart, Health insurers and medical-imaging policy—A work in progress. *New England Journal of Medicine* 360(10), 1030–1037. Copyright 2009 Massachusetts Medical Society. Reprinted with permission from Massachusetts Medical Society.

and use in the diagnostic process, and these distortions may be diverting attention and time from important tasks in the diagnostic process, such as performing a patient's clinical history and interview, conducting a physical exam, and decision making in the diagnostic process. **Thus, the committee recommends that CMS and other payers reorient relative value fees to more appropriately value the time spent with patients in evaluation and management activities.** Realigning relative value fees to better compensate clinicians for cognitive work in the diagnostic process has the potential to improve accuracy in diagnosis while also reducing incentives that drive the inappropriate utilization of diagnostic testing.

E&M payment policies and documentation guidelines also are misaligned with the goal of accurate and timely diagnosis. E&M payments penalize clinicians for spending extra time on the diagnostic process for an individual patient. There are different levels of E&M visits based on time and complexity, and practices receive better compensation if they see more patients with shorter appointment lengths. For example, in Medicare, if a clinician spends 20 minutes with a patient who is billed as a level 3 E&M visit rather than spending just 15 minutes, the clinician's practice will receive 25 percent less revenue per hour; if a clinician spends 25 minutes for a level 4 E&M visit instead of 15 minutes for a level 3 visit, the practice will receive 11 percent less revenue per hour (Miller, 2014).

Time pressures in clinical visits can contribute to various challenges in clinical reasoning and to the occurrence of errors (Durning, 2014; Kostis et al., 2007; Sarkar et al., 2012, 2014; Schiff et al., 2009; Singh et al., 2013). Although there is evidence that the lengths of clinical appointments have not generally declined,[7] there are concerns that the rising complexity of health care, the growth in patients with complicated health conditions, and increased EHR-related tasks are contributing to increased time pressures. The aging U.S. population contributes to added complexity for patient care decisions due to the need to understand the various factors that may be contributing to an older adult's health problem, such as multiple comorbidities and polypharmacy (IOM, 2008, 2013b). While unlimited time is neither the objective nor realistic, it is important to make time for effectively addressing these complex care decisions. Making more effective use of the time available will be critical, as will making improvements to the work system in which the diagnostic process occurs (such as disseminating an organizational culture that is supportive of teamwork in the diagnostic process, the better allocation of tasks, and ensuring that health information technology [health IT] is supportive of the diagnostic process).

In addition to modifying payment policies, the documentation guidelines for E&M services could also be improved to support the diagnostic process. Documentation guidelines for E&M services were created to ensure that the services performed were consistent with insurance coverage; to validate specific information, such as the site of service, the appropriateness of the care, and the accuracy of the reported information; and to prevent fraud and abuse (Berenson, 1999; CMS, 2014a). Documentation guidelines specify the extent of a patient's clinical history and interview, the physical exam, and the complexity of medical decision making involved in the E&M visit (Berenson et al., 2011; HHS, 2010). There are a number of criticisms of the documentation guidelines; the primary argument is that the level of detail required is onerous, is often irrelevant to patient care, and shifts the purpose of the medical record toward billing rather than facilitating clinical reasoning (Berenson et al., 2011; Brett, 1998; Kassirer and Angell, 1998; Kuhn et al., 2015; Schiff and Bates, 2010) (see the discussion of clinical documentation in Chapter 5).

The documentation guidelines have become an even greater concern with the broad implementation of EHRs because EHR design has focused on fulfilling documentation and legal requirements and not on facilitating the diagnostic process (Berenson et al., 2011; Schiff and Bates, 2010). EHRs

---

[7] For example, the National Ambulatory Medical Care Survey found that in 1992 most visits lasted 15 minutes or less; by 2010, only half of clinician visits were that short (Rabin, 2014).

tend to lack a cohesive patient narrative, which include nuance, details, and important contextual information that help clinicians make accurate and timely diagnoses. The orientation of EHRs to documentation, their overreliance on templates, and the copy and paste functionalities within EHRs have resulted in "EHR-generated data dumps, including repetitive documentation of elements of patients' histories and physical examinations, that merely result in electronic versions of clinically cumbersome, uninformative patient records" (Berenson et al., 2011, p. 1894). Generating documentation to support E&M coding (or higher levels of E&M coding than are warranted, which is called "upcoding") can result in inaccuracies in the patient's EHR that can contribute to diagnostic errors.

A number of payment and care delivery reforms aimed at countering the limitations of the FFS payment system are actively being considered, implemented, and evaluated (see Box 7-2). These include capitation/global payments, shared savings, bundled episodes of care, accountable care organizations, patient-centered medical homes, and pay for performance (which Medicare refers to as "value-based purchasing"). Box 7-2 includes both potential benefits of new payment models on improving diagnosis as well as some of the potential drawbacks (see also Himmelstein and Woolhandler [2014] for a discussion of the potential limitations of new payment models). Salary is not described as a payment model because the committee focused on third-party payments rather than provider organization compensation.

CMS recently announced that it plans to have 30 percent of Medicare payments based on alternative models by the end of 2016 and 50 percent of payments by the end of 2018 (Burwell, 2015). The Medicare Access and CHIP Reauthorization Act of 2015 (which repealed the sustainable growth rate) continues down the path toward alternative payment models, particularly for the payment of Medicare clinicians.[8] While the impact of alternative payment and delivery systems on quality are actively being investigated (e.g., the Blue Cross Blue Shield of Massachusetts Alternative Quality Contract, as well as patient-centered medical homes), there is very limited evidence on what impact such payment and delivery models will have on the diagnostic process and on the accuracy of diagnosis, and this represents a fundamental research need. **Thus, the committee recommends that CMS and other payers should assess the impact of payment and care delivery models on the diagnostic process, the occurrence of diagnostic errors, and learning from these errors.** Assessing the impact of payment and care delivery models, including FFS, on the diagnostic process, diagnostic errors, and learning are critical areas of focus as these models are evaluated more broadly. CMS's Innovation Center is testing

---

[8] Medicare Access and CHIP Reauthorization Act of 2015. P.L. 114-10. (April 16, 2015).

BOX 7-2
Payment and Care Delivery Reforms and
Their Potential Impact on Diagnosis

- **Global Payment, Capitation, and Per-Member Per-Month**
  - o Definition: "A single per-member per-month payment is made for all services delivered to a patient, with payment adjustments based on measured performance and patient risk" (Schneider et al., 2011, p. 13).
  - o Potential impact on diagnosis: Broader adoption could enhance provider activities that improve diagnostic accuracy and reduce diagnostic errors because the capitated, at-risk organization bears the cost of diagnostic error if there are immediate costs associated with the error. For diagnostic errors that do not necessarily lead to higher costs for the organization, investment in lowering these errors (e.g., more vigilant evidence-based cancer screening which could increase costs due to treatment of newfound cancers) may be suboptimal. The use of quality measures and reporting may incentivize organizations to detect the underuse of these screening activities, to reengineer care, to invest in electronically based decision support and artificial intelligence which could improve accuracy, to engage clinicians in ongoing activities to improve diagnostic skills, and to engage in systems approaches to mitigating harm from potential diagnostic errors.

- **Accountable Care Organizations**
  - o Definition: "Groups of providers that voluntarily assume responsibility for the care of a population of patients" (Schneider et al., 2011, p. 13).
  - o Potential impact on diagnosis: The quality of care in accountable care organizations (ACOs) is assessed through a set of quality measures, but none of them involve accuracy or timeliness of diagnosis, for the reasons described in Chapter 3. ACOs have the potential infrastructure to provide a base of activity to improve diagnostic accuracy for their constituent or affiliated clinicians. So far, most ACOs do not accept risk, so the potential of non-fee-for-service financial incentives has not yet been realized. Nevertheless, the structure of an ACO and its need to credential its members and engage in quality and safety improvement programs can provide a new source of interest and provider expertise in engaging in the problem of diagnostic errors. To date, payers have not determined that diagnostic errors are a priority quality and safety problem that needs attention. ACOs, for example, would be well positioned to administer and promote follow-up and feedback approaches and to develop a culture in which these approaches are welcomed and routine.

- **Bundled Payment or Episode-Based Payment**
  - o Definition: A "single 'bundled' payment, which may include multiple providers in multiple care settings, is made for services delivered during an episode of care related to a medical condition or procedure" (Schneider et al., 2011, p. 13).

continued

BOX 7-2 Continued

   o Potential impact on diagnosis: By definition, bundled payment would seem to apply mostly to well-established, "correct" diagnoses, for which efficiencies of care can be further gained, and it remains volume-based (i.e., the financial incentive is to produce more, efficiently provided episodes). This raises the importance of addressing appropriateness of the bundled episode procedure being performed. Appropriateness is relevant to the topic of diagnostic error in the sense of needing to determine acuity of the condition as part of the diagnostic process. For chronic conditions, episode-based payment runs the risk of non-holistic care. For example, the clinicians receiving the episode-based payment for a condition such as diabetes may not be as attuned to diagnosis and management of comorbidities that may arise in the course of management of the index condition.

- **Pay for Performance or Value-Based Purchasing**
  - o Definition: "[P]hysicians receive differential payments for meeting or missing performance benchmarks" (Schneider et al., 2011, p. 14).
  - o Potential impact on diagnosis: Theoretically this can be a useful payment tool for focusing provider attention on important quality problems that can be measured accurately and then financially rewarded and penalized. Overall, the effects of pay for performance on outcomes remain unsettled, with concerns about the effects on important elements of care that are not being measured. Current pushes for accountability neglect performance measures for diagnosis, and that is a major limitation of these approaches.

- **Patient-Centered Medical Homes**
  - o Definition: "[A] physician practice or other provider is eligible to receive additional payments if medical home criteria are met. Payment may include calculations based on quality and cost performance using a [pay for performance]-like mechanism" (Schneider et al., 2011, p. 13). Although not an inherent part of the definition, most medical home initiatives are taking place in primary care practices.

---

many of the alternative payment models and is well suited to evaluate the impact of these models on the diagnostic process and the occurrence of diagnostic errors.

While new payment models have the potential to reduce diagnostic errors, the committee also recognized that these models may also create incentives for clinicians and health care organizations that could reduce use of appropriate testing and clinician services (e.g., specialty consultations) that may inadvertently lead to greater diagnostic errors. To address these possibilities, the committee recognized that not only is direct evaluation of the impact of payment models on diagnostic errors important but

- o Potential impact on diagnosis: A well-functioning medical home, teamwork, longstanding relationships with patients as the center for care and care coordination, and ultimately, reliance on improved electronic health records and interoperability of patient information to inform clinical decision making has the potential to improve diagnostic performance. There are concerns, however, that medical home performance will be assessed using measures that do not include those related to diagnostic performance, although it is known that there is a significant problem of diagnostic error in primary care (Ely et al., 2012; Singh et al., 2013).

- **Shared Savings**
  - o Definition: "[A] payment strategy that offers incentives for providers to reduce health care spending for a defined patient population by offering them a percentage of net savings realized as a result of their efforts" (Bailit and Hughes, 2011, p. 1).
  - o Potential impact on diagnosis: As a payment method, there are no direct incentives to focus on improving diagnostic accuracy. The impact depends largely on the objectives of the underlying organization to which the payment is being applied. For example, shared savings has become the primary method for rewarding ACOs for spending less than a target spending amount. Theoretically, at least, the ACO should be interested in diagnostic accuracy if by getting the diagnosis correct, subsequent spending can be promptly reduced. So the focus would be on efforts to make correct diagnoses of acute, urgent presentations of illness in emergency departments and primary care practices and for commonly misdiagnosed conditions such as stroke and congestive heart failure. Conversely, based on incentives alone, the organization might be less interested in efforts to make accurate and timely diagnoses of conditions whose costs would not be borne for many months or years. To date, there seems to be little attention paid to diagnostic accuracy as a mechanism for achieving savings.

also there is a need for better measurement tools to identify diagnostic errors in clinical practice (see Chapters 5 and 6).

Additionally, the committee asked for input from payment and delivery experts about the potential effects of new models on diagnosis and diagnostic error. Rosenthal (2014) suggested that global payment and meaningful use incentives have the potential to improve diagnosis by promoting the adoption of diagnostic test and referral tracking systems that better connect health care professionals throughout the continuum of care. Miller (2014) suggested that the development of measures for diagnostic accuracy be developed to provide feedback and reward clinicians for diagnostic accuracy. Wennberg (2014) suggested that population-based payment models, including capitation and global budgets, have the greatest potential to reduce diagnostic errors.

Even when alternate payment and care delivery approaches to FFS are employed, they are often based on or influenced by existing coding and payment rules (Berenson et al., 2011). For example, bundled payments are combinations of current codes. Thus, the current distortions in the fee schedule and other volume-based payment approaches, such as diagnosis-related group coding, will remain a dominant component of payment and care delivery models in the near future and need to be addressed. **As long as fee schedules remain a predominant mechanism for determining clinician payment, the committee recommends that CMS and other payers should modify documentation guidelines for evaluation and management services to improve the accuracy of information in the EHR and to support decision making in the diagnostic process.**

RECOMMENDATIONS

Goal 6: Develop a reporting environment and medical liability system that facilitates improved diagnosis by learning from diagnostic errors and near misses

Recommendation 6a: The Agency for Healthcare Research and Quality (AHRQ) or other appropriate agencies or independent entities should encourage and facilitate the voluntary reporting of diagnostic errors and near misses.

Recommendation 6b: AHRQ should evaluate the effectiveness of patient safety organizations (PSOs) as a major mechanism for voluntary reporting and learning from these events and modify the PSO Common Formats for reporting of patient safety events to include diagnostic errors and near misses.

Recommendation 6c: States, in collaboration with other stakeholders (health care organizations, professional liability insurance carriers, state and federal policy makers, patient advocacy groups, and medical malpractice plaintiff and defense attorneys), should promote a legal environment that facilitates the timely identification, disclosure, and learning from diagnostic errors. Specifically, they should:
- **Encourage the adoption of communication and resolution programs with legal protections for disclosures and apologies under state laws.**

- Conduct demonstration projects of alternative approaches to the resolution of medical injuries, including administrative health courts and safe harbors for adherence to evidence-based clinical practice guidelines.

Recommendation 6d: Professional liability insurance carriers and captive insurers should collaborate with health care professionals on opportunities to improve diagnostic performance through education, training, and practice improvement approaches and increase participation in such programs.

Goal 7: Design a payment and care delivery environment that supports the diagnostic process

Recommendation 7a: As long as fee schedules remain a predominant mechanism for determining clinician payment, the Centers for Medicare & Medicaid Services (CMS) and other payers should:
- Create current procedural terminology codes and provide coverage for additional evaluation and management activities not currently coded or covered, including time spent by pathologists, radiologists, and other clinicians in advising ordering clinicians on the selection, use, and interpretation of diagnostic testing for specific patients.
- Reorient relative value fees to more appropriately value the time spent with patients in evaluation and management activities.
- Modify documentation guidelines for evaluation and management services to improve the accuracy of information in the electronic health record and to support decision making in the diagnostic process.

Recommendation 7b: CMS and other payers should assess the impact of payment and care delivery models on the diagnostic process, the occurrence of diagnostic errors, and learning from these errors.

REFERENCES

AAFP (American Association of Family Physicians). 2013. Frequently asked questions: Transitional care management. www.aafp.org/dam/AAFP/documents/practice_management/payment/TCMFAQ.pdf (accessed June 8, 2015).
ACP (American College of Physicians). 2006. Exploring the use of health courts—Addendum to "Reforming the medical professional liability system." www.acponline.org/acp_policy/policies/health_courts_reform_medical_liability_2006.pdf (accessed May 24, 2015).

ACP. 2014. *Medical liability reform: Innovative solutions for a new health care system: A position paper*. Philadelphia: American College of Physicians. www.acponline.org/acp_policy/policies/medical_liability_reform_2014.pdf (accessed June 8, 2015).

ACS (American College of Surgeons). 2015. Statement on medical liability. http://bulletin.facs.org/2015/03/statement-on-medical-liability-reform (accessed May 16, 2015).

AHRQ (Agency for Healthcare Research and Quality). 2014. Medical liability reform and patient safety initiative. www.ahrq.gov/professionals/quality-patient-safety/patient-safety-resources/resources/liability (accessed April 10, 2015).

AHRQ. 2015a. Agency for Healthcare Research and Quality: Justification of estimates for appropriations committees. www.ahrq.gov/sites/default/files/wysiwyg/cpi/about/mission/budget/2016/cj2016.pdf (accessed May 3, 2015).

AHRQ. 2015b. Common formats. www.pso.ahrq.gov/common (accessed March 28, 2015).

AHRQ. 2015c. Federally listed PSOs. www.pso.ahrq.gov/listed (accessed May 3, 2015).

AHRQ. 2015d. Medical liability reform and patient safety initiative progress report. www.ahrq.gov/professionals/quality-patient-safety/patient-safety-resources/resources/liability/medliabrep.html (accessed May 24, 2015).

AHRQ. 2015e. Patient safety organization (PSO) program: Frequently asked questions. www.pso.ahrq.gov/faq#WhatisaPSO (accessed May 3, 2015).

Allen, B., and W. T. Thorworth. 2014. Comments from the American College of Radiology. Input submitted to the Committee on Diagnostic Error in Health Care, November 5 and December 29, 2014, Washington, DC.

ASTRO (American Society for Radiation Oncology). 2014. Basics of RO coding. www.astro.org/Practice-Management/Reimbursement/Basics-of-RO-Coding.aspx (accessed March 26, 2015).

Bailit, M., and C. Hughes. 2011. *Key design elements of shared-savings payment arrangements*. The Commonwealth Fund Publication No. 1539. www.commonwealthfund.org/~/media/Files/Publications/Issue%20Brief/2011/Aug/1539_Bailit_key_design_elements_sharedsavings_ib_v2.pdf (accessed June 8, 2015).

Barach, P., and S. D. Small. 2000. Reporting and preventing medical mishaps: Lessons from non-medical near miss reporting systems. *BMJ* 320(7237):759–763.

Bendix, J. 2013. Making sense of the new transitional care codes. *Medical Economics*, March 10. http://medicaleconomics.modernmedicine.com/medical-economics/news/user-defined-tags/99495/making-sense-new-transitional-care-codes?page=full (accessed March 26, 2015).

Berenson, R. A. 1999. Evaluation and management guidelines. *New England Journal of Medicine* 340(11):889–891.

Berenson, R. A. 2005. Malpractice makes perfect. *The New Republic*, October 10. www.newrepublic.com/article/health-care-malpractice-bush-frist (accessed November 7, 2015).

Berenson, R. A. 2010. Out of whack: Pricing distortions in the medicare physician fee schedule. *Expert Voices*, September. www.nihcm.org/pdf/NIHCM-EV-Berenson_FINAL.pdf (accessed June 8, 2015).

Berenson, R. A., P. Basch, and A. Sussex. 2011. Revisiting E&M visit guidelines—A missing piece of payment reform. *New England Journal of Medicine* 364(20):1892–1895.

Blue Cross Blue Shield of North Carolina. 2015. Corporate medical policy: E-visits (online medical evaluations). www.bcbsnc.com/assets/services/public/pdfs/medicalpolicy/evisits_online_medical_evaluation.pdf (accessed June 8, 2015).

Boothman, R. C., A. C. Blackwell, D. A. Campbell Jr., E. Commiskey, and S. Anderson. 2009. A better approach to medical malpractice claims? The University of Michigan experience. *Journal of Health & Life Sciences Law* 2(2):125–159.

Boothman, R. C., S. J. Imhoff, and D. A. Campbell, Jr. 2012. Nurturing a culture of patient safety and achieving lower malpractice risk through disclosure: Lessons learned and future directions. *Frontiers of Health Services Management* 28(3):13–28.

Bovbjerg, R. R. 2010. Will the Patient Protection and Affordable Care Act address problems associated with medical malpractice? Urban Institute. www.urban.org/research/publication/will-patient-protection-and-affordable-care-act-address-problems-associated-medical-malpractice (accessed May 3, 2015).

Bovbjerg, R. R., and R. Berenson. 2012. The value of clinical practice guidelines as malpractice "safe harbors." Urban Institute. www.rwjf.org/content/dam/farm/reports/issue_briefs/2012/rwjf72667 (accessed June 8, 2015).

Bovbjerg, R. R., and F. A. Sloan. 1998. No fault for medical injury: Theory and evidence. *University of Cincinnati Law Review* 67. http://ssrn.com/abstract=147016 (accessed June 6, 2015).

Brett, A. S. 1998. New guidelines for coding physicians' services—A step backward. *New England Journal of Medicine* 339(23):1705–1708.

Burwell, S. M. 2015. Setting value-based payment goals—HHS efforts to improve U.S. health care. *New England Journal of Medicine* 372(10):897–899.

CFPS (Center for Patient Safety). 2015. National health reform provisions and PSOs. www.centerforpatientsafety.org/nationalhealthreformprovisionsandpsos (accessed November 7, 2015).

Chow, E. 2007. Health courts: An extreme makeover of medical malpractice with potentially fatal complications. *Yale Journal of Health Policy, Law, and Ethics* 7(2):387–427.

CMS (Centers for Medicare & Medicaid Services). 2013. *Telehealth services.* Department of Health and Human Services. www.cms.gov/Outreach-and-Education/Medicare-Learning-Network-MLN/MLNProducts/downloads/TelehealthSrvcsfctsht.pdf (accessed June 8, 2015).

CMS. 2014a. *Evaluation and management services guide: Official CMS information for Medicare fee-for-service providers.* Washington, DC: Centers for Medicare & Medicaid Services.

CMS. 2014b. Policy and payment changes to the Medicare physician fee schedule for 2015. www.cms.gov/newsroom/mediareleasedatabase/fact-sheets/2014-Fact-sheets-items/2014-10-31-7.html (accessed March 26, 2015).

Council of Economic Advisors. 2009. *The economic case for health care reform.* www.whitehouse.gov/assets/documents/CEA_Health_Care_Report.pdf (accessed March 17, 2015).

CRICO. 2014. *2014 annual benchmarking report: Malpractice risks in the diagnostic process.* CRICO Strategies. www.rmfstrategies.com/benchmarking (accessed June 8, 2015).

Delbanco, T., and S. K. Bell. 2007. Guilty, afraid, and alone—struggling with medical error. *New England Journal of Medicine* 357(17):1682–1683.

Donohue, G. 2014. PRI medical liability insurance. Input submitted to the Committee on Diagnostic Error in Health Care, November 25, 2014, Washington, DC.

Durning, S. J. 2014. Input submitted to the Committee on Diagnostic Error in Health Care, October 25, 2014, Washington, DC.

Edwards, S. T., and B. E. Landon. 2014. Medicare's chronic care management payment—Payment reform for primary care. *New England Journal of Medicine* 371(22):2049–2051.

Ely, J. W., L. C. Kaldjian, and D. M. D'Alessandro. 2012. Diagnostic errors in primary care: Lessons learned. *Journal of the American Board on Family Medicine* 25(1):87–97.

Evans, W. N., and B. Kim. 2006. Patient outcomes when hospitals experience a surge in admissions. *Journal of Health Economics* 25(2):365–388.

Gallagher, T. H., C. Denham, L. Leape, G. Amori, and W. Levinson. 2007. Disclosing unanticipated outcomes to patients: The art and practice. *Journal of Patient Safety* 3(3):158–165.

Gallagher, T. H., M. M. Mello, W. Levinson, M. K. Wynia, A. K. Sachdeva, L. Snyder Sulmasy, R. D. Truog, J. Conway, K. Mazor, A. Lembitz, S. K. Bell, L. Sokol-Hessner, J. Shapiro, A.-L. Puopolo, and R. Arnold. 2013. Talking with patients about other clinicians' errors. *New England Journal of Medicine* 369(18):1752–1757.

GAO (Government Accountability Office). 2010. *Patient Safety Act: HHS is in the process of implementing the act, so its effectiveness cannot yet be evaluated.* Washington, DC: Government Accountability Office.

Helmchen, L. A., M. R. Richards, and T. B. McDonald. 2010. How does routine disclosure of medical error affect patients' propensity to sue and their assessment of provider quality? Evidence from survey data. *Medical Care* 48(11):955–961.

Hendrich, A., C. K. McCoy, J. Gale, L. Sparkman, and P. Santos. 2014. Ascension health's demonstration of full disclosure protocol for unexpected events during labor and delivery shows promise. *Health Affairs* 33(1):39–45.

HHS (Department of Health and Human Services). 2010. *Improper payments for evaluation and management services cost Medicare billions in 2010.* Washington, DC: HHS Office of Inspector General.

HHS. 2014. Decision on appropriate medical malpractice payment reporting. www.citizen. org/documents/2211%20Enclosure.pdf (accessed May 16, 2015).

HHS. 2015. *Patient safety and quality improvement act of 2005 statute and rule.* www.hhs.gov/ocr/privacy/psa/regulation (accessed March 29, 2015).

Himmelstein, D. U., and S. Woolhandler. 2014. Global Amnesia: Embracing Fee-For-Non-Service—Again. *Journal of General Internal Medicine* 29(5):693.

Hoffman, J. R., and H. K. Kanzaria. (2014). Intolerance of error and culture of blame drive medical excess. *BMJ* 349:g5702.

Howard, P. 2012. The growing bipartisan support for health courts. *Health Affairs Blog*, October 2. http://healthaffairs.org/blog/2012/10/02/the-growing-bipartisan-support-for-health-courts (accessed June 8, 2015).

Howard, P., and R. G. Maine. 2013. Health courts may be best cure for what ails the liability system. *Bulletin of the American College of Surgeons*, March 2. http://bulletin.facs.org/2013/03/health-courts-best-cure (accessed June 8, 2015).

IEA (International Ergonomics Association). 2000. The discipline of ergonomics. www.iea.cc/whats/index.html (accessed April 10, 2015).

Iglehart, J. K. 2009. Health insurers and medical-imaging policy—A work in progress. *New England Journal of Medicine* 360(10):1030–1037.

IOM (Institute of Medicine). 2000. *To err is human: Building a safer health system.* Washington, DC: National Academy Press.

IOM. 2001. *Crossing the quality chasm: A new health system for the 21st century.* Washington, DC: National Academy Press.

IOM. 2002. *Fostering rapid advances in health care: Learning from system demonstrations.* Washington, DC: National Academy Press.

IOM. 2008. *Retooling for an aging America: Building the health care workforce.* Washington, DC: The National Academies Press.

IOM. 2011. *Clinical practice guidelines we can trust.* Washington, DC: The National Academies Press.

IOM. 2012. *Health IT and patient safety: Building safer systems for better care.* Washington, DC: The National Academies Press.

IOM. 2013a. *Best care at lower cost: The path to continuously learning health care in America.* Washington, DC: The National Academies Press.

IOM. 2013b. *Delivering high-quality cancer care: Charting a new course for a system in crisis.* Washington, DC: The National Academies Press.

The Joint Commission. 2005. *Health care at the crossroads: Strategies for improving the medical liability system and preventing patient injury.* The Joint Commission. www.jointcommission. org/assets/1/18/Medical_Liability.pdf (accessed June 8, 2015).

Jost, T. 2006. Health courts and malpractice claims adjudication through Medicare: Some questions. *Journal of Health Care Law & Policy* 9(2):280–290.

Kachalia, A. 2014. Legal issues in diagnostic error. Presentation to the Committee on Diagnostic Error in Health Care, August 7, 2014, Washington, DC.

Kachalia, A., and M. M. Mello. 2011. New directions in medical liability reform. *New England Journal of Medicine* 364(16):1564–1572.

Kachalia, A. B., M. M. Mello, T. A. Brennan, and D. M. Studdert. 2008. Beyond negligence: Avoidability and medical injury compensation. *Social Science and Medicine* 66(2):387–402.

Kachalia, A., S. R. Kaufman, R. Boothman, S. Anderson, K. Welch, S. Saint, M. A. Rogers. 2010. Liability claims and costs before and after implementation of a medical error disclosure program. *Annals of Internal Medicine* 153(4):213–221.

Kachalia, A., A. Little, M. Isavoran, L. M. Crider, and J. Smith. 2014. Greatest impact of safe harbor rule may be to improve patient safety, not reduce liability claims paid by physicians. *Health Affairs (Millwood)* 33(1):59–66.

Kassirer, J. P., and M. Angell. 1998. Evaluation and management guidelines—Fatally flawed. *New England Journal of Medicine* 339(23):1697–1698.

Kessler, D. P., N. Summerton, and J. R. Graham. 2006. Effects of the medical liability system in Australia, the UK, and the USA. *Lancet* 368(9531):240–246.

Kostis, W. J., K. Demissie, S. W. Marcella, Y. H. Shao, A. C. Wilson, and A. E. Moreyra. 2007. Weekend versus weekday admission and mortality from myocardial infarction. *New England Journal of Medicine* 356(11):1099–1109.

Kroft, S. H. 2014. Statement of Steven H. Kroft, MD, FASCP, American Society for Clinical Pathology (ASCP). Input submitted to the Committee on Diagnostic Error in Health Care, April 28, 2014, Washington, DC.

Kuhn, T., P. Basch, M. Barr, and T. Yackel. 2015. Clinical documentation in the 21st century: Executive summary of a policy position paper from the American College of Physicians. *Annals of Internal Medicine* 162(4):301–303.

Lembitz, A., and D. Boyle. 2014. COPIC medical liability insurance. Input submitted to the Committee on Diagnostic Error in Health Care, November 25, 2014, Washington, DC.

Localio, A. R., A. G. Lawthers, T. A. Brennan, N. M. Laird, L. E. Hebert, L. M. Peterson, J. P. Newhouse, P. C. Weiler, and H. H. Hiatt. 1991. Relation between malpractice claims and adverse events due to negligence. *New England Journal of Medicine* 325(4):245–251.

Lopez, L., J. S. Weissman, E. C. Schneider, S. N. Weingart, A. P. Cohen, and A. M. Epstein. 2009. Disclosure of hospital adverse events and its association with patients' ratings of the quality of care. *Archives of Internal Medicine* 169(20):1888–1894.

MACRMI (Massachusetts Alliance for Communication and Resolution following Medical Injury). 2015. About MACRMI. www.macrmi.info/about-macrmi/#sthash.wpQ4E35l. dpbs (accessed November 7, 2015).

Mastroianni, A. C., M. M. Mello, S. Sommer, M. Hardy, and T. H. Gallagher. 2010. The flaws in state "apology" and "disclosure" laws dilute their intended impact on malpractice suits. *Health Affairs* 29(9):1611–1619.

MedPAC (Medicare Payment Advisory Commission). 2014. Physician and other health professional payment systems. www.medpac.gov/-documents-/payment-basics/page/2 (accessed March 17, 2015).

Mello, M. M., and T. H. Gallagher. 2010. Malpractice reform—Opportunities for leadership by health care institutions and liability insurers. *New England Journal of Medicine* 362(15):1353–1356.

Mello, M. M., D. M. Studdert, A. B. Kachalia, and T. A. Brennan. 2006. "Health courts" and accountability for patient safety. *Milbank Quarterly* 84(3):459–492.

Mello M., A. Chandra, A. Gawande, and D. Studdert. 2010. National costs of the medical liability system. *Health Affairs*, 29(9):1569–1577.

Mello, M. M., A. Kachalia, and D. Studdert. 2011. *Administrative compensation for medical injuries: Lessons from three foreign systems.* Commonwealth Fund.

Mello, M. M., R. C. Boothman, T. McDonald, J. Driver, A. Lembitz, D. Bouwmeester, B. Dunlap, and T. Gallagher. 2014a. Communication-and-resolution programs: The challenges and lessons learned from six early adopters. *Health Affairs* 33(1):20–29.

Mello, M. M., D. M. Studdert, and A. Kachalia. 2014b. The medical liability climate and prospects for reform. *JAMA* 312(20):2146–2155.

MHA PSO (Michigan Health Hospital Association Patient Safety Organization). 2015. Safe tables. www.mhapso.org/safetables (accessed April 10, 2015).

Miller, H. D. 2014. How healthcare payment systems and benefit designs can support more accurate diagnosis. Input submitted to the Committee on Diagnostic Error in Health Care, December 29, 2014, Washington, DC.

National Commission on Physician Payment Reform. 2013. *Report of the National Commission on Physician Payment Reform.* http://physicianpaymentcommission.org/report (accessed March 17, 2015).

National Patient Safety Foundation's Lucian Leape Institute. 2015. Shining a Light: Safer Health Care Through Transparency. http://c.ymcdn.com/sites/www.npsf.org/resource/resmgr/LLI/Shining-a-Light_Transparency.pdf (accessed July 24, 2015).

Newman-Toker, D. E., K. M. McDonald, and D. O. Meltzer. 2013. How much diagnostic safety can we afford, and how should we decide? A health economics perspective. *BMJ Quality and Safety* 22(Suppl 2):ii11–ii20.

Nicoletti, B. 2005. How to document and bill care plan oversight. *Family Practice Management* 12(5):23–25.

ONC (Office of the National Coordinator for Health Information Technology). 2014. *Health information technology adverse event reporting: Analysis of two databases.* Washington, DC: Office of the National Coordinator for Health Information Technology.

OTA (Office of Technology Assessment). 1994. *Defensive Medicine and Medical Malpractice.* OTA-H-602. Washington, DC: U.S. Government Printing Office.

Parikh, P. D. 2014. PIAA medical liability insurance. Input submitted to the Committee on Diagnostic Error in Health Care, February 25, 2014, Washington, DC.

Peters, P. G. 2008. Health courts? *Boston University Law Review* 88:227–289.

Rabin, R. C. 2014. 15-minute visits take a toll on the doctor–patient relationship. *Kaiser Health News*, April 21. http://khn.org/news/15-minute-doctor-visits (accessed June 8, 2015).

Robeznieks, A. 2014. Malpractice claims can be kept out of court, but not the NPDB. *Modern Healthcare*, August 13. www.modernhealthcare.com/article/20140813/NEWS/308139939 (accessed June 8, 2015).

Rosenthal, M. 2014. Comments to the Institute of Medicine. Input submitted to the Committee on Diagnostic Error in Health Care, December 29, 2014, Washington, DC.

Sage, W. M., T. H. Gallagher, S. Armstrong, J. S. Cohn, T. McDonald, J. Gale, A. C. Woodward, and M. M. Mello. 2014. How policy makers can smooth the way for communication-and-resolution programs. *Health Affairs* 33(1):11–19.

Sarkar, U., D. Bonacum, W. Strull, C. Spitzmueller, N. Jin, A. Lopez, T. D. Giardina, A. N. Meyer, and H. Singh. 2012. Challenges of making a diagnosis in the outpatient setting: A multi-site survey of primary care physicians. *BMJ Quality and Safety* 21(8):641–648.

Sarkar, U., B. Simchowitz, D. Bonacum, W. Strull, A. Lopez, L. Rotteau, and K. G. Shojania. 2014. A qualitative analysis of physician perspectives on missed and delayed outpatient diagnosis: The focus on system-related factors. *Joint Commission Journal on Quality and Patient Safety* 40(10):461–470.

Schiff, G. D., and D. W. Bates. 2010. Can electronic clinical documentation help prevent diagnostic errors? *New England Journal of Medicine* 362(12):1066–1069.

Schiff, G. D., O. Hasan, S. Kim, R. Abrams, K. Cosby, B. L. Lambert, A. S. Elstein, S. Hasler, M. L. Kabongo, N. Krosnjar, R. Odwazny, M. F. Wisniewski, and R. A. McNutt. 2009. Diagnostic error in medicine: Analysis of 583 physician-reported errors. *Archives of Internal Medicine* 169(20):1881–1887.

Schiff, G., P. Griswold, B. R. Ellis, A. L. Puopolo, N. Brede, H. R. Nieva, F. Frederico, N. Leydon, J. Ling, D. Wachenheim, L. L. Leape, and M. Biondolillo. 2014. Doing right by our patients when things go wrong in the ambulatory setting. *Joint Commission Journal on Quality and Patient Safety/Joint Commission Resources* 40(2):91–96.

Schneider, E. C., P. S. Hussey, and C. Schnyer. 2011. *Payment reform: Analysis of models and performance measurement implications*. Santa Monica, CA: RAND Corporation.

SIDM (Society to Improve Diagnosis in Medicine). 2015. *$200K Breakthrough Grant Elevates Diagnostic Training*. www.improvediagnosis.org/blogpost/950784/221522/200K-Breakthrough-Grant-Elevates-Diagnostic-Training (accessed July 22, 2015).

Singh, H., T. D. Giardina, A. N. Meyer, S. N. Forjuoh, M. D. Reis, and E. J. Thomas. 2013. Types and origins of diagnostic errors in primary care settings. *JAMA Internal Medicine* 173(6):418–425.

TDCF (The Doctors Company Foundation). 2015. *Grants awarded*. www.tdcfoundation.com/Grants/index.htm (accessed July 22, 2015).

Tehrani, A., H. Lee, S. Mathews, A. Shore, M. Makary, P. Pronovost, and D. Newman-Toker. 2013. 25-year summary of U.S. malpractice claims for diagnostic errors, 1986–2010: An analysis from the National Practitioner Data Bank. *BMJ Quality and Safety* 22:672–680.

Texas Medical Association. 2013. Coding for telephone consultations. www.texmed.org/template.aspx?id=5422 (accessed April 10, 2015).

Timm, N. T. 2010. From damages caps to health courts: Continuing progress in medical malpractice reform. *Michigan State Law Review* 2010:1211–1236.

Troxel, D. 2014. The Doctors Company. Input submitted to the Committee on Diagnostic Error in Health Care, April 28, 2014, Washington, DC.

Wennberg, D. 2014. Comments for the Institute of Medicine's Committee on Diagnostic Error in Health Care. Input submitted to the Committee on Diagnostic Error in Health Care, December 29, 2014, Washington, DC.

WHO (World Health Organization). 2005. *WHO draft guidelines for adverse event reporting and learning systems*. Geneva, Switzerland: World Health Organization.

WSHA (Washington State Hospital Association). 2014. WSHA safe tables and webcasts. www.wsha.org/0518.cfm (accessed April 10, 2015).

8

A Research Agenda for the Diagnostic Process and Diagnostic Error

Progress toward improving diagnosis and reducing diagnostic error will be significantly hampered without a dedicated focus on research. A primary reason that diagnostic errors have remained an underappreciated quality challenge is the lack of information specifying the full extent of the problem. To underscore the importance of this issue, the committee sought to identify or construct an estimate of the frequency of diagnostic errors. All of the research the committee reviewed indicated that diagnostic errors are a significant and pervasive challenge, but the available research estimates were inadequate to establish a precise understanding of the incidence and nature of diagnostic errors in clinical practice today.

Absent this quantification, other issues in health care quality and safety have overshadowed diagnostic errors. And while the issue of diagnostic error has been gaining momentum in patient safety and quality improvement efforts, the relative lack of attention has resulted in substantial gaps in what is known about the diagnostic process and diagnostic error in health care today. These knowledge limitations affect not only the field of diagnosis but also the broader research enterprise. A substantial body of research relies on—and in some cases assumes that—diagnoses are correct. In research studies evaluating interventions, for example, incorrect diagnoses threaten the validity of the study outcomes and conclusions. An improved understanding of diagnosis and diagnostic error has the potential to inform and improve all areas of health research.

Thus, the committee concluded that that there is an urgent need for research on the diagnostic process and diagnostic errors. Previous chapters have highlighted the challenges to diagnosis that arise from specific elements of the health care work system. The lack of research on the diagnostic process and diagnostic error is an overarching challenge that affects all aspects of the diagnostic process and all elements within the work system. This chapter outlines the impediments to research on the diagnostic process and diagnostic error. The committee calls for a coordinated federal research agenda, committed funding, and significant public–private collaborations to enhance research in this critical area.

A FEDERAL RESEARCH AGENDA

The diagnostic process and the challenge of diagnostic errors have been neglected within the national health care research agenda (Berenson et al., 2014; Wachter, 2010; Zwaan et al., 2013). Input provided to the committee concluded that "although correct treatment presumes a correct diagnosis, federal resources devoted to diagnostic research are vastly eclipsed by those devoted to treatment" (Newman-Toker, 2014, p. 12). There are a number of reasons why diagnosis and diagnostic errors may be underrepresented in current research activities, including the dearth of sources of valid and reliable data for measuring diagnostic error, a lack of awareness of the problem, the perceived inevitability of the problem, a poor understanding of the diagnostic and clinical reasoning processes, a lack of applicable performance measures on diagnosis, and the need for financial and other resources to address the problem (Berenson et al., 2014; Croskerry, 2012).

A major barrier to research on diagnosis and diagnostic error is the disease-focused approach to medical research funding. For example, the National Institutes of Health's (NIH's) structure and funding mechanisms are often organized by disease or organ systems, which facilitates the study of these specific areas but impedes research efforts that seek to provide a more comprehensive understanding of diagnosis as a distinct research area. Newman-Toker (2014, p. 12) asserted that diagnostic research "invariably falls between rather than within individual Institute missions." As such, the topic of diagnosis, which cuts across all diseases and body parts, is not centralized within the NIH research portfolio, and available research funding for diagnosis often targets the diagnosis of specific diseases, but not diagnosis as a whole; the diagnosis of several diseases with similar presentations; or the diagnostic process itself.

Diagnosis and diagnostic error are not a focus of federal health services research efforts, with the exception of two special emphasis notices from the Agency for Healthcare Research and Quality (AHRQ) for diagnostic error which were published in 2007 and 2013, as well as 2015 grant opportunities (AHRQ, 2007, 2013, 2015a,b). AHRQ posted an R01 grant opportunity for "understanding and improving diagnostic safety in ambulatory care: incidence and contributing factors" (AHRQ, 2015a) and an R18 grant opportunity on identifying strategies and interventions to improve diagnostic safety in ambulatory care (AHRQ, 2015b).

Although these initial steps are promising, the available funding for research on diagnostic error is not in alignment with the scope of the problem or with the resources necessary to improve diagnosis. The committee concluded that there is an urgent need for dedicated, coordinated federal funding for research on diagnosis and diagnostic error. **Thus, the committee recommends that federal agencies, including the Department of Health and Human Services (HHS), the Department of Veterans Affairs (VA), and the Department of Defense (DOD), should develop a coordinated research agenda on the diagnostic process and diagnostic errors by the end of 2016.** Within HHS there are a number of agencies that have the diagnostic process and diagnostic errors within their purview, including NIH, AHRQ, the Centers for Disease Control and Prevention, and the Centers for Medicare & Medicaid Services (CMS). The VA and the DOD should also be engaged in developing this research agenda. An example of cross-governmental collaboration is the joint effort by AHRQ and the National Science Foundation to evaluate how industrial and systems engineering contribute to better health care delivery. Following a workshop that outlined a research agenda, these agencies released a joint grant solicitation to fill the gaps identified during the course of the workshop (Valdez, 2010).

Given the potential for federal research in diagnosis and diagnostic error to fall between institutional missions, federal agencies need to collaborate to develop a coordinated national research agenda that addresses diagnosis and diagnostic error. **Because of the urgent need for research in these areas, federal agencies should commit dedicated funding to implementing this research agenda.** Overall federal investment in biomedical and health services research is declining (Moses et al., 2015), and the committee recognizes that funding for diagnosis and diagnostic error will likely draw resources away from other important priorities. However, given the consistent lack of resources for research on diagnosis, and the potential for diagnostic errors to contribute to significant patient harm, the committee concluded that this prioritization is necessary in order to achieve broader improvements in the quality and safety of health care. Furthermore, because much of health care (both in research and in clinical practice) relies on correct diagnoses, research in this area is likely to enhance the effectiveness of other efforts (e.g., those focused on treatment and management), and it could also potentially lead to cost savings by preventing diagnostic errors, inappropriate treatment, and related adverse events.

PUBLIC–PRIVATE COLLABORATION ON RESEARCH

In addition to federal-level research on diagnosis and diagnostic errors, there is an important role for public–private collaboration and coordination among the federal government, foundations, industry, and other organizations. Collaborative funding efforts help extend the existing financial resources and reduce duplications in research efforts. Interested parties can unite around areas of mutual interest and spearhead progress. Foundations, industry, and other stakeholders can make important contributions—financially and within their areas of expertise—to enhance knowledge in this area. **Thus, the committee recommends that the federal government should pursue and encourage opportunities for public–private partnerships among a broad range of stakeholders, such as the Patient-Centered Outcomes Research Institute (PCORI), foundations, the diagnostic testing and health information technology (health IT) industries, health care organizations, and professional liability insurers to support research on the diagnostic process and diagnostic errors.**

The scientific literature includes descriptions of various types of collaborative models that have been employed to share information, resources, and capabilities (Altshuler et al., 2010; Portilla and Alving, 2010). Organizations like Grantmakers in Health coordinate corporate and foundation funding efforts to improve health and health care delivery (GIH, 2015). An example of a public–private partnership that could be leveraged is the National Center for Interprofessional Practice and Education, which takes a cross-cutting view of health systems and health care professional education (NCIPE, 2015). Another example is the CMS Innovation Center's Health Care Payment Learning and Action Network, launched in the spring of 2015 (CMS, 2015). This model will support HHS's efforts to move from paying for volume to paying for the value of services provided (Burwell, 2015). As a part of this effort, organizations can collaborate to generate evidence. In line with Recommendation 7b, this could include generating evidence about how payment models influence the diagnostic process and the occurrence of diagnostic errors.

Zwaan and colleagues (2013) outlined potential research opportunities broadly, classified into three areas: the epidemiology of diagnostic errors, the causes of diagnostic error, and error prevention strategies. The Society to Improve Diagnosis in Medicine has formed a research committee to bring together multidisciplinary perspectives in order to advance a research agenda that seeks to address critical gaps in the evidence base (SIDM, 2015). Building on this work, the committee identified additional areas of research that could help shape a national research agenda on diagnosis and diagnostic error (see Box 8-1). This list is not exhaustive;

BOX 8-1
Potential Areas of Research

Patient and Family Engagement and the Diagnostic Process
- Effective strategies for partnering with patients in the diagnostic process; approaches for reaching diverse population groups, including those who are diverse in language, culture, and individual values, preferences, and needs.
- Development of patient-focused educational resources and shared decision-making tools/strategies in the diagnostic process.
- Patient-centered priorities in reducing diagnostic errors.
- Identification of multiple perspectives to better understand and mitigate diagnostic error (including the patient, family, primary care clinicians, specialists, other health care professionals, organizational leaders, risk management perspectives, and others).
- The impact of patient variables on the diagnostic process and outcomes.
- Disparities in accurate and timely diagnosis among populations at highest risk, including those with health literacy limitations, socioeconomic disadvantages, limited English proficiency, and racial/ethnic minority populations.

Health Care Professional Education and Training
- How health care professional schools currently train and evaluate students for diagnostic competency.
- Effective practices to teach and evaluate clinical reasoning.
- The use of simulation training to improve diagnostic performance.
- Etiology of cognitive errors (inadequate knowledge and shortcomings in cognitive processes).
- Components of intra- and interprofessional training that improve the diagnostic process.

Health Information Technology (Health IT)
- How health IT can be better leveraged to support the identification of diagnostic errors by analyzing large quantities of data to find trends, patterns, and anomalies that would not be visible otherwise.
- Development of strategies for the identification and remediation of health IT functionality and usability issues affecting diagnosis (difficulties navigating, seeing, understanding, or interacting with user interfaces/displays).
- Investigation of how health IT can be leveraged to narrow the gap between patients' actual health literacy level and that required to navigate the diagnostic process.
- Examination of the impact of computer-assisted diagnosis technology on diagnostic accuracy in medical imaging.
- Evaluation of the relationship between the amount of clinical context provided by diagnostic test orders and diagnostic error.

continued

BOX 8-1 Continued

- Development of health IT tools to efficiently extract information from the electronic health record that is relevant to an individual patient's specific diseases and conditions, allowing the clinicians to expend more of their efforts on information integration and interpretation to provide a personalized diagnosis.
- Potential for artificial intelligence, big data, and analytics approaches to improve the diagnostic process and identify diagnostic errors and near misses.

Identification, Analysis, and Reduction of Diagnostic Errors
- National studies/surveys of health care organizations to document:
  - Current approaches and progress in the identification of diagnostic errors.
  - Evidence to improve diagnosis and reduce diagnostic errors.
  - The relationship between diagnostic variance and patient outcomes.
- A national effort to capture diagnostic delays and errors could be considered as a part of ongoing surveillance through the National Center for Health Statistics, such as the National Ambulatory Medical Care Survey and the National Hospital Ambulatory Medical Care Survey.
- Longitudinal analysis of diagnostic errors to determine when improvement efforts are succeeding.
- Disease-specific analyses of diagnostic errors and near misses.
- Development of tools and methods that can identify diagnostic errors in practice.
  - The necessary structures (Are the right tools in place to increase the likelihood of accurate and timely diagnoses?), processes (Are the appropriate steps undertaken to ensure that a diagnosis is accurate and timely?), and patient outcomes (Are both clinical outcomes and patient-reported outcomes about how the diagnostic error affected them noted?).
  - Variations research (similar to geographic variations research to identify variability of diagnostic accuracy across regions, organizations, health care professionals, settings of care, etc.).

---

instead, it is meant to highlight some of the issues that were raised during committee discussions. The committee concluded that it was not feasible to prioritize specific research areas in diagnosis and diagnostic error; such prioritization will require additional time and effort beyond the scope of the study.

Because this has been an underemphasized area in research and health care delivery, there are many promising avenues for research. Chapter 3 describes the committee's proposed five purposes of measurement; re-

- The specific elements of diagnostic error associated with different settings of care (including inpatient, outpatient, extended care, home, and community settings).
- Methods to assess the diagnostic performance of diagnostic team members.
- Assessment of the elements of organizational culture that promote improved diagnostic performance.
- Effective and cost-effective approaches for identifying diagnostic errors.
- Identification of priority conditions for which known approaches to improve diagnostic accuracy and timeliness would have a high impact.
- Mitigation of potential adverse consequences related to assessing diagnostic errors.
- Identification of tools that can measure interventions.

Work System Improvements
- Research on the work system factors that contribute to poor diagnostic performance, diagnostic errors, and near misses in current practice.
- Research exploring the generalizability of findings on teamwork, culture, leadership, and education from other disciplines and from broader health care quality and patient safety settings to the diagnostic process.
- Identification of cultural and other organizational characteristics of health care organizations that improve diagnosis and reduce diagnostic errors.
- Interventions that redesign the work system and assess their effects on diagnosis.

External Environment
- Impact of payment, care delivery models, and coding practices on the diagnostic process and the accuracy of diagnosis.
- Economic consequences of diagnostic errors for patients and their families, health care organizations, and the nation.
- Mechanisms to improve voluntary reporting.
- Alternative approaches to medical liability to improve disclosure, learning, and the prevention of diagnostic errors.

search in each of these areas could be very helpful. Additional research could better define the scope of the problem, identify vulnerabilities in the diagnostic process, describe the work system factors that contribute to errors, and evaluate interventions. Further measurement research could advance efforts to assess diagnostic performance in education and training environments and could consider issues related to measurement for accountability. An important area of research will be the economic impact of diagnostic errors. Today, there is limited information about the economic consequences of diagnostic errors for patients and their families, for health care organizations, and for the country as a whole.

As discussed in Chapter 4, it is also critical to carry out more research on teamwork in the diagnostic process, patient engagement, and health care professional education. There has been limited research on teamwork in the diagnostic process, and future research efforts could help identify best practices to facilitate and support such teamwork. Furthermore, diagnostic research that includes patient and family perspectives will be critical to increasing the effectiveness of interventions, because patient actions are often needed to achieve correct diagnoses, especially in outpatient settings (Gandhi et al., 2006). To better enable patient and family engagement in the diagnostic process, further research could also elaborate on methods and tools that effectively engage patients and their families as true partners. In the area of health care professional education, research on methods to assess diagnostic competencies among health care professionals and best practices for developing clinical reasoning and other competencies essential to the diagnostic process is warranted.

Chapter 5 describes the use of health IT in the diagnostic process. A major area of research is understanding how to effectively leverage health IT to support all diagnostic team members in the diagnostic process, especially in supporting clinical reasoning tasks. For example, a better understanding of the performance diagnostic decision support tools in clinical practice is needed. In addition, research that identifies the potential adverse effects of health IT on the diagnostic process can be helpful to ensure the safe design, implementation, and use of health IT. Given the growth of mobile health applications and wearable technologies, research could also provide information on how these can be effectively incorporated in the diagnostic process.

In Chapter 6, the committee calls on health care organizations to begin monitoring the diagnostic process and to identify, learn from, and reduce diagnostic errors in clinical practice. Because there has been limited collection of this information in clinical practice, health care organizations will need to experiment and assess which approaches are effective for monitoring the diagnostic process and identifying, analyzing, and reducing diagnostic errors. Further research on developing systematic feedback mechanisms on diagnostic performance and research on best practices for the delivery of this feedback to individuals, care teams, and leadership will also be necessary. Research can also inform the design of a health care organization's work system so that it supports the work and activities of the diagnostic process.

Chapter 7 describes how voluntary reporting, medical liability, and payment and care delivery can influence the diagnostic process. There are several topics that deserve research in this area, including demonstration projects to evaluate how alternative approaches to medical liability—such as administrative health courts and safe harbors for adherence to evidence-based clinical practice guidelines—influence the occurrence and disclosure of diagnostic errors and also influence the analysis of and learning from these errors. As mentioned previously, there is also a need to understand how payment and care delivery influence the diagnostic process, diagnostic errors, and learning.

Achieving progress in reducing diagnostic errors and improving diagnosis will require an emphasis on collaboration. Collaborative research in diagnosis and diagnostic error will necessitate the involvement of multiple disciplines, and it will benefit from the use of multiple and mixed methods (Creswell et al., 2011). For instance, qualitative approaches such as cognitive work analyses of the human factors/ergonomics discipline could provide in-depth information on the types of diagnostic errors identified by health services researchers (Bisantz and Roth, 2007). This type of multidisciplinary mixed-methods research can provide the type of information that is needed to further quantify and understand the nature of diagnostic errors.

RECOMMENDATION

Goal 8: Provide dedicated funding for research on the diagnostic process and diagnostic errors

Recommendation 8a: Federal agencies, including the Department of Health and Human Services, the Department of Veterans Affairs, and the Department of Defense, should:
- **Develop a coordinated research agenda on the diagnostic process and diagnostic errors by the end of 2016.**
- **Commit dedicated funding to implementing this research agenda.**

Recommendation 8b: The federal government should pursue and encourage opportunities for public–private partnerships among a broad range of stakeholders, such as the Patient-Centered Outcomes Research Institute, foundations, the diagnostic testing and health information technology industries, health care organizations, and professional liability insurers to support research on the diagnostic process and diagnostic errors.

REFERENCES

AHRQ (Agency for Healthcare Research and Quality). 2007. Special emphasis notice (SEN): AHRQ announces interest in research on diagnostic errors in ambulatory care settings. http://grants.nih.gov/grants/guide/notice-files/NOT-HS-08-002.html (accessed May 5, 2015).

AHRQ. 2013. AHRQ announces interest in research to improve diagnostic performance in ambulatory care settings. http://grants.nih.gov/grants/guide/notice-files/NOT-HS-13-009.html (accessed February 4, 2015).

AHRQ. 2015a. Understanding and improving diagnostic safety in ambulatory care: Incidence and contributing factors (R01). http://grants.nih.gov/grants/guide/pa-files/PA-15-180.html (accessed May 3, 2015).

AHRQ. 2015b. Understanding and improving diagnostic safety in ambulatory care: Strategies and interventions (R18). http://grants.nih.gov/grants/guide/pa-files/PA-15-179.html (accessed May 3, 2015).

Altshuler, J. S., E. Balogh, A. D. Barker, S. L. Eck, S. H. Friend, G. S. Ginsburg, R. S. Herbst, S. J. Nass, C. M. Streeter, and J. A. Wagner. 2010. Opening up to precompetitive collaboration. *Science Translational Medicine* 2(52):52cm26.

Berenson, R. A., D. K. Upadhyay, and D. R. Kaye. 2014. Placing diagnosis errors on the policy agenda. *Timely Analysis of Immediate Health Policy Issues*. Washington, DC: Urban Institute. www.urban.org/sites/default/files/alfresco/publication-pdfs/413104-Placing-Diagnosis-Errors-on-the-Policy-Agenda-brief.pdf (accessed June 9, 2015).

Bisantz, A., and E. Roth. 2007. Analysis of cognitive work. *Reviews of Human Factors and Ergonomics* 3(1):1–43.

Burwell, S. M. 2015. Setting value-based payment goals—HHS efforts to improve U.S. Health care. *New England Journal of Medicine* 372(10):897–899.

CMS (Centers for Medicare & Medicaid Services). 2015. Health care payment learning and action network. http://innovation.cms.gov/initiatives/Health-Care-Payment-Learning-and-Action-Network (accessed May 5, 2015).

Creswell, J. W., A. C. Klassen, V. L. Plano-Clark, and K. C. Smith. 2011. Best practices for mixed methods research in the health sciences. Office of Behavioral and Social Sciences Research. http://obssr.od.nih.gov/mixed_methods_research (accessed May 27, 2015).

Croskerry, P. 2012. Perspectives on diagnostic failure and patient safety. *Healthcare Quarterly* 15(Special issue):50–56.

Gandhi, T. K., A. Kachalia, E. J. Thomas, A. L. Puopolo, C. Yoon, T. A. Brennan, and D. M. Studdert. 2006. Missed and delayed diagnoses in the ambulatory setting: A study of closed malpractice claims. *Annals of Internal Medicine* 145(7):488–496.

GIH (Grantmakers in Health). 2015. Grantmakers in Health. www.gih.org (accessed May 26, 2015).

Moses, H., 3rd, D. H. Matheson, S. Cairns–Smith, B. P. George, C. Palisch, and E. R. Dorsey. 2015. The anatomy of medical research: U.S. and international comparisons. *JAMA* 313(2):174–189.

NCIPE (National Center for Interprofessional Practice and Education). 2015. *National Center for Interprofessional Practice and Education*. https://nexusipe.org (accessed May 27, 2015).

Newman-Toker, D. 2014. Prioritization of diagnostic error problems and solutions: Concepts, economic modeling, and action plan. Presentation to the Committee on Diagnostic Error in Health Care, August 7, 2014, Washington, DC.

Portilla, L. M., and B. Alving. 2010. Reaping the benefits of biomedical research: Partnerships required. *Science Translational Medicine* 2(35):35cm17.

SIDM (Society to Improve Diagnosis in Medicine). 2015. Diagnostic error resources. www.improvediagnosis.org/?page=SafetyToolkit (accessed March 15, 2015).

Valdez, R. S. 2010. *Industrial and systems engineering and health care: Critical areas of research—Final report*. Rockville, MD: Agency for Healthcare Research and Quality.

Wachter, R. M. 2010. Why diagnostic errors don't get any respect—and what can be done about them. *Health Affairs (Millwood)* 29(9):1605–1610.

Zwaan, L., G. D. Schiff, and H. Singh. 2013. Advancing the research agenda for diagnostic error reduction. *BMJ Quality & Safety* 22(Suppl 2):ii52–ii57.

9

The Path to Improve Diagnosis and Reduce Diagnostic Error

Illuminating the blind spot of diagnostic error and improving diagnosis in health care will require a significant reenvisioning of the diagnostic process and widespread commitment to change. Diagnostic error is a complex and multifaceted problem; there is no single solution that is likely to achieve the changes that are needed. To address this challenge and to improve diagnosis for patients and their families, the committee makes eight recommendations. This chapter highlights the overarching conclusions from the committee's deliberations and presents these recommendations.

OVERARCHING CONCLUSIONS

Several major conclusions emerged from the committee's discussions. The first conclusion is that urgent change is needed to address the issue of diagnostic error, which poses a major challenge to health care quality. Diagnostic errors persist throughout all settings of care, involve common and rare diseases, and continue to harm an unacceptable number of patients. Yet, diagnosis—and, in particular, the occurrence of diagnostic errors—is not a major focus in health care practice or research. The result of this inattention is significant: It is likely that most people will experience at least one diagnostic error in their lifetime, sometimes with devastating consequences.

The committee drew this conclusion based on its collective assessment of the available evidence describing the epidemiology of diagnostic errors. In every research area that the committee evaluated, diagnostic er-

355

rors were a consistent quality and safety challenge. For example, a recent study estimated that 5 percent of U.S. adults who seek outpatient care experience a diagnostic error, and the researchers who conducted the study noted that this is likely a conservative estimate (Singh et al., 2014). Postmortem examination research that spans several decades has consistently shown that diagnostic errors contribute to around 10 percent of patient deaths (Shojania et al., 2002, 2003). The Harvard Medical Practice Study, which reviewed medical records, found diagnostic errors in 17 percent of the adverse events occurring in hospitalized patients (Leape et al., 1991), and a more recent study in the Netherlands found that diagnostic errors comprised 6.4 percent of hospital adverse events (Zwaan et al., 2010). Analyses of malpractice claims data indicate that diagnostic errors are the leading type of paid claims, represent the highest proportion of total payments, and are almost twice as likely to have resulted in the patient's death compared to other claims (Tehrani et al., 2013).

However, the committee concluded that the available research estimates were not adequate to extrapolate a specific estimate or range of the incidence of diagnostic errors within clinical practice today. There is even less information available with which to assess the frequency and severity of harm related to diagnostic errors. Part of the challenge is the variety of settings in which these errors can occur, including hospitals, emergency departments, a variety of outpatient settings (such as primary and specialty care settings and retail clinics), and long-term care settings (such as nursing homes and rehabilitation centers), combined with the complexity of the diagnostic process itself. Although there are more data available to examine diagnostic errors in some of these settings, there are wide gaps in the information and great variability in the amount and quality of information available. In addition, aggregating data from various research methods—such as postmortem examinations, medical record reviews, and malpractice claims—is problematic. Each method captures information about different subgroups in the population, different dimensions of the problem, and different insights into the frequency and causes of diagnostic error. Nonetheless, the committee concluded that, taken together, the evidence suggests that diagnostic errors are a significant and common challenge in health care necessitating urgent attention.

The second conclusion is that it is very important to consider diagnosis from a patient-centered perspective, as patients bear the ultimate risk of harm from diagnostic errors. Thus, patients should be recognized as vital partners in the diagnostic process, and the health care system needs to encourage and support their engagement and to facilitate respectful learning from diagnostic errors. The committee's definition of diagnostic error—*the failure to (a) establish an accurate and timely explanation of the patient's health problem(s) or (b) communicate that explanation to the patient*—reflects a patient-centered approach and highlights the key role of communication among the patient and the health care professionals involved in the diagnostic process. The term "explanation" is included in the definition to highlight the manner in which a diagnosis is conveyed to a patient such that it facilitates patient understanding and aligns with a patient's level of health literacy.

The committee concluded that a sole focus on reducing diagnostic errors will not achieve the extensive change that is needed. Reducing diagnostic errors will require a broader focus on *improving diagnosis* in health care. This conclusion reflects the input provided to the committee by Gary Klein, a senior scientist at MacroCognition, who argued that improvements in diagnosis will require balancing two interdependent efforts: reducing diagnostic errors and improving diagnostic performance (Klein, 2014). Related input from David Newman-Toker, an associate professor at Johns Hopkins University, suggested that improving diagnostic performance will require addressing both diagnostic quality and efficiency in order to achieve high-value diagnostic performance (Newman-Toker, 2014; Newman-Toker et al., 2013). Thus, many of the recommendations focus on improving diagnosis and the diagnostic process as well on the identification and mitigation of diagnostic errors.

To provide a framework for this dual focus, the committee developed a conceptual model to articulate the diagnostic process, identify the factors that influence this process, and identify opportunities to improve the diagnostic process and outcomes. This conceptual model highlights the committee's conclusion that diagnosis is a team-based process that occurs within the context of a broader system. This system involves the dynamic interaction of the participants in the diagnostic process (which are influenced by the participants' cognitive, perceptual, and affective factors), the tasks that they perform, the technology and tools they utilize, the organization and physical environment in which diagnosis takes place, and the external environmental factors involved, such as oversight processes, error reporting, medical liability, and the payment and care delivery environment.

RECOMMENDATIONS

The committee's recommendations focus on achieving eight goals to improve diagnosis and reduce diagnostic error (see Box 9-1). These recommendations are meant to be applicable to all diagnostic team members and settings of care; thus, some of the committee's recommendations are intentionally broad. Given the early state of the field, the committee also sought to develop recommendations that were not overly proscriptive. Importantly, the evidence base for some recommendations stems from

---

BOX 9-1
Goals for Improving Diagnosis and Reducing Diagnostic Error

- Facilitate more effective teamwork in the diagnostic process among health care professionals, patients, and their families
- Enhance health care professional education and training in the diagnostic process
- Ensure that health information technologies support patients and health care professionals in the diagnostic process
- Develop and deploy approaches to identify, learn from, and reduce diagnostic errors and near misses in clinical practice
- Establish a work system and culture that supports the diagnostic process and improvements in diagnostic performance
- Develop a reporting environment and medical liability system that facilitates improved diagnosis by learning from diagnostic errors and near misses
- Design a payment and care delivery environment that supports the diagnostic process
- Provide dedicated funding for research on the diagnostic process and diagnostic errors

---

the broader patient safety and quality improvement literature. Making connections to previous efforts is important, given the limited focus on diagnosis and its relevance to overall health care quality. Patients and patient advocates have much to offer on how to implement the committee's recommendations. Leveraging the expertise, power, and influence of the patient community will help spur progress.

Facilitate More Effective Teamwork in the Diagnostic Process Among Health Care Professionals, Patients, and Their Families

The diagnostic process is a collaborative activity. Making accurate and timely diagnoses requires teamwork among health care professionals, patients, and their family members. The committee's focus on teamwork in diagnosis grew out of the recognition that too often diagnosis is characterized as a solitary activity, taking place exclusively within an individual physician's mind. While the task of integrating relevant information and communicating a diagnosis to a patient is often the responsibility of an individual clinician, the diagnostic process ideally involves collaboration among multiple health care professionals, the patient, and the patient's family. Consistent with the committee's conclusion, recent reports in the

literature make the case that the diagnostic process is a team-based endeavor (Graedon and Graedon, 2014; Haskell, 2014; Henriksen and Brady,
2013; McDonald, 2014; Schiff, 2014a). For example, Schiff noted that the
new paradigm for diagnosis is that it is carried out by a well-coordinated
team of people working together through reliable processes; in this view,
diagnosis is the collective work of the team of health care professionals
and the patient and his or her family (Schiff, 2014a).

Patients and their families are critical partners in the diagnostic process. The goal of patient engagement in diagnosis is to improve patient
care and outcomes by enabling patients and their families to contribute
valuable input that will facilitate an accurate and timely diagnosis and
improve shared decision making about the path of care. There are indications, however, that patients and families are not routinely engaged as
true partners in the diagnostic process and that they face challenges in engaging in the diagnostic process (Haskell, 2014; Julavits, 2014; McDonald,
2014). Two of the more significant challenges involve unfamiliarity with
the diagnostic process and health care environments that are not supportive of patient engagement.

The committee identified several opportunities to improve patient
and family engagement in the diagnostic process. First, patients and their
families could benefit from having a better overall understanding of the
diagnostic process. Learning opportunities that describe what to expect
during this process, the roles of specific diagnostic team members, and
materials that facilitate patient and family participation in the process
could all be helpful. For example, the National Patient Safety Foundation,
the Society to Improve Diagnosis in Medicine, and Kaiser Permanente
have developed resources to help patients partner with their clinicians
to receive a correct diagnosis (Kaiser Permanente, 2012; NPSF and SIDM,
2014). Health care organizations and health care professionals have the
responsibility to create environments that are receptive to and supportive
of patient engagement in the diagnostic process. This includes recognizing that patients and their families have varying needs, values, and
preferences in regard to engagement and being responsive to the desired
level of involvement. Furthermore, the health care environments need
to encourage patients and families to share feedback about their experiences with diagnosis and their concerns about diagnostic errors and near
misses. Although there are limited systematic mechanisms for patients
to provide feedback to health care professionals about the accuracy of
their diagnoses, establishing opportunities to provide patient feedback is
critical to improving diagnostic performance (Schiff, 2008). This feedback
could also become a routine aspect of assessing patient satisfaction.

An important opportunity to improve engagement is through the use
of health information technology (health IT) tools that make a patient's

health information more accessible and transparent, including clinical notes and diagnostic testing results. The Office of the National Coordinator for Health Information Technology's Meaningful Use 2 requirements include patient's having access to their electronic health information, such as medication lists, diagnostic test results, allergies, and clinical problem lists; organizations have begun to employ patient portals in order to provide patients with access to this information (Adler-Milstein et al., 2014; Bruno et al., 2014; Furukawa et al., 2014; HealthIT.gov, 2015). The OpenNotes initiative, which is available to almost 5 million patients, has promoted even greater transparency of a patient's health information by inviting patients to view the notes recorded by health care professionals during the patients' clinical visit. Initiatives like OpenNotes may promote patient engagement in the diagnostic process and also serve as a mechanism for patients and their families to identify and avert diagnostic errors (Bell et al., 2014; Delbanco et al., 2010, 2012).

Health care professionals and organizations can also involve patients and their families in organizational learning efforts aimed at analyzing the causes of diagnostic errors and identifying interventions that could improve the diagnostic process. Patients and their families have unique insight into the diagnostic process, their outcomes, and the occurrence of diagnostic errors; thus, their perspectives are critical to improving the diagnostic process (Etchegaray et al., 2014; Gertler et al., 2014; Weingart et al., 2005). When a diagnostic error occurs, health care organizations can identify opportunities to involve a patient and his or her family in efforts to learn from the error, using mechanisms such as root cause analyses, morbidity and mortality conferences, and patient and family advisory councils (AHRQ, 2014c; Gertler et al., 2014; Zimmerman and Amori, 2007).

In addition to patient engagement, the committee highlighted the roles of health care professionals in the diagnostic process and the need for improved intra- and interprofessional collaboration. Depending on a patient's health problem, the diagnostic process can involve various types of health care professionals, such as primary care clinicians (physicians, advance practice nurses [APNs], physician assistants [PAs]), physicians in a broad range of specialties (including radiology, pathology, and other disease-focused areas), nurses, technologists, therapists, social workers, pharmacists, and patient navigators. For simplicity, the committee's conceptual model articulates two main types of health care professionals: diagnosticians, or those who make diagnoses, such as physicians, APNs, and PAs; and the health care professionals who support the diagnostic process. Inadequate teamwork and communication are major contributors to medical errors, including diagnostic errors (Baker et al., 2006; CRICO, 2014; Dingley et al., 2008; Singh et al., 2008). Because a patient's diagnosis can hinge on the successful collaboration among these health care professionals, it is important that all health care professionals are well-prepared and supported to engage in diagnostic teamwork.

Recognition that interprofessional education and training is critical to the delivery of high-quality care has been gaining widespread traction; however, health care professionals are still not adequately prepared for this team-based practice (IOM, 2014; Patel et al., 2009; Pecukonis et al., 2008; Schmitt et al., 2011). Opportunities for interprofessional training have been slow to materialize because of a host of different issues, including logistical challenges, deep-rooted cultural differences among the health care professions, differences in educational curricula and trajectory, and costs (Josiah Macy Jr. Foundation and Carnegie Foundation for the Advancement of Teaching, 2010). Furthermore, intraprofessional collaboration can be difficult to achieve in practice, and the way that physicians are prepared today may be hindering their ability to engage in teamwork and cooperation (Hughes and Salas, 2013). For example, the traditional hierarchy among medical students, residents, and experienced physicians may prevent the more junior clinicians from speaking up about a potential error (Sorra et al., 2014).

In addition, the roles of some health care professionals who participate in the diagnostic process have been insufficiently recognized in current practice. For example, the fields of pathology and radiology are critical to diagnosis, but these health care professionals have sometimes been referred to as ancillary services and are not always engaged as full members of the diagnostic team despite their significant contributions to diagnosis. Enhanced collaboration has the potential to improve all aspects of the diagnostic testing process, including test ordering, analysis and interpretation, reporting and communicating the results, and subsequent decision making (Allen and Thorwarth, 2014; Epner, 2015; Kroft, 2014). One opportunity to better integrate these health care professionals into the diagnostic process is the diagnostic management team model; these integrated teams feature collaboration among pathologists, radiologists, and the treating health care professionals in order to ensure that the correct diagnostic tests are ordered and that the results are correctly interpreted and acted upon (Govern, 2013).[1]

In addition, nurses are often not recognized as collaborators in the diagnostic process, despite their critical roles in ensuring proper communication and care coordination among the health care professionals and between the professionals and the patient and his or her family; monitoring the patient's condition over time to see if the patient's course of treatment aligns with the working diagnosis; and identifying and preventing potential diagnostic errors. Depending on a particular patient's needs,

---

[1] Personal communication, M. Laposata, August 8, 2014.

many other health care professionals can play key roles in the diagnostic process, and they also need to be engaged to improve diagnosis.

Goal 1: Facilitate more effective teamwork in the diagnostic process among health care professionals, patients, and their families

Recommendation 1a: In recognition that the diagnostic process is a dynamic team-based activity, health care organizations should ensure that health care professionals have the appropriate knowledge, skills, resources, and support to engage in teamwork in the diagnostic process. To accomplish this, they should facilitate and support:
- Intra- and interprofessional teamwork in the diagnostic process.
- Collaboration among pathologists, radiologists, other diagnosticians, and treating health care professionals to improve diagnostic testing processes.

Recommendation 1b: Health care professionals and organizations should partner with patients and their families as diagnostic team members and facilitate patient and family engagement in the diagnostic process, aligned with their needs, values, and preferences. To accomplish this, they should:
- Provide patients with opportunities to learn about the diagnostic process.
- Create environments in which patients and their families are comfortable engaging in the diagnostic process and sharing feedback and concerns about diagnostic errors and near misses.
- Ensure patient access to electronic health records (EHRs), including clinical notes and diagnostic testing results, to facilitate patient engagement in the diagnostic process and patient review of health records for accuracy.
- Identify opportunities to include patients and their families in efforts to improve the diagnostic process by learning from diagnostic errors and near misses.

Enhance Health Care Professional Education and Training in the Diagnostic Process

Getting the right diagnosis depends on all health care professionals receiving appropriate education and training. There are indications, however, that health care professionals, including diagnosticians, are not prepared to function optimally in the diagnostic process (Brush,

2014; Dhaliwal, 2014; Durning, 2014; Richardson, 2007; ten Cate, 2014; Trowbridge et al., 2013). Education and training-related challenges include methods that have not kept pace with advances in the learning sciences[2] and have an insufficient focus on areas critical to the diagnostic process. Numerous experts in health care professional education provided input to the committee; a common theme of this input was that health care professional education and training is not adequately preparing individuals to become skilled diagnosticians. One of the criticisms is that current approaches to education do not take advantage of advances in the learning sciences, which have found that learners need to develop a deep conceptual understanding of their content area and to have opportunities to reflect on their knowledge; furthermore, educators need to consider factors such as the learning environment, building on prior knowledge, and focusing on learning in addition to teaching. The lack of feedback—or information on the accuracy of a clinician's diagnosis—in the current training environment can result in few opportunities to reflect on one's state of knowledge. This can lead to poorly calibrated clinicians who are unaware of their diagnostic performance and overly confident in their diagnoses (Berner and Graber, 2008). In addition, the authenticity of the learning environment can affect the acquisition of diagnostic skills, and a better alignment of training environments with clinical practice can improve the development of diagnostic skills. For example, clinicians often learn from case studies that reflect prototypical cases, but they are faced with the complexities of real patient cases in their clinical practice (Papa, 2014).

It was not within the committee's charge to define the specific curriculum for all health care professionals; the content of the curriculum and training will need to be tailored to the needs of specific health care professionals. However, the committee highlighted several areas that are important to the diagnostic process. Opportunities to improve the content of health care professional education and training in the diagnostic process include placing a greater emphasis on teamwork and communication with patients, their families, and other health care professionals; providing more training in the ordering of diagnostic testing and in the application of these results to subsequent decision making; and offering more training in the use of health IT. In addition, current health care professional education and training underemphasizes clinical reasoning, including critical thinking skills and decision making in the diagnostic process (Brush, 2014; Durning, 2014; Richardson, 2014; ten Cate, 2014). Although diagnosticians are trained to make diagnoses, few programs

---

[2] The learning sciences study how people learn in order to optimize education and training.

feature explicit training in various aspects of clinical reasoning, such as the dual process theory, heuristics, and biases. This lack of focus on clinical reasoning and on understanding the cognitive contributions to decision making represents a major gap in health care professional education for all diagnostic team members. Among the strategies proposed to improve clinical reasoning education and training are instruction and practice on generating and refining a differential diagnosis; developing an appreciation of how diagnostic errors occur and of the strategies to mitigate them; engaging in metacognition and debiasing strategies; and fostering intuition and progressive problem solving (Eva and Norman, 2005; Gigerenzer, 2000; Gigerenzer and Goldstein, 1996; Hirt and Markman, 1995; Hodges et al., 2001; Marewski and Gigerenzer, 2012; Mumma and Steven, 1995; Mussweiler et al., 2000; Redelmeier, 2005; Trowbridge et al., 2013; Wegwarth et al., 2009).

Oversight processes, such as education and training program accreditation, licensure, and certification, can help ensure that health care professionals achieve and maintain competency in the diagnostic process. Many accreditation organizations already include skills important for diagnostic performance in their accreditation requirements, but diagnostic competencies need to be a larger priority within those requirements. Organizations responsible for health care professional licensure and certification can help ensure that individual health care professionals have achieved and maintain competency in the skills essential for diagnosis. For example, the American Board of Medical Specialties, which grants board certification in more than 150 medical specialties and subspecialties, could use its certification processes to assess competencies in the diagnostic process both in initial board certification and in maintenance of certification efforts.

Goal 2: Enhance health care professional education and training in the diagnostic process

Recommendation 2a: Educators should ensure that curricula and training programs across the career trajectory:
- **Address performance in the diagnostic process, including areas such as clinical reasoning; teamwork; communication with patients, their families, and other health care professionals; appropriate use of diagnostic tests and the application of these results on subsequent decision making; and use of health information technology.**
- **Employ educational approaches that are aligned with evidence from the learning sciences.**

Recommendation 2b: Health care professional certification and accreditation organizations should ensure that health care professionals have and maintain the competencies needed for effective performance in the diagnostic process, including the areas listed above.

Ensure That Health Information Technologies Support Patients and Health Care Professionals in the Diagnostic Process

Health IT plays a critical role in the diagnostic process and includes such technologies as electronic health records (EHRs), health information exchanges, laboratory and medical imaging information systems, clinical decision support, patient engagement tools, computerized provider order entry, and medical devices. When health IT tools support the diagnostic team members and tasks in the diagnostic process and reflect human-centered design principles, health IT has the potential to improve diagnosis and reduce diagnostic errors. For example, health IT can facilitate timely access to information; improve communication among health care professionals, patients, and their families; aid in clinical reasoning and decision making; and help provide feedback and follow-up in the diagnostic process (El-Kareh et al., 2013; Schiff and Bates, 2010). Despite this potential, there have been few demonstrations that health IT improved diagnosis in clinical practice. Indeed, many experts are concerned that current health IT tools are not effectively facilitating the diagnostic process and that they may even be contributing to diagnostic errors (Basch, 2014; Berenson et al., 2011; El-Kareh et al., 2013; Kuhn et al., 2015; Ober, 2015; ONC, 2014; Schiff and Bates, 2010; Verghese, 2008).

The major challenges of health IT in the diagnostic process include problems with the usefulness and usability of health IT tools, poor integration into clinical workflow, difficulty sharing information among diagnostic team members and settings, limitations in supporting clinical reasoning in the diagnostic process, and a lack of opportunities to measure diagnostic errors through health IT tools. In particular, clinicians have expressed concern that clinical documentation in EHRs is not promoting high-quality diagnosis, but is instead aimed at meeting billing and legal requirements, forcing clinicians to "focus on ticking boxes rather than on thoughtfully documenting their clinical thinking" (Schiff and Bates, 2010, p. 1066) (see also Recommendation 7). Collaboration among health IT vendors, the Office of the National Coordinator for Health Information Technology (ONC), and users is warranted to ensure that health IT tools are better aligned with the diagnostic process.

Another health IT–related challenge in the diagnostic process is the lack of interoperability, or the inability for different IT systems and software applications to communicate, exchange data, and use information effectively (Basch, 2014; CHCF, 2014; HIMSS, 2014). Because the diagnostic process occurs over time and can involve multiple health care professionals across different care settings, the free flow of information is critical. In order for health care professionals to develop a complete picture of a patient's health problem, it is crucial that all relevant health information is available and easily accessible. However, progress toward achieving health interoperability has been slow (CHCF, 2014). Only 30 percent of clinicians and hospitals are able to exchange clinical data with other clinicians electronically (Adler-Milstein and Jha, 2014). Similarly, a recent survey of office-based physicians found that while 67 percent were able to view lab results electronically, only 42 percent were able to incorporate lab results into their EHR, and only 31 percent of the physicians exchanged patient clinical summaries with other clinicians (Patel et al., 2013). Challenges to interoperability include the inconsistent and slow adoption of standards, particularly among organizations that are not subject to EHR certification programs, as well as a lack of incentives, such as a business model that generates revenue for health IT vendors via fees associated with transmitting and receiving data (Adler-Milstein, 2015; CHCF, 2014).

Among the federal efforts to improve interoperability are programs to support the development of flexible interoperability standards and meaningful use incentives. Given the importance of interoperability to diagnosis, ONC can play a critical role in accelerating progress toward interoperability by ensuring that health IT vendors meet these requirements by 2018. This recommendation is in line with the recent legislation that repealed the sustainable growth rate, which included a provision that declared it a national objective to "achieve widespread exchange of health information through interoperable certified electronic health records technology nationwide by December 31, 2018."[3]

Improving interoperability across different health care organizations as well as across laboratory and radiology information systems will be critical to improving the diagnostic process. One challenge will be specifying the scope of interoperable information. For example, the interface between EHRs and laboratory and radiology information systems typically has limited clinical information, and the lack of sufficient patient information makes it difficult for a pathologist or radiologist to determine whether diagnostic testing is appropriate or to understand the context for interpreting findings (Epner, 2014, 2015). Another emerging challenge is establishing interoperability between EHRs and patient-facing health IT, including health-related mobile health applications such as those that

---

[3] Medicare Access and CHIP Reauthorization Act of 2015. P.L. 114-10. (April 16, 2015).

keep track of physical activity and glucose levels (Dehling et al., 2015; Marceglia et al., 2015; Otte-Trojel et al., 2014).

Patient safety risks in the diagnostic process related to the use of health IT are another important concern because there is growing recognition that the use of health IT can result in adverse events (IOM, 2012; ONC, 2014). Health IT safety risks have been identified in the context of the sociotechnical system (including technology, people, workflow, organizational factors, and external environment) that can dynamically interact and contribute to adverse events (IOM, 2012; Sittig and Singh, 2010). A number of health IT–related patient safety risks may affect the occurrence of diagnostic errors. For example, two areas of increased concern are clinical documentation and the use of the copy and paste functionality of EHRs. While the use of copy and paste functionality may increase efficiency by saving time spent retyping or reentering information, it carries with it a number of risks, including redundancy that contributes to lengthy notes and cognitive overload as well as the propagation of inaccurate, outdated, or incomprehensible information (AHIMA, 2014; The Joint Commission, 2015; Kuhn et al., 2015).

Unfortunately, contractual provisions, designed to protect vendors' intellectual property interests and liability from unsafe use of health IT products end up limiting the free exchange of information about health IT–related patient safety risks (IOM, 2012). Specifically, "some vendors require contract clauses that force [health IT] system purchasers to adopt vendor-defined policies that prevent the disclosure of errors, bugs, design flaws, and other [health IT] software-related hazards" (Goodman et al., 2011, p. 77). These contractual barriers among health IT vendors and users may propagate safety risks and pose significant challenges to the use of data for future patient safety and quality improvement research (IOM, 2012). Thus, the Institute of Medicine (IOM) report *Health IT and Patient Safety* recommended that "the Secretary of the Department of Health and Human Services [HHS] should ensure insofar as possible that health IT vendors support the free exchange of information about health IT experiences and issues and not prohibit sharing of such information, including details (e.g., screenshots) relating to patient safety" (IOM, 2012, pp. 7 and 128). The committee endorses this recommendation and adds that the Secretary of HHS should require health IT vendors to permit and support the free exchange of information on users' experiences with health IT design and implementation that contribute to adverse effects on the diagnostic process. Health IT users can discuss these patient safety concerns in appropriate forums, such as the forthcoming ONC National Patient Safety Center or patient safety organizations (PSOs) (RTI International, 2014; Sittig et al., 2015). The Agency for Healthcare Research and Quality (AHRQ) has developed a Common Format reporting form for health IT adverse events, and HHS is beginning to evaluate patient safety events related to health IT (ONC, 2014; RTI International, 2014).

Because the safety of health IT is critical for improvements to the diagnostic process, health IT vendors need to proactively monitor their products in order to identify potential adverse events, which could contribute to diagnostic errors and challenges in the diagnostic process (Carayon et al., 2011). To ensure that these vendors' products are unlikely to contribute to diagnostic errors and adverse events, independent, routine third-party evaluations of health IT products used in the diagnostic process need to be performed. If health IT products have the potential to contribute to diagnostic errors or have other adverse effects on the diagnostic process, health IT vendors have a responsibility to communicate this information to their users in a timely manner.

Goal 3: Ensure that health information technologies support patients and health care professionals in the diagnostic process

Recommendation 3a: Health information technology (health IT) vendors and the Office of the National Coordinator for Health Information Technology (ONC) should work together with users to ensure that health IT used in the diagnostic process demonstrates usability, incorporates human factors knowledge, integrates measurement capability, fits well within clinical workflow, provides clinical decision support, and facilitates the timely flow of information among patients and health care professionals involved in the diagnostic process.

Recommendation 3b: ONC should require health IT vendors to meet standards for interoperability among different health IT systems to support effective, efficient, and structured flow of patient information across care settings to facilitate the diagnostic process by 2018.

Recommendation 3c: The Secretary of the Department of Health and Human Services should require health IT vendors to:
- **Routinely submit their products for independent evaluation and notify users about potential adverse effects on the diagnostic process related to the use of their products.**
- **Permit and support the free exchange of information about real-time user experiences with health IT design and implementation that adversely affect the diagnostic process.**

Develop and Deploy Approaches to Identify, Learn from, and Reduce Diagnostic Errors and Near Misses in Clinical Practice

Diagnostic errors are an understudied and underappreciated quality challenge in health care organizations (Graber, 2005; Wachter, 2010). Very few health care organizations have focused on the identification of diagnostic errors and near misses in clinical practice (Graber et al., 2014; Kanter, 2014; Singh, 2014; Trowbridge, 2014). In a presentation to the committee, Paul Epner reported that the Society to Improve Diagnosis in Medicine "know[s] of no effort initiated in any health system to routinely and effectively assess diagnostic performance" (Epner, 2014). Thus, "the true prevalence of diagnostic error is unknown" (Singh et al., 2008, p. 489). The paucity of attention on diagnostic errors in clinical practice has been attributed to a number of factors. Two major contributors are the lack of effective measurement of diagnostic error and the difficulty in detecting these errors in clinical practice (Berenson et al., 2014; Graber et al., 2012; Singh and Sittig, 2015). Additional factors may include a health care organization's competing priorities in patient safety and quality improvement, the perception that diagnostic errors are inevitable or that they are too difficult to address, and the lack of financial resources to address this problem (Croskerry, 2003; Graber, 2005; Graber et al., 2014; Henriksen, 2014; Singh and Sittig, 2015). These challenges make it difficult to identify, analyze, and learn from diagnostic errors in clinical practice.

Compared to diagnostic errors, other types of medical errors—including medication errors, surgical errors, and health care–acquired infections—have historically received more attention within health care organizations (Graber et al., 2014; Kanter, 2014). This is partly attributable to the lack of focus on diagnostic errors within national patient safety and quality improvement efforts. For example, AHRQ's Patient Safety Indicators and The Joint Commission's list of specific sentinel events do not focus on diagnostic errors (The Joint Commission, 2014; Schiff et al., 2005). The National Quality Forum's Serious Reportable Events include 29 endorsed events, but only one of those is closely tied to diagnostic error: "Patient death or serious injury resulting from a failure to follow up or communicate laboratory, pathology, or radiology test results" (NQF, 2011, p. 10). The neglect of diagnostic performance measures for accountability purposes means that hospitals today could meet standards for high-quality care and be rewarded through public reporting and pay-for-performance initiatives even if they have major challenges with diagnostic accuracy (Wachter, 2010).

Identifying diagnostic errors within clinical practice is critical to improving the quality of diagnosis for patients; however, measurement has become an "unavoidable obstacle to progress" (Singh, 2013, p. 789). The lack of comprehensive information on diagnostic errors within clinical practice perpetuates the belief that these errors are uncommon or unavoidable and impedes progress on reducing diagnostic errors. Improving diagnosis will likely require a concerted effort among all health care organizations and across all settings of care to better identify diagnostic errors and near misses, to learn from them, and, ultimately, to take steps to improve the diagnostic process. In addition to identifying near misses and errors, health care organizations can also benefit from evaluating factors that are contributing to improved diagnostic performance.

Given the nascent field of measurement of the diagnostic process, bottom-up experimentation will be necessary to develop approaches for monitoring the diagnostic process and identifying diagnostic errors and near misses. It is unlikely that any one specific method will be successful at identifying all diagnostic errors and near misses; some approaches may be more appropriate than others for specific organizational settings, types of diagnostic errors, or for identifying factors that contributed to these errors. It may be necessary for health care organizations to use a variety of methods to develop a better sense of their diagnostic performance (Shojania, 2010). Medical record reviews, medical malpractice claims analysis, health insurance claims analysis, and second reviews in diagnostic testing may be more pragmatic approaches for health care organizations because they leverage readily available data sources. Patient surveys may also be an important mechanism for health care organizations to consider; this is in line with the committee's recommendation to create environments in which patients and their families feel comfortable sharing their feedback and concerns about diagnostic error. It is important to note that many of these methods are just beginning to be applied to diagnostic error detection in clinical practice; very few are validated or available for widespread use in clinical practice (Bhise and Singh, 2015; Graber, 2013; Singh and Sittig, 2015).

Beyond identifying diagnostic errors and near misses, organizational learning to improve diagnostic performance and reduce diagnostic errors will require a focus on understanding where in the diagnostic process these errors occurred, the work system factors that contributed to their occurrence, what the outcomes were, and how these errors may be prevented or mitigated. Health care organizations can employ formal error analysis and other risk assessment methods to understand the work system factors that underlie these events, including analytical methods employed in human factors and ergonomics research. Once health care organizations have a better understanding of diagnostic errors within their organization, they will need to implement and evaluate interventions to prevent or mitigate these errors.

Accreditation organizations and Medicare conditions of participation should ensure that health care organizations' programs are achieving improvements in the quality and safety of diagnosis, including appropriate monitoring, careful analysis of diagnostic errors, and system changes in response to these errors and near misses.

Postmortem examinations are an important method for identifying diagnostic errors because these examinations can, in many cases, determine the cause of death and reveal discrepancies between premortem and postmortem clinical findings (Shojania et al., 2002). However, the number of postmortem examinations performed in the United States has declined substantially since the 1960s because of a range of medical, legal, social, and economic factors (Lundberg, 1998; Shojania et al., 2002).

The committee concluded that a new approach to increasing the use of postmortem examinations is warranted. The committee weighed the relative merits of increasing the number of postmortem examinations conducted throughout the United States versus a more targeted approach. The current requirements for postmortem examinations under the Medicare conditions of participation already state that postmortem examinations should be performed when there is an unusual death or a death of medical-legal and educational interest, and the committee concluded that health care organizations should continue to perform the examinations in these circumstances. In addition, the committee concluded that it is appropriate to have a limited number of highly qualified health care systems participate in conducting routine postmortem exams that produce research-quality information about the incidence and nature of diagnostic errors. To accomplish this, a subset of health care systems that reflect a broad array of different settings of care could receive funding to perform postmortem examinations in a representative sample of patient deaths.[4] This approach will likely provide better epidemiologic data and represent an advance over current selection methods for performing postmortem examinations, because clinicians do not seem to be able to predict cases in which diagnostic errors will be found (Shojania et al., 2002, 2003). The committee recognizes that the data collected from health care systems that are highly qualified to conduct routine postmortem examinations may not be representative of all systems of care. However, the committee concluded that this approach is more feasible given the financial and workforce demands of conducting postmortem examinations.

These health care organizations could also investigate how new, minimally invasive postmortem approaches compare with full-body postmor-

---

[4] Not all patients' next of kin will consent to the performance of a postmortem examination; these systems can characterize the frequency with which the request for a postmortem examination is refused and better describe the risk of response bias in results.

tem examinations. Less invasive approaches include medical imaging, laparoscopy, biopsy, histology, and cytology. Given the advances in molecular diagnostics and advanced imaging techniques, these new approaches could provide useful insights on diagnostic error and may be more acceptable options for patients' next of kin. Further understanding the benefits and limitations of minimally invasive approaches may provide critical information moving forward. If successful approaches to minimally invasive postmortem examinations are found, they could play a role in reestablishing the practice of routine postmortem investigation in medicine.

Health care organizations can also implement mechanisms that improve systematic feedback at all levels. Feedback entails informing individuals, teams, or organizations about their diagnostic performance, including their successes, near misses, and diagnostic errors. The committee received substantial input indicating that there are limited opportunities for feedback on diagnostic performance. Feedback can help clinicians assess how well they are performing in the diagnostic process, correct overconfidence, identify when remediation efforts are needed, and reduce the likelihood of repeated mistakes. Feedback on diagnostic performance can also provide opportunities for organizational learning and improvements to the work system of health care organizations. Characteristics of effective feedback mechanisms include being actionable, timely, individualized, and nonpunitive (Hysong et al., 2006). Health care organizations also need to be aware of the factors that can impede the provision of feedback, such as the fragmentation of the health care system, resistance to critical feedback from clinicians, and the lack of time for follow-up (Schiff, 2008).

There are many opportunities to provide feedback in clinical practice. Methods to monitor the diagnostic process and identify diagnostic errors and near misses can be leveraged as mechanisms to provide feedback. Feedback opportunities include disseminating postmortem examination results to clinicians who were involved in the patient's care; sharing the results of patient surveys, medical record reviews, or information gained through follow-up with the health care professionals; using patient-actors or simulated care scenarios to assess and inform health care professionals' diagnostic performance; and others. Because patients and their families have unique insights into the diagnostic process and the occurrence of diagnostic error, following up with patients and their families about their experiences and outcomes will be an important source of feedback (Schiff, 2008). Another example of feedback is RADPEER, a program developed by the American College of Radiology that allows anonymous peer review of previous image interpretations to be conducted during the interpretation of current images. Summary statistics of these reviews are made available to participating groups, and they can be used as feedback to improve individual and group practice performance (Allen and Thorwarth, 2014). Morbidity and mortality conferences, root cause analyses, departmental meetings, and WalkRounds provide additional opportunities for feedback to different groups in health care.

There is also an opportunity to improve diagnosis by engaging health care professional societies in identifying areas within their specialties to reduce diagnostic errors and improve diagnostic performance. This can facilitate improvements in diagnosis based on intrinsic motivation and professionalism rather than other incentives or disincentives. Efforts to improve diagnosis can include both improving the quality and safety of diagnosis and increasing efficiency and value by minimizing inappropriate diagnostic testing. This effort could be modeled on Choosing Wisely, which was initiated by the American Board of Internal Medicine Foundation to encourage patient and health care professional communication as a means to ensure high-quality, high-value care. The initiative invited each health care professional society to identify a list of five services (i.e., tests, treatments, procedures) that are commonly used in practice but may be unnecessary or not supported by the evidence as improving patient care. These lists were made publicly available as a way of encouraging discussions about appropriate care between patients and health care professionals. Choosing Wisely received widespread national media attention and engaged more than 50 health care professional societies (Choosing Wisely, 2014). A major lesson from the Choosing Wisely initiative was the importance of beginning with a small group of founding organizations and then expanding membership. Engaging consumer groups as the initiative progressed was also an important component. Another factor in the initiative's success was that it allowed flexibility within limits; participating health care professional societies and boards were given flexibility in identifying their "Top 5" services, but items on each list had to be evidence-based and within the purview of that particular society.

A similar effort engaging health care professional societies could focus on prioritizing diagnostic errors. Early efforts on prioritization could focus on identifying the most common diagnostic errors and "don't miss" health conditions, such as those that present the greatest likelihood for diagnostic errors and harm (Newman-Toker, 2014; Newman-Toker et al., 2013). Each organization could be asked to identify five high-priority areas to improve diagnosis. These groups could be given latitude in how they chose to identify their targets, as in Choosing Wisely. Efforts to improve diagnosis can include both improving the quality and safety of diagnosis and increasing efficiency and value, such as identifying inappropriate diagnostic testing. Another approach may be for societies to identify "low-hanging fruit," or targets that are easily remediable, as a high priority. This strategy could increase the likelihood of creating early wins that may contribute to the long-term success of this type of effort. Some groups might identify particular actions, tools, or approaches to reduce diagnostic errors with a particular diagnosis within their specialties (such as checklists, second reviews, or decision support tools).

This could also be an opportunity for health care professional societies to collaborate, especially on diagnoses that may be missed due to an inappropriate isolation of symptoms. For example, urologists, primary care clinicians, and neurologists could collaborate to make the diagnosis of normal pressure hydrocephalus (whose symptoms include frequent urination, balance problems, and memory loss) a "not to be missed" diagnosis (McDonald, 2014).

Goal 4: Develop and deploy approaches to identify, learn from, and reduce diagnostic errors and near misses in clinical practice

Recommendation 4a: Accreditation organizations and the Medicare conditions of participation should require that health care organizations have programs in place to monitor the diagnostic process and identify, learn from, and reduce diagnostic errors and near misses in a timely fashion. Proven approaches should be incorporated into updates of these requirements.

Recommendation 4b: Health care organizations should:
- Monitor the diagnostic process and identify, learn from, and reduce diagnostic errors and near misses as a component of their research, quality improvement, and patient safety programs.
- Implement procedures and practices to provide systematic feedback on diagnostic performance to individual health care professionals, care teams, and clinical and organizational leaders.

Recommendation 4c: The Department of Health and Human Services should provide funding for a designated subset of health care systems to conduct routine postmortem examinations on a representative sample of patient deaths.

Recommendation 4d: Health care professional societies should identify opportunities to improve accurate and timely diagnoses and reduce diagnostic errors in their specialties.

Establish a Work System and Culture That Supports the Diagnostic Process and Improvements in Diagnostic Performance

Testimony to the committee indicated that the work systems of many health care organizations could do a better job of supporting the diagnostic process (Gandhi, 2014; Kanter, 2014; Sarter, 2014; Schiff, 2014b). Health care organizations influence the work system in which diagnosis occurs and play a role in implementing changes to improve diagnosis and avert diagnostic errors.

The committee focused on organizational culture as well as the leadership and management of an organization as key characteristics for ensuring continuous learning and improvements to the diagnostic process. Organizational culture refers to an organization's norms of behavior and the shared basic assumptions and values that sustain those norms (Kotter, 2012; Schein, 2004). Health care organizations are responsible for developing a culture that promotes a safe place for all health care professionals to identify and learn from diagnostic errors. Organizational leaders and managers can facilitate this culture and set the priorities to achieve progress in improving diagnostic performance and reducing the occurrence of diagnostic errors.

Some aspects of culture in health care organizations, such as an emphasis on quality, safety, professionalism, and the intrinsic motivation of health care professionals, promote diagnostic performance. There are other aspects of culture that do not promote improved diagnostic performance, such as an emphasis on blame and punishment and a lack of emphasis on team-based care. A recent survey of more than 400,000 staff at 653 hospitals found that fewer than half of all surveyed staff members perceived that their organization had a nonpunitive response to error (AHRQ, 2014a). A culture that emphasizes discipline and punishment for those who make mistakes presents a significant barrier to the reporting of errors, which in turn thwarts the learning process. Cultural taboos on providing feedback to colleagues can further hinder efforts to identify and learn from diagnostic errors. To improve diagnosis, health care organizations need to develop nonpunitive cultures that promote open discussion and feedback on diagnostic performance (Gandhi, 2014; Kanter, 2014; Thomas, 2014). Organizations can support learning and continual improvement in diagnostic performance by implementing a just culture (Kanter, 2014; Khatri et al., 2009; Larson, 2002; Marx, 2001; Milstead, 2005) or by adapting the traits of high reliability organizations, which operate in high-stakes conditions but maintain high safety levels (such as those found in nuclear power and aviation industries) (Chassin and Loeb, 2011; Singh, 2014; Thomas, 2014; Weick and Sutcliffe, 2011). The involvement of supportive and committed leadership is another component of successful attempts to improve culture (Chassin, 2013; Hines et al., 2008; IOM, 2013; Kotter, 1995, 2012).

Collaboration among organizational leaders is critical to achieving a health care organization's quality goals, as well as successful change initiatives (Dixon-Woods et al., 2011; Firth-Cozens, 2004; Gandhi, 2014; Kotter, 1995; Larson, 2002; Moran and Brightman, 2000; Silow-Carroll et al., 2007). Leaders communicate the priorities of the organization, set expectations, and ensure that the rules, policies, and resources encourage and support the improvement of diagnostic performance. In many health care organizations, organizational leaders have not yet focused significant attention on improving diagnosis and reducing diagnostic errors (Gandhi, 2014; Graber, 2005; Henriksen, 2014; Wachter, 2010; Zwaan et al., 2013). However, facilitating change will require their support and involvement, and it may also include prioritizing diagnosis and supporting senior managers in implementing policies and practices that support continued learning and improved diagnostic performance, adopting a continuously learning culture, raising awareness of the quality and safety challenges related to diagnostic error, and dispelling the myth that diagnostic errors are inevitable (Leape, 2010; Wachter, 2010).

Many components of the work system are under the purview of health care organizations. Thus, organizations can implement changes that ensure a work system that supports the diagnostic process. One principle that health care organizations can apply to the design of the diagnostic work system is "error recovery," which refers to the early identification of an error so that actions can be taken to mitigate or avert negative effects resulting from the error (IOM, 2000). There are a variety of opportunities for health care organizations to improve error recovery and resiliency in the diagnostic process. For example, improved patient access to clinical notes and diagnostic testing results is one form of error recovery; this access gives patients the opportunity to identify and correct errors in their medical records that could lead to a diagnostic error, potentially before any harm results. Thoughtful use of redundancies, such as second reviews of anatomic pathology specimens and medical images, consultations, and second opinions in challenging cases or complex care environments, is also a form of error recovery that health care organizations can consider.

In addition, organizations can ensure that workforce staffing and supervision policies support human performance and address patient safety risks caused by fatigue (including decision fatigue), sleep deprivation, and sleep debt (IOM, 2009). Health care organizations can also focus on improvements in workflow design, care transitions, and settings of care that are prone to diagnostic errors (such as emergency departments and outpatient settings). Technologies that support the diagnostic process, such as clinical decision support, can also be considered.

Health care organizations can ensure that the design and characteristics of the physical environments in which diagnosis takes place support the diagnostic process. Elements of the physical environment, including layout, distractions, noise, and lighting, can have an impact on human performance and, thereby, the quality and safety of care (Carayon, 2012; Hogarth, 2010; Reiling et al., 2008). Although the impact of the physical environment on diagnostic error has not been well studied, there are indications that it may be an important contributor to diagnostic performance. For example, the emergency department has been described as a challenging environment in which to make accurate and timely diagnoses because of the presence of high-acuity illness, incomplete information, time constraints, and frequent interruptions and distractions (Croskerry and Sinclair, 2001). Cognitive performance is vulnerable to distractions and interruptions, which influence the likelihood of error. Other physical environment factors that are likely to influence the diagnostic process include the placement of health IT used in the diagnostic process, the presence of noise that interferes with clinical reasoning and communication among the diagnostic team, and the amount of space available for team members to complete tasks related to the diagnostic process.

Health care organizations can also make concerted efforts to address diagnostic challenges related to fragmentation within the broader health care system. Although improved teamwork and interoperability will help with systemic fragmentation in health care, organizations need to recognize that patients may traverse organizational boundaries, and this has the potential to contribute to diagnostic errors and failures to learn from them. It is important to develop approaches within health care organizations to identify potential vulnerabilities to fragmentation. For example, the committee heard testimony that one important area to address is strengthening communication with pathologists and radiologists to improve diagnostic test selection and result interpretation. Closed-loop reporting systems that ensure test results or specialist findings are reported back to the treating health care professional in a timely manner are one mechanism that can be used to reduce diagnostic errors (Lacson et al., 2014).

Goal 5: Establish a work system and culture that supports the diagnostic process and improvements in diagnostic performance

Recommendation 5: Health care organizations should:

- Adopt policies and practices that promote a nonpunitive culture that values open discussion and feedback on diagnostic performance.
- Design the work system in which the diagnostic process occurs to support the work and activities of patients, their families, and health care professionals and to facilitate accurate and timely diagnoses.
- Develop and implement processes to ensure effective and timely communication between diagnostic testing health care professionals and treating health care professionals across all health care delivery settings.

Develop a Reporting Environment and Medical Liability System That Facilitates Improved Diagnosis by Learning from Diagnostic Errors and Near Misses

Reporting

The committee concluded that there is a need for safe places where health care organizations and professionals can share and learn from their experiences with diagnostic errors, near misses, and adverse events. Performing analyses of these events presents the best opportunity to learn from such experiences and to implement changes to improve the diagnostic process. *To Err Is Human* (2000) recommended that reporting systems be used to collect this information. Various groups, including individual states, The Joint Commission, the Department of Veterans Affairs, and AHRQ have developed a number of reporting systems, which collect different types of information for different purposes. Characteristics of successful reporting systems include: "reporting is safe for the individuals who report, reporting leads to a constructive response, expertise and adequate financial resources are available to allow for meaningful analysis of reports, and the reporting system must be capable of disseminating information on hazards and recommendations for changes" (WHO, 2005, p. 49; see also Barach and Small, 2000). In contrast, systems that focus on punishing individuals will prevent people from reporting because they fear that their reports may be used as evidence of fault, could precipitate lawsuits, or could result in disciplinary action by state medical boards and employers (IOM, 2012; WHO, 2005). Thus, there is a need for safe environments, without the threat of legal discovery or disciplinary action, where diagnostic errors, adverse events, and near misses can be analyzed and learned from in order to improve the quality of diagnosis and prevent future diagnostic errors.

It is often difficult to create environments where diagnostic errors, near misses, and adverse events can be shared and discussed. Health care organizations and clinicians have been challenged by the limitations of the inconsistent and individual peer review processes that have been enacted by various states for the protection of information relating to adverse events and medical errors, for the external use of such information, and for the benefits they receive from reporting. In response to this challenge, *To Err Is Human* recommended that "Congress should pass legislation to extend peer review protections to data related to patient safety and quality improvement that are collected and analyzed by health care organizations for internal use or shared with others solely for purposes of improving safety and quality" (IOM, 2000, p. 10). In 2005, the Patient Safety and Quality Improvement Act (PSQIA) was passed by Congress; it provides privilege and confidentiality protections to health care organizations that share specific patient safety information with federally listed patient safety organizations (PSOs) (HHS, 2015). The PSO program, which is overseen by AHRQ, is an important national tool for increasing voluntary error reporting and analysis.

The PSO program enables public or private organizations to be listed as PSOs provided they meet certain qualifications articulated in the Patient Safety Rule (AHRQ, 2015d). If health care organizations or health care professionals join a specific PSO, they can then voluntarily send patient safety data to the PSO for analysis and feedback on how to improve care. Additionally, PSOs can send de-identified patient safety data to patient safety databases overseen by AHRQ. The intent of the program is for AHRQ to analyze the aggregated data and to publish reports based on those analyses (GAO, 2010).

Progress in implementing the PSO program has been slow, and there is very limited information about the impact of PSOs on learning about and improving the quality and safety of care. The Government Accountability Office concluded in 2010 that it was too early to evaluate the effectiveness of the program (GAO, 2010). Currently, there are more than 80 PSOs (AHRQ, 2015c), and the PSO network is active, as evidenced by the PSOs' websites, which share information with their members about strategies to mitigate patient safety events. A provision in the Affordable Care Act will likely increase the number of hospitals that join PSOs; hospitals with more than 50 beds will be required to join a PSO by January 2017 in order to contract with health plans in insurance exchanges (CFPS, 2015; CMS, 2013).

AHRQ has developed Common Formats, or generic- and event-specific forms, to encourage standardized event reporting among PSOs (AHRQ, 2015b). However, these formats are voluntary, and some organizations are implementing them variably or using legacy reporting formats

(ONC, 2014). In addition, there are no common formats for diagnostic errors (PSO Privacy Protection Center, 2014); in order to promote voluntary reporting efforts, common formats for diagnostic errors and near misses are needed. AHRQ could begin with common formats for high-priority areas such as the most frequent diagnostic errors and "don't miss" health conditions that may result in significant patient harm, such as stroke, acute myocardial infarction, and pulmonary embolism.

In 2015, AHRQ noted that no data were submitted to the network of patient safety databases for aggregation and analysis because the data have not been of sufficient quality or volume to ensure accuracy and de-identification. In addition, fewer than half of PSOs (27 of 76) signed data use agreements with AHRQ by the end of 2014; signing a user agreement is a requirement for sending data to be aggregated for analysis (AHRQ, 2015a). There are also concerns that the federal privilege protections extended by PSQIA are not shielding organizations from state reporting requirements. A recent ruling by the Kentucky Supreme Court found that information that a hospital is required to generate under state law is not protected by PSQIA, even if it is shared with a PSO.[5] This type of court decision could undermine the creation of a safe environment to share this information and prevent voluntary submissions to PSOs.

Given that the PSO program has potential to improve learning about diagnostic errors and to expedite the implementation of solutions and adoption of best practices, it is important to evaluate whether the program is meeting the statutory objectives of PSQIA, namely, that the PSO program is creating opportunities to examine and learn from medical errors, including diagnostic errors.

The committee is concerned that a number of challenges that the current program is facing may limit its ability to facilitate much-needed voluntary reporting, analysis, and learning from diagnostic errors and near misses. Because of this concern, the committee recognizes that additional federal efforts across HHS—including AHRQ—as well as the involvement of other independent entities may need to be considered in order to prioritize voluntary event reporting for diagnostic errors and near misses. For example, the IOM report *Health IT and Patient Safety: Building Safer Systems for Better Care* made a recommendation for a new entity, akin to the National Transportation Safety Board, that could investigate patient deaths, serious injuries, and potentially unsafe conditions, and report the results of these activities (IOM, 2012).

Smaller-scale or more localized efforts to encourage voluntary reporting of diagnostic errors and near misses could also be implemented. For example, at the level of a health care organization, quality and patient

---

[5] *Tibbs v. Bunnel*, Ky., 2012-SC-000603-MR (August 21, 2014).

safety committees can analyze and learn from diagnostic errors, as these activities may be protected from disclosure by state statutes.

Medical Liability

The two core functions of the medical liability system are to compensate negligently injured patients and to promote quality by encouraging clinicians and organizations to avoid medical errors. Although the medical liability environment may act as a generalized deterrent to medical errors, it is not well aligned with the promotion of high-quality, safe care. Concerns over medical liability prevent clinicians from disclosing medical errors to patients and their families despite calls from numerous groups about the ethical necessity of full disclosure and a requirement for The Joint Commission accreditation (Hendrich et al., 2014; Sage et al., 2014). In spite of this, clinicians often struggle to fulfill this responsibility: There is limited guidance for clinicians concerning how to disclose this information effectively; a number of factors, including embarrassment, inexperience, lack of confidence, and mixed messages from risk managers and health care organizations, can discourage clinicians from making disclosures to patients and their families (Gallagher et al., 2007, 2013; The Joint Commission, 2005).

The current tort-based system for resolving medical liability disputes sets up barriers to improvements in quality and patient safety and stifles continuous learning. Medical malpractice reform could be designed to permit patients and health care professionals to become allies in trying to make health care safer by encouraging transparency with regard to errors. Such an approach would allow patients to be promptly and fairly compensated for any injuries that were avoidable, while turning errors into lessons to improve subsequent performance (AHRQ, 2014b; Berenson, 2005; Kachalia and Mello, 2011).

Diagnostic errors are a leading type of malpractice claim, and these claims are more likely to be associated with patient deaths than other types of medical errors (Tehrani et al., 2013). Reforming the medical liability system, therefore, has the potential to improve learning from diagnostic errors and increase the disclosure of diagnostic errors to patients and their families as well as to lead to fairer treatment in the medical injury resolution processes. There have been many calls for changes to the medical liability system. Traditional mechanisms to reform the liability system—such as imposing barriers to bringing lawsuits, limiting compensation, and changing the way that damage awards are paid—have not contributed to improvements in either compensating negligently injured patients or deterring unsafe care (Mello et al., 2014). Thus, the committee concluded that stakeholders need to consider alternative approaches to improving the legal environment and promoting learning from diagnostic errors. Similarly, *To Err Is Human* concluded that alternative approaches to the resolution of medical injuries could resolve the incentive to hide medical injuries, and in 2002, the IOM proposed state-level demonstration projects to explore alternative approaches to the current liability system that are patient-centered and focused on patient safety (IOM, 2000, 2002).

Although enthusiasm for alternative approaches to the current medical liability system is growing, in general progress has been slow, especially toward more fundamental changes to the medical liability system. Thus, the committee took both a pragmatic and an aspirational approach to considering changes to medical liability that would promote the improved disclosure of diagnostic errors as well as opportunities to learn from these errors. A number of alternative approaches to the current medical liability system were evaluated, and the committee concluded that the most promising approaches include communication and resolution programs (CRPs), the use of evidence-based clinical practice guidelines as safe harbors, and administrative health courts. CRPs represent a more pragmatic approach in that they are the more likely to be implemented in the current medical liability climate, and they have a strong focus on improving patient safety as well as reducing litigation. States, in collaboration with other stakeholders, should encourage the adoption of CRPs with legal protections for disclosures and apologies under state laws. Safe harbors for adherence to evidence-based clinical practice guidelines and administrative health courts are challenging in regard to implementation, and more information is needed about their impact on improving diagnosis. Thus, further demonstrations of these two approaches are warranted.

CRPs are principled comprehensive patient safety programs in which health care professionals and organizations openly discuss adverse outcomes with patients and proactively seek resolution while promoting patient-centeredness, learning, and quality improvement. CRPs rely on creating transparent health care cultures in which the early reporting of adverse events is the norm and is coupled with systems-based event analysis that is designed to understand the root causes of adverse events and to develop plans for preventing recurrences. Improved transparency surrounding diagnostic errors can help foster an improved culture of reporting, which can in turn promote learning about and identification of interventions to improve the safety and quality of diagnosis (Mello et al., 2014). Although CRPs do not require legislative changes, CRP adoption could be facilitated through changes to state laws, such as laws protecting disclosures and apologies (Sage et al., 2014). In addition, a national collaborative of CRPs could help accelerate the spread of CRPs and widely disseminate learning from these programs.

Safe harbors for following evidence-based clinical guidelines have the potential to raise the quality of health care by creating an incentive (liability protection) for clinicians to follow evidence-based clinical practice guidelines. Unlike the case with other approaches to improving the medical liability environment, input to the committee suggested that safe harbors would offer direct opportunities to improve diagnosis (Kachalia, 2014). However, there are few clinical practice guidelines available for diagnosis, and implementing safe harbors for adherence to these guidelines is administratively complex.

Administrative health courts have been proposed as a way to provide injured patients with expedited compensation decisions for certain types of medical errors and to promote the disclosure of medical errors (such as diagnostic errors). Administrative health courts provide a nonjudicial process of handling medical injuries in which cases are filed through an administrative process. The goal in using these courts is to quickly and equitably compensate patients who have experienced avoidable injuries without requiring the patients to prove negligence in an adversarial proceeding (Berenson, 2005). The establishment of these courts would represent a fundamental change that would promote a more open environment for identifying, studying, and learning from errors. However, implementing administrative health courts would pose a number of challenges, including the need for legislative action, the courts' operational complexity, and resistance from stakeholders who are strongly committed to preserving the current tort-based system.

Risk Management

Professional liability insurance carriers and health care organizations that participate in a captive insurance program or other self-insurance arrangement have a vested interest in improving diagnosis. Many of these carriers and organizations are actively exploring opportunities to improve diagnosis and reduce diagnostic errors. Given their expertise in understanding the contributors to diagnostic errors, they bring an important perspective to efforts to improve diagnosis, both those focused on individual health care professionals and those focused on the work system components that may contribute to diagnostic errors. The expertise of health professional liability insurance carriers needs to be leveraged to improve the diagnostic process. Improved collaboration between health professional liability insurance carriers and health care professionals and organizations could help to identify resources, prioritize areas of concern, and devise interventions. Collaboration among health care professional educators and professional liability insurance carriers could also be helpful in developing interventions for trainees.

Goal 6: Develop a reporting environment and medical liability system that facilitates improved diagnosis by learning from diagnostic errors and near misses

Recommendation 6a: The Agency for Healthcare Research and Quality (AHRQ) or other appropriate agencies or independent entities should encourage and facilitate the voluntary reporting of diagnostic errors and near misses.

Recommendation 6b: AHRQ should evaluate the effectiveness of patient safety organizations (PSOs) as a major mechanism for voluntary reporting and learning from these events and modify the PSO Common Formats for reporting of patient safety events to include diagnostic errors and near misses.

Recommendation 6c: States, in collaboration with other stakeholders (health care organizations, professional liability insurance carriers, state and federal policy makers, patient advocacy groups, and medical malpractice plaintiff and defense attorneys), should promote a legal environment that facilitates the timely identification, disclosure, and learning from diagnostic errors. Specifically, they should:
- Encourage the adoption of communication and resolution programs with legal protections for disclosures and apologies under state laws.
- Conduct demonstration projects of alternative approaches to the resolution of medical injuries, including administrative health courts and safe harbors for adherence to evidence-based clinical practice guidelines.

Recommendation 6d: Professional liability insurance carriers and captive insurers should collaborate with health care professionals on opportunities to improve diagnostic performance through education, training, and practice improvement approaches and increase participation in such programs.

Design a Payment and Care Delivery Environment That Supports the Diagnostic Process

Fee-for-service (FFS) payment, the predominant form of payment for health care services in the United States, pays health care professionals for each service they provide. FFS payment has long been recognized for its inability to incentivize well-coordinated, high-quality, and efficient health care (Council of Economic Advisors, 2009; IOM, 2001, 2013; National Commission on Physician Payment Reform, 2013). There is relatively little information about the impact of payment on the diagnostic process. However, the committee concluded that it is likely to have an impact, and several payment experts who provided input to the committee helped elaborate on some of the likely consequences (Miller, 2014; Rosenthal, 2014; Wennberg, 2014).

In general, FFS payment may not incentivize a high-quality, efficient diagnostic process because the more services the diagnostic process takes, the more remuneration will result. There is no disincentive for ordering unnecessary diagnostic testing that could lead to false positive results and diagnostic errors (Miller, 2014; Wennberg, 2014). There is also a financial incentive to provide treatment to patients rather than determining that a patient does not have a health problem; thus, inappropriate diagnoses are better compensated than determining that a patient does not have a health problem. Likewise, accuracy in the diagnostic process is not incentivized by FFS payment: Clinicians who interpret diagnostic tests or provide a diagnosis during a patient visit receive payment regardless of whether the work was done adequately to support accurate interpretation and diagnosis and regardless of whether the interpretations and diagnoses were accurate (Miller, 2014).

Given the importance of team-based care in the diagnostic process, the lack of financial incentives in FFS payment to coordinate care can contribute to challenges in diagnosis and diagnostic errors, particularly delays in diagnosis (Allen and Thorwarth, 2014; Kroft, 2014; Miller, 2014; Rosenthal, 2014). FFS Medicare and most commercial payers do not pay for a clinician's time spent contacting other clinicians by phone or e-mail to facilitate the diagnostic process, for example, by helping determine the appropriate diagnostic testing procedures for a patient. In addition, clinicians are not reimbursed for proactive outreach to patients to obtain diagnostic testing, schedule visits with specialists, or make follow-up appointments (Miller, 2014). To improve teamwork and care coordination in the diagnostic process, new current procedural terminology (CPT) codes can be developed and compensated, such as codes for communication among treating clinicians, pathologists, and radiologists about diagnostic testing ordering, interpretation, and the subsequent decision making. These codes could be modeled on existing Medicare codes that compensate clinicians' time for coordination and planning activities, such as the codes for radiation therapy planning, post-discharge transitional care coordination, and complex chronic care coordination (ASTRO, 2014; Bendix, 2013; CMS, 2014b; Edwards and Landon, 2014).

The Medicare physician fee schedule sets payment rates based on relative value units that are meant to reflect the level of time, effort, skill, and stress associated with providing each service (MedPAC, 2014). Fee schedule services can include evaluation and management services ("E&M services," such as office, inpatient, or emergency department visits), diagnostic testing, and other procedures. For all medical specialties, there are well-documented fee schedule distortions that result in more generous payments (in relation to the costs of production) for procedures and also for diagnostic testing interpretations compared to E&M services (Berenson, 2010; National Commission on Physician Payment Reform, 2013). These distortions have coincided with a large growth in diagnostic testing in health care: For example, the percent of patients presenting to the emergency department with dizziness who underwent computed tomography scans rose from 9 percent in 1995 to 40 percent in 2013, although there has been no increase in diagnoses of stroke or other neurologic diseases (Iglehart, 2009; Newman-Toker et al., 2013).

The lower relative value afforded to E&M services versus procedure-oriented care is an obstacle to improved diagnostic performance. E&M services reflect the cognitive expertise and skills that all clinicians have and use in the diagnostic process, and the distortions may be diverting attention and time from important tasks in the diagnostic process, such as performing a patient's clinical history and interview, conducting a physical exam, and thoughtful decision making in the diagnostic process. Realigning relative value fees to better compensate clinicians for the cognitive work in the diagnostic process has the potential to improve accuracy in diagnosis while reducing the incentives that drive inappropriate utilization of diagnostic testing in the diagnostic process.

E&M payment policies and documentation guidelines are also misaligned with the goal of accurate and timely diagnosis. E&M payments penalize clinicians for spending extra time on the diagnostic process for individual patients. There are different levels of E&M visits based on time and complexity, and clinicians receive better compensation if they see more patients with shorter appointment lengths. For example, in Medicare if a clinician spends 20 minutes instead of 15 minutes with a patient billed as a level 3 E&M visit, the clinician will receive 25 percent less revenue per hour; if a clinician spends 25 minutes for a level 4 E&M visit instead of 15 minutes for a level 3 visit, the clinician will receive 11 percent less revenue per hour (Miller, 2014). Time pressures in clinical visits can contribute to challenges in clinical reasoning and to the occurrence of errors (Durning, 2014; Evans and Kim, 2006; Kostis et al., 2007; Sarkar et al., 2012, 2014; Schiff et al., 2009; Singh et al., 2013). Documentation guidelines for E&M services were created to ensure that the services performed were consistent with the insurance coverage; to validate specific information, such as the site of service, the appropriateness of the care, and the accuracy of the reported information; and to prevent fraud and abuse (Berenson, 1999; CMS, 2014a). Documentation guidelines also specify the extent of a patient's clinical history and physical exam and the complexity of the medical decision making involved in the E&M visit (Berenson et al., 2011; HHS, 2010). There are a number of criticisms of the documentation guidelines. The primary criticism is that the level of detail required is onerous, often irrelevant to patient care, and shifts the purpose of the medical record toward billing rather than on facilitating clinical reasoning (Berenson et al., 2011; Brett, 1998; Kassirer and Angell, 1998; Kuhn et al., 2015; Schiff and Bates, 2010).

The documentation guidelines have become an even greater concern with the broad implementation of EHRs because EHR design emphasizes fulfilling documentation and legal requirements rather than facilitating the diagnostic process (Berenson et al., 2011; Schiff and Bates, 2010). The orientation of EHRs to documentation, their overreliance on templates, and their copy and paste functionalities have resulted in "EHR-generated data dumps, including repetitive documentation of elements of patients' histories and physical examinations, that merely result in electronic versions of clinically cumbersome, uninformative patient records" (Berenson et al., 2011, p. 1894). Generating documentation to support E&M coding (or assigning higher levels of E&M coding than warranted—known as "upcoding") can result in inaccuracies in the patient's EHR that can contribute to diagnostic errors.

A number of payment and care delivery reforms to counter the limitations of the FFS payment system are now actively being considered, implemented, and evaluated. These include capitation/global payments, shared savings, bundled episodes of care, accountable care organizations, patient-centered medical homes, and pay for performance (which in Medicare is labeled "value-based purchasing"). The Centers for Medicare & Medicaid Services (CMS) recently announced that it plans "to have 30 percent of Medicare fee-for-service payments tied to quality or value through alternative payment models by the end of 2016, and 50 percent of payments by the end of 2018" (Burwell, 2015). Legislation that repealed the sustainable growth rate also continues down the path toward alternative payment models, particularly for the payment of Medicare clinicians.[6] There is very limited evidence concerning the impact of payment and delivery models on the diagnostic process and the accuracy of diagnosis, and this represents a fundamental research need. Assessing the impact of payment and care delivery models, including FFS, on the diagnostic process, diagnostic errors, and learning are critical areas of focus as these models are evaluated.

The committee asked for input from payment and delivery experts

---

[6] Medicare Access and CHIP Reauthorization Act of 2015. P.L. 114-10. (April 16, 2015).

about the potential effects of new models on diagnosis and diagnostic error. Rosenthal (2014) suggested that global payment and meaningful use incentives have the potential to improve diagnosis by promoting the adoption of diagnostic test and referral tracking systems that better connect health care professionals throughout the continuum of care. Miller (2014) suggested that the development of measures for diagnostic accuracy could be used to also provide feedback and reward clinicians for diagnostic accuracy. Wennberg (2014) suggested that population-based payment models, including capitation and global budgets, have the greatest potential to reduce diagnostic errors. While new payment models have the potential to reduce diagnostic errors, these models may also create incentives for clinicians and health care organizations that could reduce use of appropriate testing and clinician services (e.g., specialty consultations) that may inadvertently lead to greater diagnostic errors. Thus, research in this area will be helpful in assessing the impact of payment and care delivery models on diagnosis.

Even when alternate payment and care delivery approaches to FFS are employed, they are often based on or influenced by existing coding and payment rules (Berenson et al., 2011). For example, bundled payments are combinations of current codes. Thus, the current distortions in the fee schedule and other volume-based payment approaches, such as diagnosis-related group coding, will remain a dominant component of payment and care delivery models in the near future and need to be addressed.

Goal 7: Design a payment and care delivery environment that supports the diagnostic process

Recommendation 7a: As long as fee schedules remain a predominant mechanism for determining clinician payment, the Centers for Medicare & Medicaid Services (CMS) and other payers should:
- **Create current procedural terminology codes and provide coverage for additional evaluation and management activities not currently coded or covered, including time spent by pathologists, radiologists, and other clinicians in advising ordering clinicians on the selection, use, and interpretation of diagnostic testing for specific patients.**
- **Reorient relative value fees to more appropriately value the time spent with patients in evaluation and management activities.**
- **Modify documentation guidelines for evaluation and management services to improve the accuracy of information in**

the electronic health record and to support decision making in the diagnostic process.

Recommendation 7b: CMS and other payers should assess the impact of payment and care delivery models on the diagnostic process, the occurrence of diagnostic errors, and learning from these errors.

Provide Dedicated Funding for Research on the Diagnostic Process and Diagnostic Errors

The diagnostic process and the challenge of diagnostic errors have been neglected within the national health care research agenda (Berenson et al., 2014; Wachter, 2010; Zwaan et al., 2013). Input provided to the committee concluded that "although correct treatment presumes a correct diagnosis, federal resources devoted to diagnostic research are vastly eclipsed by those devoted to treatment" (Newman-Toker, 2014, p. 12). There are a number of reasons why diagnosis and diagnostic errors may be underrepresented in current research activities, including a lack of awareness or the perceived inevitability of the problem, attitudes and a culture that encourage inaction and tolerance of errors, poorly understood characteristics of the diagnostic and clinical reasoning processes, and the lack of financial and other resources needed to address the problem (Berenson et al., 2014; Croskerry, 2012).

A major barrier to research on diagnosis and diagnostic error is the current disease-focused approach to medical research funding. For example, the structure and funding mechanisms of the National Institutes of Health (NIH) are often organized by disease or organ systems, which facilitates the study of these specific areas but impedes research efforts that seek to provide a more comprehensive understanding of diagnosis as a distinct research area. Newman-Toker (2014, p. 12) asserted that diagnostic research "invariably falls between rather than within individual Institute missions." As such, the topic of diagnosis, which cuts across various diseases and body parts, is not centralized within the NIH research portfolio, and available research funding for diagnosis often targets specific diseases but not diagnosis as a whole or the diagnosis of several diseases with similar presentations. Diagnosis and diagnostic error are not a focus of federal health services' research efforts, with the exception of two special emphasis notices from AHRQ for diagnostic error in 2007 and 2013, as well as 2015 grant opportunities (AHRQ, 2007, 2013, 2015e,f). AHRQ posted an R01 grant opportunity for "understanding and improving diagnostic safety in ambulatory care: incidence and contributing factors" (AHRQ, 2015e) and an R18 grant opportunity for identifying strategies and interventions to improve diagnostic safety in ambulatory care (AHRQ, 2015f).

Although these initial steps are promising, the committee concluded that there is an urgent need for dedicated, coordinated federal funding for research on diagnosis and diagnostic error. Given the potential for federal research for diagnosis and diagnostic error to fall between institutional missions, federal agencies need to collaborate to develop a national research agenda that addresses diagnosis and diagnostic error by 2016. Zwaan and colleagues (2013) outlined potential research opportunities that were broadly classified into three categories: the epidemiology of diagnostic errors, the causes of diagnostic error, and error prevention strategies. The Society to Improve Diagnosis in Medicine has formed a research committee to bring together multidisciplinary perspectives to advance a research agenda derived from critical gaps in the evidence base. Building on this work, the committee identified additional areas of research that could help shape a national research agenda on diagnosis and diagnostic error (see Chapter 8).

The federal government should commit dedicated funding to implementing this research agenda. Because federal investments in biomedical and health services research are declining (Moses et al., 2015), the committee recognizes that funding for diagnosis and diagnostic error will likely draw federal resources away from other important priorities. However, given the consistent lack of resources for research on diagnosis and the potential for diagnostic errors to contribute significant patient harm, the committee concluded that this is necessary for broader improvements to the quality and safety of health care. In addition, improving diagnosis could also lead to potential cost savings by preventing diagnostic errors, inappropriate treatment, and related adverse events.

In addition to federal-level research on diagnosis and diagnostic errors, there is an important role for public–private collaboration and coordination among the federal government, foundations, industry, and other organizations. Collaborative funding efforts help extend the existing financial resources and reduce duplications in research efforts. Interested parties can unite around mutual interests and spearhead progress toward a specific cause. Foundations and industry can make important contributions—financially and within their areas of expertise—to the field of diagnosis and diagnostic errors that can enhance the medical community's knowledge in this area. Various types of collaborative models that have been employed to share information, resources, and capabilities have been described in the literature (Altshuler et al., 2010; Portilla and Alving, 2010).

Goal 8: Provide dedicated funding for research on the diagnostic process and diagnostic errors

Recommendation 8a: Federal agencies, including the Department of Health and Human Services, the Department of Veterans Affairs, and the Department of Defense, should:
- **Develop a coordinated research agenda on the diagnostic process and diagnostic errors by the end of 2016.**
- **Commit dedicated funding to implementing this research agenda.**

Recommendation 8b: The federal government should pursue and encourage opportunities for public–private partnerships among a broad range of stakeholders, such as the Patient-Centered Outcomes Research Institute, foundations, the diagnostic testing and health information technology industries, health care organizations, and professional liability insurers to support research on the diagnostic process and diagnostic errors.

REFERENCES

Adler-Milstein, J. 2015. America's health IT transformation: Translating the promise of electronic health records into better care. Paper presented at U.S. Senate Committee on Health, Education, Labor and Pensions, March 17. www.help.senate.gov/imo/media/doc/Adler-Milstein.pdf (accessed June 5, 2015).

Adler-Milstein, J., and A. Jha. 2014. Health information exchange among U.S. hospitals: Who's in, who's out and why? *Healthcare* 2(1):26–32.

Adler-Milstein, J., C. M. DesRoches, M. F. Furukawa, C. Worzala, D. Charles, P. Kralovec, S. Stalley, and A. K. Jha. 2014. More than half of U.S. hospitals have at least a basic EHR, but stage 2 criteria remain challenging for most. *Health Affairs (Millwood)* 33(9):1664–1671.

AHIMA (American Health Information Management Association). 2014. Appropriate use of the copy and paste functionality in electronic health records. www.ahima.org/topics/ehr (accessed March 27, 2015).

AHRQ (Agency for Healthcare Research and Quality). 2007. Special emphasis notice (SEN): AHRQ announces interest in research on diagnostic errors in ambulatory care settings. http://grants.nih.gov/grants/guide/notice-files/NOT-HS-08-002.html (accessed May 5, 2015).

AHRQ. 2013. AHRQ announces interest in research to improve diagnostic performance in ambulatory care settings. http://grants.nih.gov/grants/guide/notice-files/NOT-HS-13-009.html (accessed February 4, 2015).

AHRQ. 2014a. Hospital survey on patient safety culture: 2014 user comparative database report: Chapter 5. Overall results. www.ahrq.gov/professionals/quality-patient-safety/patientsafetyculture/hospital/2014/hosp14ch5.html (accessed February 25, 2014).

AHRQ. 2014b. Medical Liability Reform & Patient Safety Initiative. www.ahrq.gov/professionals/quality-patient-safety/patient-safety-resources/resources/liability (accessed April 9, 2015).

AHRQ. 2014c. Patient and family advisory councils. https://cahps.ahrq.gov/quality-improvement/improvement-guide/browse-interventions/Customer-Service/Listening-Posts/Advisory-Councils.html (accessed May 26, 2015).

AHRQ. 2015a. Agency for Healthcare Research and Quality: Justification of estimates for appropriations committees. www.ahrq.gov/sites/default/files/wysiwyg/cpi/about/mission/budget/2016/cj2016.pdf (accessed May 3, 2015).

AHRQ. 2015b. Common formats. www.pso.ahrq.gov/common (accessed March 28, 2015).

AHRQ. 2015c. Federally-listed PSOs. www.pso.ahrq.gov/listed (accessed May 3, 2015).

AHRQ. 2015d. Patient Safety Organization (PSO) Program: Frequently asked questions. www.pso.ahrq.gov/faq#WhatisaPSO (accessed May 3, 2015).

AHRQ. 2015e. Understanding and improving diagnostic safety in ambulatory care: Incidence and contributing factors (R01). http://grants.nih.gov/grants/guide/pa-files/PA-15-180.html (accessed May 3, 2015).

AHRQ. 2015f. Understanding and improving diagnostic safety in ambulatory care: Strategies and interventions (R18). http://grants.nih.gov/grants/guide/pa-files/PA-15-179.html (accessed May 3, 2015).

Allen, B. and W. T. Thorworth. 2014. Input submitted to the Committee on Diagnostic Error in Health Care, November 5 and December 29, 2014, Washington, DC.

Altshuler, J. S., E. Balogh, A. D. Barker, S. L. Eck, S. H. Friend, G. S. Ginsburg, R. S. Herbst, S. J. Nass, C. M. Streeter, and J. A. Wagner. 2010. Opening up to precompetitive collaboration. *Science Translational Medicine* 2(52):52cm26.

ASTRO (American Society for Radiation Oncology). 2014. Basics of RO coding. www.astro.org/Practice-Management/Reimbursement/Basics-of-RO-Coding.aspx (accessed March 26, 2015).

Baker, D. P., R. Day, and E. Salas. 2006. Teamwork as an essential component of high-reliability organizations. *Health Services Research* 41(4p2):1576–1598.

Barach, P., and S. D. Small. 2000. Reporting and preventing medical mishaps: Lessons from non-medical near miss reporting systems. *BMJ* 320(7237):759–763.

Basch, P. 2014. ONC's 10-year roadmap towards interoperability requires changes to the meaningful use program. http://healthaffairs.org/blog/2014/11/03/oncs-10-year-roadmap-towards-interoperability-requires-changes-to-the-meaningful-use-program (accessed March 27, 2015).

Bell, S., M. Anselmo, J. Walker, and T. Delbanco. 2014. Information on OpenNotes. Input submitted to the Committee on Diagnostic Error in Health Care, December 2, 2014, Washington, DC.

Bendix, J. 2013. Making sense of the new transitional care codes. http://medicaleconomics.modernmedicine.com/medical-economics/news/user-defined-tags/99495/making-sense-new-transitional-care-codes?page=full (accessed March 26, 2015).

Berenson, R. A. 1999. Evaluation and management guidelines. *New England Journal of Medicine* 340(11):889; author reply 890–891.

Berenson, R. A. 2005. Malpractice makes perfect. *The New Republic*, October 10. www.newrepublic.com/article/health-care-malpractice-bush-frist (accessed May 26, 2015).

Berenson, R. A. 2010. Out of whack: Pricing distortions in the Medicare physician fee schedule. *Expert Voices*, September. www.nihcm.org/pdf/NIHCM-EV-Berenson_FINAL.pdf (accessed June 8, 2015).

Berenson, R. A., P. Basch, and A. Sussex. 2011. Revisiting E&M visit guidelines—A missing piece of payment reform. *New England Journal of Medicine* 364(20):1892–1895.

Berenson, R. A., D. K. Upadhyay, and D. R. Kaye. 2014. *Placing diagnosis errors on the policy agenda*. Washington, DC: Urban Institute. www.urban.org/research/publication/placing-diagnosis-errors-policy-agenda (accessed June 7, 2015).

Berner, E. S., and M. L. Graber. 2008. Overconfidence as a cause of diagnostic error in medicine. *American Journal of Medicine* 121(5):S2–S23.

Bhise, V., and H. Singh. 2015. Measuring diagnostic safety of inpatients: Time to set sail in uncharted waters. *Diagnosis* 2(1):1–2.

Brett, A. S. 1998. New guidelines for coding physicians' services—A step backward. *New England Journal of Medicine* 339(23):1705–1708.

Bruno, M. A., J. M. Petscavage-Thomas, M. J. Mohr, S. K. Bell, and S. D. Brown. 2014. The "open letter": Radiologists' reports in the era of patient web portals. *Journal of the American College of Radiology* 11(9):863–867.

Brush, J. E. 2014. Forming good habits to decrease diagnostic error: A case for likelihood ratios. Input submitted to the Committee on Diagnostic Error in Health Care, October 21, 2014, Washington, DC.

Burwell, S. M. 2015. Setting value-based payment goals—HHS efforts to improve U.S. health care. *New England Journal of Medicine* 372(10):897–899.

Carayon, P. 2012. The physical environment in health care. In C. J. Alvarado (ed.), *Handbook of human factors and ergonomics in health care and patient safety* (pp. 215–234). Boca Raton, FL: Taylor & Francis Group.

Carayon, P., H. Faye, A. S. Hundt, B.–T. Karsh, and T. Wetterneck, T. 2011. Patient safety and proactive risk assessment. In Y. Yuehwern (ed.), *Handbook of Healthcare Delivery Systems* (pp. 12–1–12–15.). Boca Raton, FL: Taylor & Francis.

CFPS (Center for Patient Safety). 2015. National health reform provisions and PSOs. www.centerforpatientsafety.org/nationalhealthreformprovisionsandpsos (accessed November 7, 2015).

Chassin, M. R. 2013. Improving the quality of health care: What's taking so long? *Health Affairs (Millwood)* 32(10):1761–1765.

Chassin, M. R., and J. M. Loeb. 2011. The ongoing quality improvement journey: Next stop, high reliability. *Health Affairs (Millwood)* 30(4):559–568.

CHCF (California HealthCare Foundation). 2014. Ten years in: Charting the progress of health information exchange in the U.S. www.chcf.org/~/media/MEDIA%20LIBRARY%20Files/PDF/T/PDF%20TenYearsProgressHIE.pdf (accessed February 9, 2015).

Choosing Wisely. 2014. Lists. www.choosingwisely.org/doctor-patient-lists (accessed May 26, 2015).

CMS (Centers for Medicare & Medicaid Services). 2013. Patient Protection and Affordable Care Act; HHS Notice of Benefit and Payment Parameters for 2015. *Federal Register.* www.federalregister.gov/articles/2013/12/02/2013-28610/patient-protection-and-affordable-care-act-hhs-notice-of-benefit-and-payment-parameters-for-2015 (accessed November 12, 2015).

CMS. 2014a. *Evaluation and management services guide: Official CMS information for Medicare fee-for-service providers.* Washington, DC: CMS.

CMS. 2014b. Policy and payment changes to the Medicare physician fee schedule for 2015. www.cms.gov/newsroom/mediareleasedatabase/fact-sheets/2014-Fact-sheets-items/2014-10-31-7.html (accessed March 26, 2015).

Council of Economic Advisors. 2009. *The economic case for health care reform.* www.whitehouse.gov/assets/documents/CEA_Health_Care_Report.pdf (accessed March 17, 2015).

CRICO. 2014. Analysis of Diagnosis-Related Medical Malpractice Claims. Input submitted to the Committee on Diagnostic Error in Health Care, August 4, 2014, Washington, DC.

Croskerry, P. 2003. The importance of cognitive errors in diagnosis and strategies to minimize them. *Academic Medicine* 78(8):775–780.

Croskerry, P. 2012. Perspectives on diagnostic failure and patient safety. *Healthcare Quarterly* 15(Special issue):50–56.

Croskerry, P., and D. Sinclair. 2001. Emergency medicine: A practice prone to error. *Canadian Journal of Emergency Medicine* 3(4):271–276.

Dehling, T., F. Gao, S. Schneider, and A. Sunyaev. 2015. Exploring the far side of mobile health: Information security and privacy of mobile health apps on iOS and Android. *JMIR mHealth and uHealth* 3(1):e8.

Delbanco, T., J. Walker, J. D. Darer, J. G. Elmore, H. J. Feldman, S. G. Leveille, J. D. Ralston, S. E. Ross, E. Vodicka, and V. D. Weber. 2010. Open notes: doctors and patients signing on. *Annals of Internal Medicine* 153(2):121–125.

Delbanco, T., J. Walker, S. K. Bell, J. D. Darer, J. G. Elmore, N. Farag, H. J. Feldman, R. Mejilla, L. Ngo, J. D. Ralston, S. E. Ross, N. Trivedi, E. Vodicka, and S. G. Leveille. 2012. Inviting patients to read their doctors' notes: A quasi-experimental study and a look ahead. *Annals of Internal Medicine* 157(7):461–470.

Dhaliwal, G. 2014. Blueprint for diagnostic excellence. Presentation to the Committee on Diagnostic Error in Health Care, November 21, 2014, Washington, DC.

Dingley, C., K. Daugherty, M. K. Derieg, and R. Persing. 2008. Improving patient safety through provider communication strategy enhancements. In *Advances in Patient Safety: New Directions and Alternative Approaches (Vol. 3: Performance and Tools)*. Rockville, MD: Agency for Healthcare Research and Quality. www.ahrq.gov/professionals/quality-patient-safety/patient-safety-resources/resources/advances-in-patient-safety-2/vol3/Advances-Dingley_14.pdf (accessed June 11, 2015).

Dixon-Woods, M., C. Bosk, E. Aveling, C. Goeschel, and P. Pronovost. 2011. Explaining Michigan: Developing an ex-post theory of a quality improvement program. *Milbank Quarterly* 89(2):167–205.

Durning, S. J. 2014. Submitted input. Input submitted to the Committee on Diagnostic Error in Health Care, October 24, 2014, Washington, DC.

Edwards, S. T., and B. E. Landon. 2014. Medicare's chronic care management payment—Payment reform for primary care. *New England Journal of Medicine* 371(22):2049–2051.

El-Kareh, R., O. Hasan, and G. Schiff. 2013. Use of health information technology to reduce diagnostic error. *BMJ Quality and Safety* 22(Suppl 2):ii40–ii44.

Epner, P. 2014. An Overview of Diagnostic Error in Medicine. Presentation to the Committee on Diagnostic Error in Health Care, April 28, 2014, Washington, DC.

Epner, P. 2015. Written input. Input submitted to the Committee on Diagnostic Error in Health Care, January 13, 2015, Washington, DC.

Etchegaray, J. M., M. J. Ottosen, L. Burress, W. M. Sage, S. K. Bell, T. H. Gallagher, and E. J. Thomas. 2014. Structuring patient and family involvement in medical error event disclosure and analysis. *Health Affairs (Millwood)* 33(1):46–52.

Eva, K. W., and G. R. Norman. 2005. Heuristics and biases—A biased perspective on clinical reasoning. *Medical Education* 39(9):870–872.

Evans, W. N., and B. Kim. 2006. Patient outcomes when hospitals experience a surge in admissions. *Journal of Health Economics* 25(2):365–388.

Firth-Cozens, J. 2004. Organisational trust: The keystone to patient safety. *Quality & Safety in Health Care* 13(1):56–61.

Furukawa, M. F., J. King, V. Patel, C. J. Hsiao, J. Adler-Milstein, and A. K. Jha. 2014. Despite substantial progress in EHR adoption, health information exchange and patient engagement remain low in office settings. *Health Affairs (Millwood)* 33(9):1672–1679.

Gallagher, T., C. Denham, L. Leape, G. Amori, and W. Levinson. 2007. Disclosing unanticipated outcomes to patients: The art and practice. *Journal of Patient Safety* 3:158–165.

Gallagher, T. H., M. M. Mello, W. Levinson, M. K. Wynia, A. K. Sachdeva, L. Snyder Sulmasy, R. D. Truog, J. Conway, K. Mazor, A. Lembitz, S. K. Bell, L. Sokol-Hessner, J. Shapiro, A.-L. Puopolo, and R. Arnold. 2013. Talking with patients about other clinicians' errors. *New England Journal of Medicine* 369(18):1752–1757.

Gandhi, T. 2014. Focus on diagnostic errors: understanding and prevention. Presentation to the Committee on Diagnostic Error in Health Care, August 7, 2014, Washington, DC.

GAO (Government Accountability Office). 2010. *Patient Safety Act: HHS is in the process of implementing the act, so its effectiveness cannot yet be evaluated.* GAO 10-281. Washington, DC: Government Accountability Office.

Gertler, S. A., Z. Coralic, A. Lopez, J. C. Stein, and U. Sarkar. 2014. Root cause analysis of ambulatory adverse drug events that present to the emergency department. *Journal of Patient Safety.* February 27 [Epub ahead of print].

Gigerenzer, G. 2000. *Adaptive thinking: Rationality in the real world.* New York: Oxford University Press.

Gigerenzer, G., and D. G. Goldstein. 1996. Reasoning the fast and frugal way: Models of bounded rationality. *Psychology Review* 103:650–669.

Goodman, K. W., E. S. Berner, M. A. Dente, B. Kaplan, R. Koppel, D. Rucker, D. Z. Sands, and P. Winkelstein. 2011. Challenges in ethics, safety, best practices, and oversight regarding HIT vendors, their customers, and patients: A report of an AMIA special task force. *Journal of the American Medical Informatics Association* 18(1):77–81.

Govern, P. 2013. Diagnostic management efforts thrive on teamwork. http://news.vanderbilt.edu/2013/03/diagnostic-management-efforts-thrive-on-teamwork (accessed May 26, 2015).

Graber, M. L. 2005. Diagnostic errors in medicine: A case of neglect. *Joint Commission Journal on Quality and Patient Safety* 31(2):106–113.

Graber, M. L. 2013. The incidence of diagnostic error in medicine. *BMJ Quality and Safety* 22(Suppl 2):ii21–ii27.

Graber, M. L., R. M. Wachter, and C. K. Cassel. 2012. Bringing diagnosis into the quality and safety equations. *JAMA* 308(12):1211–1212.

Graber, M., R. Trowbridge, J. Myers, C. A. Umscheid, W. Strull, and M. Kanter. 2014. The next organizational challenge: Finding and addressing diagnostic error. *Joint Commission Journal on Quality and Patient Safety* 40(3):102–110.

Graedon, T., and J. Graedon. 2014. Let patients help with diagnosis. *Diagnosis* 1(1):49–51.

Haskell, H. 2014. What's in a story? Lessons from patients who have suffered diagnostic failure. *Diagnosis* 1(1):53–54.

HealthIT.gov. 2015. Patient ability to electronically view, download & transmit (VDT) health information. www.healthit.gov/providers-professionals/achieve-meaningful-use/core-measures-2/patient-ability-electronically-view-download-transmit-vdt-health-information (accessed March 15, 2015).

Hendrich, A., C. K. McCoy, J. Gale, L. Sparkman, and P. Santos. 2014. Ascension health's demonstration of full disclosure protocol for unexpected events during labor and delivery shows promise. *Health Affairs (Millwood)* 33(1):39–45.

Henriksen, K. 2014. Improving diagnostic performance: some unrecognized obstacles. *Diagnosis* 1(1):35–38.

Henriksen, K., and J. Brady. 2013. The pursuit of better diagnostic performance: A human factors perspective. *BMJ Quality & Safety* 22(Suppl 2):ii1–ii5.

HHS (Department of Health and Human Services). 2010. *Improper payments for evaluation and management services cost Medicare billions in 2010.* Washington, DC: HHS Office of Inspector General.

HHS. 2015. Patient Safety and Quality Improvement Act of 2005 Statute and Rule. www.hhs.gov/ocr/privacy/psa/regulation (accessed March 29, 2015).

HIMSS (Healthcare Information and Management Systems Society). 2014. What is interoperability? www.himss.org/library/interoperability-standards/what-is-interoperability (accessed February 9, 2015).

Hines, S., K. Luna, J. Lofthus, M. Marquardt, and D. Stelmokas. 2008. *Becoming a high reliability organization: Operational advice for hospital leaders*. Rockville, MD: Agency for Healthcare Research and Quality.

Hirt, E., and K. Markman. 1995. Multiple explanation: A consider-an-alternative strategy for debiasing judgments. *Journal of Personality and Social Psychology* 69:1069–1086.

Hodges, B., G. Regehr, and D. Martin. 2001. Difficulties in recognizing one's own incompetence: Novice physicians who are unskilled and unaware of it. *Academic Medicine* 76(10 Suppl):S87–S89.

Hogarth, R. 2010. On the learning of intuition. In H. Plessner, C. Betsch, and T. Betsch (eds.), *Intuition in judgment and decision making* (pp. 91–105). New York: Taylor & Francis.

Hughes, A. M., and E. Salas. 2013. Hierarchical medical teams and the science of teamwork. *AMA Journal of Ethics* 15(6):529–533. http://virtualmentor.ama-assn.org/2013/06/msoc1-1306.html (accessed May 26, 2015).

Hysong, S. J., R. G. Best, and J. A. Pugh. 2006. Audit and feedback and clinical practice guideline adherence: Making feedback actionable. *Implementation Science* 1(9). www.implementationscience.com/content/pdf/1748-5908-1-9.pdf (accessed June 10, 2015).

Iglehart, J. K. 2009. Health insurers and medical-imaging policy—A Work in Progress. *New England Journal of Medicine* 360(10):1030–1037.

IOM (Institute of Medicine). 2000. *To err is human: Building a safer health system*. Washington, DC: National Academy Press.

IOM. 2001. *Crossing the quality chasm: A new health system for the 21st century*. Washington, DC: National Academy Press.

IOM. 2002. *Fostering rapid advances in health care: Learning from system demonstrations*. Washington, DC: The National Academies Press.

IOM. 2009. *Resident duty hours: Enhancing sleep, supervision, and safety*. Washington, DC: The National Academies Press.

IOM. 2012. *Health IT and patient safety: Building safer systems for better care*. Washington, DC: The National Academies Press.

IOM. 2013. *Best care at lower cost: The path to continuously learning health care in America*. Washington, DC: The National Academies Press.

IOM. 2014. *Graduate medical education that meets the nation's health needs*. Washington, DC: The National Academies Press.

The Joint Commission. 2005. *Health care at the crossroads: Strategies for improving the medical liability system and preventing patient injury*. The Joint Commission. www.jointcommission.org/assets/1/18/Medical_Liability.pdf (accessed April 9, 2015).

The Joint Commission. 2014. Sentinel event policy and procedures. www.jointcommission.org/Sentinel_Event_Policy_and_Procedures (accessed June 11, 2015).

The Joint Commission. 2015. *Preventing copy-and-paste errors in the EHR*. www.jointcommission.org/issues/article.aspx?Article=bj%2B%2F2w37MuZrouWveszI1weWZ7ufX%2FP4tLrLI85oCi0%3D (accessed March 27, 2015).

Josiah Macy Jr. Foundation and Carnegie Foundation for the Advancement of Teaching. 2010. *Educating nurses and physicians: Towards new horizons. Advancing inter-professional education in academic health centers, conference summary*. June 16–18, 2010, Palo Alto, California.

Julavits, H. 2014. Diagnose this! How to be your own best doctor. *Harper's* April:25–35.

Kachalia, A. 2014. Legal issues in diagnostic error. Presentation to the Committee on Diagnostic Error in Health Care, August 7, 2014, Washington, DC.

Kachalia, A., and M. M. Mello. 2011. New directions in medical liability reform. *New England Journal of Medicine* 364(16):1564–1572.

Kaiser Permanente. 2012. Smart Partners About Your Health, edited by Kaiser Permanente.

Kanter, M. 2014. Diagnostic errors—Patient safety. Presentation to the Committee on Diagnostic Error in Health Care, August 7, 2014, Washington, DC.

Kassirer, J. P., and M. Angell. 1998. Evaluation and management guidelines—Fatally flawed. *New England Journal of Medicine* 339(23):1697–1698.

Khatri, N., G. D. Brown, and L. L. Hicks. 2009. From a blame culture to a just culture in health care. *Health Care Management Review* 34(4):312–322.

Klein, G. 2014. A naturalistic perspective. Input submitted to the Committee on Diagnostic Error in Health Care, December 20, 2014, Washington, DC.

Kostis, W. J., K. Demissie, S. W. Marcella, Y. H. Shao, A. C. Wilson, and A. E. Moreyra. 2007. Weekend versus weekday admission and mortality from myocardial infarction. *New England Journal of Medicine* 356(11):1099–1109.

Kotter, J. 1995. Leading change: Why transformation efforts fail. *Harvard Business Review* 73(2):59-67.

Kotter, J. 2012. The key to changing organizational culture. *Forbes*, September 27. www.forbes.com/sites/johnkotter/2012/09/27/the-key-to-changing-organizational-culture (accessed March 9, 2015).

Kroft, S. H. 2014. Statement of Steven H. Kroft, MD, FASCP, American Society for Clinical Pathology (ASCP). Presentation to the Committee on Diagnostic Error in Health Care, April 28, 2014, Washington, DC.

Kuhn, T., P. Basch, M. Barr, and T. Yackel. 2015. Clinical documentation in the 21st century: Executive summary of a policy position paper from the American College of Physicians. *Annals of Internal Medicine* 162(4):301–303.

Lacson, R., L. M. Prevedello, K. P. Andriole, S. D. O'Connor, C. Roy, T. Gandhi, A. K. Dalal, L. Sato, and R. Khorasani. 2014. Four-year impact of an alert notification system on closed-loop communication of critical test results. *American Journal of Roentgenology* 203(5):933–938.

Larson, E. B. 2002. Measuring, monitoring, and reducing medical harm from a systems perspective: A medical director's personal reflections. *Academic Medicine* 77(10):993–1000.

Leape., L. L. 2010. Q&A with Lucian Leape, M.D., adjunct professor of health policy, Harvard University. www.commonwealthfund.org/publications/newsletters/states-in-action/2010/jan/january-february-2010/ask-the-expert/ask-the-expert (accessed September 23, 2014).

Leape, L. L., T. A. Brennan, N. Laird, A. G. Lawthers, A. R. Localio, B. A. Barnes, L. Hebert, J. P. Newhouse, P. C. Weiler, and H. Hiatt. 1991. The nature of adverse events in hospitalized patients: Results of the Harvard Medical Practice Study II. *New England Journal of Medicine* 324(6):377–384.

Lundberg, G. D. 1998. Low-tech autopsies in the era of high-tech medicine: Continued value for quality assurance and patient safety. *JAMA* 280(14):1273–1274.

Marceglia, S., P. Fontelo, and M. J. Ackerman. 2015. Transforming consumer health informatics: Connecting CHI applications to the health-IT ecosystem. *Journal of the American Medical Informatics Association* 22(e1):e210–e212.

Marewski, J. N., and G. Gigerenzer. 2012. Heuristic decision making in medicine. *Dialogues Clinical Neuroscience* 14(1):77–89.

Marx, D. A. 2001. Patient safety and the "just culture": A primer for health care executives. Medical Event Reporting System–Transfusion Medicine. www.safer.healthcare.ucla.edu/safer/archive/ahrq/FinalPrimerDoc.pdf (accessed June 7, 2015).

McDonald, K. M. 2014. The diagnostic field's players and interactions: From the inside out. *Diagnosis* 1(1):55–58.

MedPAC (Medicare Payment Advisory Commission). 2014. Physician and other health professional payment system. www.medpac.gov/-documents-/payment-basics/page/2 (accessed March 17, 2015).

Mello, M. M., D. M. Studdert, and A. Kachalia. 2014. The medical liability climate and prospects for reform. *JAMA* 312(20):2146–2155.

Miller, H. D. 2014. How healthcare payment systems and benefit designs can support more accurate diagnosis. Input submitted to the Committee on Diagnostic Error in Health Care, December 29, 2014, Washington, DC.

Milstead, J. A. 2005. The culture of safety. *Policy, Politics, & Nursing Practice* 6(1):51–54.

Moran, J. W., and B. K. Brightman. 2000. Leading organizational change. *Journal of Workplace Learning* 12(2):66–74.

Moses, H., 3rd, D. H. Matheson, S. Cairns-Smith, B. P. George, C. Palisch, and E. R. Dorsey. 2015. The anatomy of medical research: U.S. and international comparisons. *JAMA* 313(2):174–189.

Mumma, G., and W. Steven. 1995. Procedural debiasing of primary/anchoring effects in clinical-like judgments. *Journal of Clinical Psychology* 51:841–853.

Mussweiler, T., F. Strack, and T. Pfeiffer. 2000. Overcoming the inevitable anchoring effect: Considering the opposite compensates for selective accessibility. *Personality and Social Psychology Bulletin* 26(9):1142–1150.

National Commission on Physician Payment Reform. 2013. *Report of the National Commission on Physician Payment Reform*. Washington, DC: National Commission on Physician Payment Reform. http://physicianpaymentcommission.org/report (accessed March 17, 2015).

Newman-Toker, D. 2014. Prioritization of diagnostic error problems and solutions: Concepts, economic modeling, and action plan. Presentation to the Committee on Diagnostic Error in Health Care, August 7, 2014, Washington, DC.

Newman-Toker, D. E., K. M. McDonald, and D. O. Meltzer. 2013. How much diagnostic safety can we afford, and how should we decide? A health economics perspective. *BMJ Quality and Safety* 22(Suppl 2):ii11–ii20.

NPSF (National Patient Safety Foundation) and SIDM (Society to Improve Diagnosis in Medicine). 2014. Checklist for getting the right diagnosis. www.npsf.org/?page=rightdiagnosis and http://c.ymcdn.com/sites/www.npsf.org/resource/collection/930A0426-5BAC-4827-AF94-1CE1624CBE67/Checklist-for-Getting-the-Right-Diagnosis.pdf (accessed June 26, 2015).

NQF (National Quality Forum.) 2011. *Serious reportable events in healthcare—2011 update: A consensus report*. Washington, DC: National Quality Forum. www.qualityforum.org/projects/hacs_and_sres.aspx (accessed June 11, 2015).

Ober, K. P. 2015. The electronic health record: Are we the tools of our tools? *The Pharos* 78(1):8–14.

ONC (Office of the National Coordinator for Health Information Technology). 2014. *Health information technology adverse event reporting: Analysis of two databases*. Washington, DC: Office of the National Coordinator for Health Information Technology.

Otte-Trojel, T., A. de Bont, J. van de Klundert, and T. G. Rundall. 2014. Characteristics of patient portals developed in the context of health information exchanges: Early policy effects of incentives in the meaningful use program in the United States. *Journal of Medical Internet Research* 16(11):e258.

Papa, F. 2014. A response to the IOM's ad hoc committee on Diagnostic Error in Health Care. Input submitted to the Committee on Diagnostic Error in Health Care, October 24, 2014, Washington, DC.

Patel, V., N. Yoskowitz, and J. Arocha. 2009. Towards effective evaluation and reform in medical education: A cognitive and learning sciences perspective. *Advances in Health Sciences Education* 14(5):791–812.

Patel, V., M. J. Swain, J. King, and M. F. Furukawa. 2013. Physician capability to electronically exchange clinical information, 2011. *American Journal of Managed Care* 19(10):835–843.

Pecukonis, E., O. Doyle, and D. L. Bliss. 2008. Reducing barriers to interprofessional train-ing: Promoting interprofessional cultural competence. *Journal of Interprofessional Care* 22(4):417–428.

Portilla, L. M., and B. Alving. 2010. Reaping the benefits of biomedical research: Partnerships required. *Science Translational Medicine* 2(35):35cm17.

PSO (Patient Safety Organization) Privacy Protection Center. 2014. AHRQ Common For-mats. www.psoppc.org/web/patientsafety (accessed August 10, 2015).

Redelmeier, D. A. 2005. Improving patient care. The cognitive psychology of missed diag-noses. *Annals of Internal Medicine* 142(2):115–120.

Reiling, J., G. Hughes, and M. Murphy. 2008. Chapter 28: The impact of facility design on patient safety. In R. G. Hughes (ed.), *Patient safety and quality: An evidence-based handbook for nurses* (pp. 700–725). Rockville, MD: Agency for Healthcare Research and Quality.

Richardson, W. S. 2007. We should overcome the barriers to evidence-based clinical diagno-sis! *Journal of Clinical Epidemiology* 60(3):217–227.

Richardson, W. S. 2014. Twenty suggestions that could improve clinical diagnosis and reduce diagnostic error. Input submitted to the Committee on Diagnostic Error in Health Care, October 23, 2014, Washington, DC.

Rosenthal, M. 2014. Comments to the Institute of Medicine Committee on Diagnostic Error in Health Care. Input submitted to the Committee on Diagnostic Error in Health Care, December 29, 2014, Washington, DC.

RTI International. 2014. RTI International to develop road map for health IT safety center. www.rti.org/newsroom/news.cfm?obj=FCC8767E-C2DA-EB8B-AD7E2F778E6CB91A (accessed March 27, 2015).

Sage, W. M., T. H. Gallagher, S. Armstrong, J. S. Cohn, T. McDonald, J. Gale, A. C. Woodward, and M. M. Mello. 2014. How policy makers can smooth the way for communication-and-resolution programs. *Health Affairs (Millwood)* 33(1):11–19.

Sarkar, U., D. Bonacum, W. Strull, C. Spitzmueller, N. Jin, A. Lopez, T. D. Giardina, A. N. Meyer, and H. Singh. 2012. Challenges of making a diagnosis in the outpatient setting: A multi-site survey of primary care physicians. *BMJ Quality and Safety* 21(8):641–648.

Sarkar, U., B. Simchowitz, D. Bonacum, W. Strull, A. Lopez, L. Rotteau, and K. G. Shojania. 2014. A qualitative analysis of physician perspectives on missed and delayed outpatient diagnosis: The focus on system-related factors. *Joint Commission Journal on Quality and Patient Safety* 40(10):461–470.

Sarter, N. 2014. Use(r)-centered design of health IT: Challenges and lessons learned. Pre-sentation to the Committee on Diagnostic Error in Health Care, August 7, 2014, Wash-ington, DC.

Schein, E. H. 2004. *Organizational culture and leadership*, 3rd ed. San Francisco, CA: John Wiley & Sons.

Schiff, G. D. 2008. Minimizing diagnostic error: The importance of follow-up and feedback. *American Journal of Medicine* 121(5):S38–S42.

Schiff, G. D. 2014a. Diagnosis and diagnostic errors: Time for a new paradigm. *BMJ Quality and Safety* 23(1):1–3.

Schiff, G. D. 2014b. Presentation to IOM Committee on Diagnostic Error in Health Care. Presentation to the Committee on Diagnostic Error in Health Care, August 7, 2014, Washington, DC.

Schiff, G. D., and D. W. Bates. 2010. Can electronic clinical documentation help prevent diagnostic errors? *New England Journal of Medicine* 362(12):1066–1069.

Schiff, G. D., S. Kim, R. Abrams, K. Cosby, A. S. Elstein, S. Hasler, N. Krosnjar, R. Odwanzy, M. F. Wisniewsky, and R. A. McNutt. 2005. *Diagnosing diagnosis errors: Lessons from a multi-institutional collaborative project for the diagnostic error evaluation and research project investigators.* Rockville, MD: Agency for Healthcare Research and Quality. www.ahrq.gov/qual/advances (accessed June 10, 2015).

Schiff, G. D., O. Hasan, S. Kim, R. Abrams, K. Cosby, B. L. Lambert, A. S. Elstein, S. Hasler, M. L. Kabongo, N. Krosnjar, R. Odwazny, M. F. Wisniewski, and R. A. McNutt. 2009. Diagnostic error in medicine: Analysis of 583 physician-reported errors. *Archives of Internal Medicine* 169(20):1881–1887.

Schmitt, M., A. Blue, C. A. Aschenbrener, and T. R. Viggiano. 2011. Core competencies for interprofessional collaborative practice: reforming health care by transforming health professionals' education. *Academic Medicine* 86(11):1351.

Shojania, K. G. 2010. The elephant of patient safety: What you see depends on how you look. *Joint Commission Journal of Quality and Patient Safety* 36(9):399–401.

Shojania, K. G., E. C. Burton, K. M. McDonald, and L. Goldman. 2002. Autopsy as an outcome and performance measure. Rockville, MD: Agency for Healthcare Research and Quality.

Shojania, K. G., E. C. Burton, K. M. McDonald, and L. Goldman. 2003. Changes in rates of autopsy-detected diagnostic errors over time: A systematic review. *JAMA* 289(21):2849–2856.

Silow-Carroll, S., T. Alteras, and J. A. Meyer. 2007. *Hospital quality improvement: Strategies and lessons from U.S. hospitals.* www.commonwealthfund.org/publications/fund-reports/2007/apr/hospital-quality-improvement--strategies-and-lessons-from-u-s--hospitals (accessed June 7, 2015).

Singh, H. 2013. Diagnostic errors: Moving beyond "no respect" and getting ready for prime time. *BMJ Quality & Safety* 22(10):789–792.

Singh, H. 2014. Building a robust conceptual foundation for defining and measuring diagnostic errors. Presentation to the Committee on Diagnostic Error in Health Care, August 7, 2014, Washington, DC.

Singh, H., and D. F. Sittig. 2015. Advancing the science of measurement of diagnostic errors in healthcare: The Safer Dx framework. *BMJ Quality & Safety* 24:103–110.

Singh, H., A. D. Naik, R. Rao, and L. A. Petersen. 2008. Reducing diagnostic errors through effective communication: Harnessing the power of information technology. *Journal of General Internal Medicine* 23(4):489–494.

Singh, H., T. D. Giardina, A. N. D. Meyer, S. N. Forjuoh, M. D. Reis, and E. J. Thomas. 2013. Types and origins of diagnostic errors in primary care settings. *JAMA Internal Medicine* 173(6):418–425.

Singh, H., A. N. D. Meyer, and E. J. Thomas. 2014. The frequency of diagnostic errors in outpatient care: Estimations from three large observational studies involving US adult populations. *BMJ Quality & Safety* 23(9). doi: 10.1136/bmjqs-2013-002627.

Sittig, D. F., and H. Singh. 2010. A new sociotechnical model for studying health information technology in complex adaptive healthcare systems. *Quality and Safety in Health Care* 19(Suppl 3):i68–i74.

Sittig, D. F., D. C. Classen, and H. Singh. 2015. Patient safety goals for the proposed Federal Health Information Technology Safety Center. *Journal of the American Medical Informatics Association* 22(2):472–478.

Sorra, J., T. Famolaro, N. D. Yount, S. A. Smith, S. Wilson, and H. Liu. 2014. *Hospital Survey on Patient Safety Culture—2014 user comparative database report.* AHRQ Publication No. 14-0019-EF. Rockville, MD: Agency for Healthcare Research and Quality.

Tehrani, A., H. Lee, S. Mathews, A. Shore, M. Makary, P. Pronovost, and D. Newman-Toker. 2013. 25-year summary of U.S. malpractice claims for diagnostic errors 1986–2010: An analysis from the National Practitioner Data Bank. *BMJ Quality and Safety* 22:672–680.

ten Cate, O. 2014. Advice to the Institute of Medicine Committee on Diagnostic Error. Input submitted to the Committee on Diagnostic Error in Health Care, November 28, 2014, Washington, DC.

Thomas, E. J. 2014. Safety culture and diagnostic error: A rising tide lifts all boats. Presentation to the Committee on Diagnostic Error in Health Care, November 5, 2014, Washington, DC.

Trowbridge, R. 2014. Diagnostic performance: Measurement and feedback. Paper presented to the Committee on Diagnostic Error in Health Care, August 7, 2014, Washington, DC.

Trowbridge, R., G. Dhaliwal, and K. Cosby. 2013. Educational agenda for diagnostic error reduction. *BMJ Quality and Safety* 22(Suppl 2):ii28–ii32.

Verghese, A. 2008. Culture shock—patient as icon, icon as patient. *New England Journal of Medicine* 359(26):2748–2751.

Wachter, R. M. 2010. Why diagnostic errors don't get any respect—And what can be done about them. *Health Affairs (Millwood)* 29(9):1605–1610.

Wegwarth, O., W. Gaissmaier, and G. Gigerenzer. 2009. Smart strategies for doctors and doctors-in-training: Heuristics in medicine. *Medical Education* 43(8):721–728.

Weick, K. E., and K. M. Sutcliffe. 2011. Business organizations must learn to operate "mindfully" to ensure high performance. www.bus.umich.edu/FacultyResearch/Research/ManagingUnexpected.htm (accessed May 26, 2015).

Weingart, S. N., O. Pagovich, D. Z. Sands, J. M. Li, M. D. Aronson, R. B. Davis, D. W. Bates, and R. S. Phillips. 2005. What can hospitalized patients tell us about adverse events? Learning from patient-reported incidents. *Journal of General Internal Medicine* 20(9):830–836.

Wennberg, D. 2014. Comments for the Institute of Medicine's Committee on Diagnostic Error in Health Care. Input submitted to the Committee on Diagnostic Error in Health Care, December 29, 2014, Washington, DC.

WHO (World Health Organization). 2005. *WHO draft guidelines for adverse event reporting and learning systems.* Geneva, Switzerland: WHO.

Zimmerman, T. M., and G. Amori. 2007. Including patients in root cause and system failure analysis: Legal and psychological implications. *Journal of Healthcare Risk Management* 27(2):27–34.

Zwaan, L., M. de Bruijne, C. Wagner, A. Thijs, M. Smits, G. van der Wal, and D. R. Timmermans. 2010. Patient record review of the incidence, consequences, and causes of diagnostic adverse events. *Archives of Internal Medicine* 170(12):1015–1021.

Zwaan, L., G. D. Schiff, and H. Singh. 2013. Advancing the research agenda for diagnostic error reduction. *BMJ Quality & Safety* 22(Suppl 2):ii52–ii57.

Appendix A

Glossary

Active error—an error involving frontline clinicians (sometimes referred to as an error occurring at the "sharp end" of patient safety) (IOM, 2000).

Adverse event—"an event that results in unintended harm to the patient by an act of commission or omission rather than by the underlying disease or condition of the patient" (IOM, 2004, p. 32).

Burnout—condition due to occupational stress resulting from demanding and emotional relationships between health care professionals and patients that is marked by emotional exhaustion, a negative attitude toward one's patients, and the belief that one is no longer effective at work with patients (Bakker et al., 2005).

Calibration—the process of a clinician becoming aware of his or her diagnostic abilities and limitations through feedback.

Clinical decision support (CDS)—a health information technology component that "provides clinicians, staff, patients or other individuals with knowledge and person-specific information, intelligently filtered or presented at appropriate times, to enhance health and health care. CDS encompasses a variety of tools to enhance decision making in the clinical workflow. These tools include computerized alerts and reminders to care providers and patients; clinical guidelines; condition-specific order sets; focused patient data reports and summaries; documentation templates;

diagnostic support; and contextually relevant reference information, among other tools" (HealthIT.gov, 2014).

Clinical reasoning—"the cognitive process that is necessary to evaluate and manage a patient's medical problems" (Barrows, 1980, p. 19).

Clinician survey—a questionnaire (written, telephone, interview, Web-based) that obtains clinicians' self-reports about diagnostic errors they have made or what they know about diagnostic errors made by other clinicians.

Cognitive autopsy—a form of cognitive and affective root cause analysis that focuses on factors that can affect cognition such as ambient conditions, physical state (fatigue), and cognitive heuristics (Croskerry, 2005).

Cognitive bias—a predisposition to think in a way that leads to systematic failures in judgment. Cognitive biases often result from heuristics that fail in a predictable manner, but they can also be caused by affect and motivation (Kahneman, 2011).

Communication and resolution program (CRP)—a program that encourages "the disclosure of unanticipated care outcomes to affected patients and their families and proactively seek[s] resolutions, which may include providing an apology; an explanation; and, where appropriate, an offer of reimbursement, compensation, or both" (Mello et al., 2014, p. 20).

Defensive medicine—"occurs when doctors order tests, procedures, or visits, or avoid high-risk patients or procedures, primarily (but not necessarily solely) to reduce their exposure to malpractice liability" (OTA, 1994, p. 13).

Diagnosis—the explanation of a patient's health problem.

Diagnostic error—the failure to (a) establish an accurate and timely explanation of the patient's health problem(s) or (b) communicate that explanation to the patient.

Diagnostic management team—a group of diagnostic specialists (pathologists, radiologists, and other diagnosticians) that offer participating health care professionals assistance in selecting appropriate diagnostic tests and interpreting diagnostic test results (Govern, 2013).

Diagnostic process—a complex, patient-centered, collaborative activity that involves information gathering and clinical reasoning with the goal of determining a patient's health problem.

Dual process theory—a model of cognition that proposes two processes—fast, intuitive system 1, and slow, analytic system 2 processes—are responsible for human reasoning and decision making.

Electronic health record (EHR)—a real-time, patient-centered record that contains information about a patient's medical history, diagnoses, medications, immunization dates, allergies, radiology images, and lab and test results (HealthIT.gov, 2013).

Error—"failure of a planned action to be completed as intended (i.e., error of execution) and the use of a wrong plan to achieve an aim (i.e., error of planning) [commission]. It also includes failure of an unplanned action that should have been completed (omission)" (IOM, 2004, p. 330).

Error recovery—the early identification of an error so that actions can be taken to reduce or avert negative effects resulting from the error (IOM, 2000).

Feedback—information on the accuracy of diagnosis and diagnostic performance that is provided to individual health care professionals, care teams, or organizational leaders.

Harm—"hurtful or adverse outcomes of an action or event, whether temporary or permanent" (IOM, 2011, p. 240).

Health information technology (health IT)—"a technical system of computers and software that operates in the context of a larger sociotechnical system; that is, a collection of hardware and software working in concert within an organization that includes people, processes, and technology" (IOM, 2012, p. 2).

Health literacy—"the degree to which individuals have the capacity to obtain, process, and understand basic health information and services needed to make appropriate health care decisions and services needed to prevent or treat illness" (HRSA, 2015).

Heuristic—a special type of system 1 process that can facilitate decision making but can also lead to errors. Sometimes referred to as cognitive strategies or mental shortcuts, heuristics are automatically and unconsciously employed during reasoning and decision making (Cosmides, 1996; Cosmides and Tooby, 1994; Gigerenzer, 2000; Gigerenzer and Goldstein, 1996; Klein, 1998, 2003; Lipshitz et al., 2001).

Human factors (or ergonomics)—"the scientific discipline concerned with the understanding of interactions among humans and other elements of a system, and the profession that applies theory, principles, data, and methods to design in order to optimize human well-being and overall system performance. Ergonomists contribute to the design and evaluation of tasks, jobs, products, environments, and systems in order to make them compatible with the needs, abilities, and limitations of people" (IEA, 2000).

Integrated practice unit—a group of clinicians and non-clinicians who are responsible for the comprehensive care of a specific medical condition and the associated complications, or a set of closely related conditions (Porter, 2010).

Interoperability—the ability of different information technology systems and software applications to communicate, exchange data, and use the information that has been exchanged (HIMSS, 2014).

Inter-rater reliability—the degree to which two or more independent raters can consistently and systematically apply a rubric to assign scores to observations (or participants) based on a preestablished scoring protocol (or rubric) (Stemler, 2007).

Intra-rater reliability—the degree of agreement among multiple repetitions of a scoring protocol performed by a single rater.

Latent error—"errors in the design, organization, training, or maintenance that lead to operator errors and whose effects typically lie dormant in the system for lengthy periods of time" (IOM, 2000, p. 210). Latent errors are more removed from the control of frontline clinicians and can include failures in organizations and design that enable active errors to cause harm (often called the "blunt end" of patient safety) (AHRQ, 2015; IOM, 2000).

Learning sciences—the multidisciplinary science that studies how people learn in order to optimize education and training.

Morbidity and mortality (M&M) conferences—forums that allow clinicians to discuss and learn from errors that have occurred within an organization.

Near miss—a failure in the diagnostic process that does not lead to a diagnostic error.

Overdiagnosis—"when a condition is diagnosed that would otherwise not go on to cause symptoms or death" (Welch and Black, 2010, p. 605).

Patient portal—"Secure, online patient access to health information and serves as an interface to provide useful information to both patients and health professionals" (IOM, 2012, p. 118).

Patient safety—"freedom from accidental injury; ensuring patient safety involves the establishment of operational systems and processes that minimize the likelihood of errors and maximizes the likelihood of intercepting them when they occur" (IOM, 2000, p. 211); the prevention of harm caused by errors of commission and omission (IOM, 2004).

Patient survey—a questionnaire (written, telephone, interview, Web-based) that obtains patients' self-reports about diagnostic errors they have experienced or their awareness of diagnostic errors experienced by others.

Postmortem examination (autopsy)—"an external and internal examination of the body after death using review of medical records, surgical techniques, microscopy, and laboratory analysis. It is performed by a pathologist, a medical doctor specially trained for the procedure who is able to recognize the effects of disease on the body" (CAP, 2014).

Quality of care—"degree to which health services for individuals and populations increase the likelihood of desired health outcomes and are consistent with current professional knowledge" (IOM, 1990, p. 128).

Root cause analysis—"a structured method used to analyze serious adverse events. Initially developed to analyze industrial accidents, [root cause analysis] is now widely deployed as an error analysis tool in health care" (AHRQ, 2012).

Safe—"avoiding injuries to patients from the care that is intended to help them" (IOM, 2001, p. 39).

Safe care—"involves making evidence-based clinical decisions to maximize the health outcomes of an individual and to minimize the potential for harm. Both errors of commission and omission should be avoided" (IOM, 2004, p. 334).

Second review—a process used in pathology and radiology in which a second health care professional reviews the same information as the first health care professional in order to detect discrepancies in results that may be indicative of error.

Simulation—"allows researchers and practitioners to test new clinical processes and enhance individual and team skills before encountering patients. Many simulation applications involve mannequins that present with symptoms and respond to the simulated treatment, analogous to flight simulators used by pilots" (AHRQ, 2014).

Standardized patient—"a person carefully recruited and trained to take on the characteristics of a real patient thereby affording the student an opportunity to learn and to be evaluated on learned skills in a simulated clinical environment" (Johns Hopkins, 2015).

System—"set of interdependent elements interacting to achieve a common aim. These elements may be both human and nonhuman (equipment, technologies, etc.)" (IOM, 2000, p. 211).

System 1—fast (nonanalytical, intuitive) automatic cognitive processes that require very little working memory capacity and are often triggered by stimuli or result from overlearned associations or implicitly learned activities.

System 2—slow (analytical, reflective) cognitive processes that place a heavy load on working memory and involve hypothetical and counterfactual reasoning (Evans and Stanovich, 2013; Stanovich and Toplak, 2012).

Usability—"the extent to which a product can be used by specified users to achieve specified goals with effectiveness, efficiency and satisfaction in a specified context of use" (ISO, 1998).

Voluntary reporting—"those reporting systems for which the reporting of patient safety events is voluntary (not mandatory). Generally, reports on all types of events are accepted" (IOM, 2004, p. 335).

Workflow—the sequence of physical and cognitive tasks performed by various people within and between work environments (Carayon et al., 2010).

REFERENCES

AHRQ (Agency for Healthcare Research and Quality). 2012. Patient safety primers: Root cause analysis. http://psnet.ahrq.gov/primer.aspx?primerID=10 (accessed April 11, 14, 2014).

AHRQ. 2014. Improving patient safety through simulation research. www.ahrq.gov/research/findings/factsheets/errors-safety/simulproj11/index.html (accessed April 10, 2015).

AHRQ. 2015. Patient safety network: Patient safety primers. Systems approach. http://psnet.ahrq.gov/primer.aspx?primerID=21 (accessed May 8, 2015).

Bakker, A. B., P. M. Le Blanc, and W. B. Schaufeli. 2005. Burnout contagion among intensive care nurses. *Journal of Advanced Nursing* 51(3):276–287.

Barrows, H. S. 1980. *Problem-based learning: An approach to medical education*. New York: Springer Publishing Company.

CAP (College of American Pathologists). 2014. Autopsy. www.cap.org/apps//cap.portal?_nfpb=true&cntvwrPtlt_actionOverride=%2Fportlets%2FcontentViewer%2Fshow&_windowLabel=cntvwrPtlt&cntvwrPtlt%7BactionForm.contentReference%7D=committees%2Fautopsy%2Fautopsy_index.html&_state=maximized&_pageLabel=cntvwr (accessed April 10, 2015).

Carayon, P., B. T. Karsh, R. Cartmill, et al. 2010. *Incorporating health information technology into workflow redesign: Request for information summary report*. Rockville, MD: Agency for Healthcare Research and Quality.

Cosmides, L. 1996. Are humans good intuitive statisticians after all? Rethinking some conclusions from the literature on judgment under uncertainty. *Cognition* 58(1):1–73.

Cosmides, L., and J. Tooby. 1994. Better than rational: Evolutionary psychology and the invisible hand. *American Economic Review* 84(2):327–332.

Croskerry, P. 2005. Diagnostic failure: A cognitive and affective approach. *Advances in Patient Safety* 2:241–254.

Evans, J. S. B. T., and K. E. Stanovich. 2013. Dual-process theories of higher cognition: Advancing the debate. *Perspectives on Psychological Science* 8(3):223–241.

Gigerenzer, G. 2000. *Adaptive thinking: Rationality in the real world*. New York: Oxford University Press.

Gigerenzer, G., and D. G. Goldstein. 1996. Reasoning the fast and frugal way: Models of bounded rationality. *Psychology Review* 103:650–669.

Govern, P. 2013. Diagnostic management efforts thrive on teamwork. http://news.vanderbilt.edu/2013/03/diagnostic-management-efforts-thrive-on-teamwork (accessed February 11, 2015).

HealthIT.gov. 2013. Learn EHR basics. www.healthit.gov/providers-professionals/learn-ehr-basics (accessed March 11, 2014).

HealthIT.gov. 2014. Clinical decision support. www.healthit.gov/policy-researchers-implementers/clinical-decision-support-cds (accessed April 9, 2014).

HIMSS (Healthcare Information and Management Systems Society). 2014. What is interoperability? www.himss.org/library/interoperability-standards/what-is-interoperability (accessed February 9, 2015).

HRSA (Health Resources and Services Administration). 2015. About health literacy. www.hrsa.gov/publichealth/healthliteracy/healthlitabout.html (accessed August 10, 2015).

IEA (International Ergonomics Association). 2000. The discipline of ergonomics. www.iea.cc/whats/index.html (accessed April 10, 2015).

IOM (Institute of Medicine). 1990. *Medicare: A strategy for quality assurance, Volume II*. Washington, DC: National Academy Press.

IOM. 2000. *To err is human: Building a safer health system*. Washington, DC: National Academy Press.

IOM. 2001. *Crossing the quality chasm: A new health system for the 21st century*. Washington, DC: National Academy Press.

IOM. 2004. *Patient safety: Achieving a new standard for care*. Washington, DC: The National Academies Press.

IOM. 2011. *Finding what works in health care: Standards for systematic reviews*. Washington, DC: The National Academies Press.

IOM. 2012. *Health IT and patient safety: Building safer systems for better care*. Washington, DC: The National Academies Press.

ISO (International Organization for Standardization). 1998. *Ergonomic requirements for office work with visual display terminals (VDTS)—Part 11: Guidance on usability*. www.iso.org/obp/ui/#iso:std:iso:9241:-11:ed-1:v1:en (accessed February 25, 2015).

Johns Hopkins. 2015. Standardized patient program. www.hopkinsmedicine.org/simulation_center/training/standardized_patient_program (accessed April 10, 2015).

Kahneman, D. 2011. *Thinking fast and slow*. New York: Farrar, Strauss and Giroux.

Klein, G. 1998. *Sources of power: How people make decisions*. Cambridge, MA: MIT Press.

Klein, G. 2003. *The power of intuition*. New York: Doubleday.

Lipshitz, R., G. Klein, J. Orasanu, and E. Salas. 2001. Taking stock of naturalistic decision making. *Journal of Behavioral Decision Making* 14(5):331–352.

Mello, M. M., R. C. Boothman, T. McDonald, J. Driver, A. Lembitz, D. Bouwmeester, B. Dunlap, and T. Gallagher. 2014. Communication-and-resolution programs: The challenges and lessons learned from six early adopters. *Health Affairs* 33(1):20–29.

OTA (Office of Technology Assessment). 1994. Defensive Medicine and Medical Malpractice, OTA-H-602. Washington, DC: U.S. Government Printing Office.

Porter, M. E. 2010. What is value in health care? *New England Journal of Medicine* 363(26):2477–2481.

Stanovich, K. E., and M. E. Toplak. 2012. Defining features versus incidental correlates of type 1 and type 2 processing. *Mind & Society* 11(1):3–13.

Stemler, S. E. 2007. Interrater reliability. In N. J. Salkind (ed.), *Encyclopedia of Measurement and Statistics*. Thousand Oaks, CA: Sage Publications.

Welch, H. G., and W. C. Black. 2010. Overdiagnosis in cancer. *Journal of the National Cancer Institute* 102(9):605–613.

Appendix B

Committee Member and Staff Biographies

COMMITTEE MEMBER BIOGRAPHIES

John R. Ball, M.D., J.D. (*Chair*), is an executive vice president emeritus of the American College of Physicians and the American Society for Clinical Pathology. He is a graduate of Emory University, received a J.D. and an M.D. from Duke University, and was a Robert Wood Johnson Clinical Scholar at George Washington University. After a residency in internal medicine at Duke University, he held several health policy positions in the U.S. Public Health Service and was a senior policy analyst in the Office of Science and Technology Policy, Executive Office of the President. Dr. Ball originated the Washington office of the American College of Physicians and served as its executive vice president for 8 years. He subsequently was president and chief executive officer of Pennsylvania Hospital and an executive vice president and chief executive officer of the American Society for Clinical Pathology. In retirement, he has recently served as interim president of the Milbank Memorial Fund, on whose board he also serves. He is also a member of the board of Mission Health System in Asheville, North Carolina, where he resides. Dr. Ball was elected a member of the National Academy of Medicine in 1992.

Elisabeth Belmont, Esq., serves as the corporate counsel for MaineHealth, which is ranked among the nation's top 100 integrated health care delivery networks and has combined annual revenues of nearly $2 billion. She has significant experience in the defense of professional liability claims and educates health care providers on using "lessons learned" from such claims to inform quality improvement and patient safety initiatives to minimize medical errors. Ms. Belmont's practice also focuses on electronic health information network strategy development and implementation to support innovations in care delivery and payment models as well as the use of "big data" to enhance care processes and clinical outcomes. She has participated in a number of national initiatives where quality improvement, patient safety, and health information technology intersect, including events sponsored by the Department of Health and Human Services (HHS) Office of the National Coordinator for Health Information Technology, HHS Office of the Inspector General, American Health Lawyers Association, American Society of Healthcare Risk Management, and American Association for the Advancement of Science. Ms. Belmont is a member of the Board on Health Care Services of the Institute of Medicine of the National Academies. She co-chairs the National Quality Forum's Health IT Patient Safety Measures Standing Committee. Additionally, Ms. Belmont serves as a member of the Editorial Advisory Board of Bloomberg BNA's *Health Law* Reporter. Ms. Belmont is a past president of the American Health Lawyers Association, a former chair of the association's health information and technology practice group, and a former chair of the association's Quality in Action Task Force. She also served as principal investigator for a research study funded by the American Society of Healthcare Risk Management, Minimizing Electronic Health Record–related Serious Safety Events and Related Medical Malpractice Liability. Ms. Belmont is the recipient of numerous honors, including being named by *Modern Healthcare* as 1 of the 2007 Top 25 Most Powerful Women in Healthcare and being selected to receive the 2014 David J. Greenburg Service Award. She is a nationally recognized author and lecturer on a myriad of health law topics.

Robert A. Berenson, M.D., is an Institute Fellow at the Urban Institute. He is an expert in health care policy, particularly Medicare, with experience practicing medicine, serving in senior positions in two administrations, and helping organize and manage a successful preferred provider organization. His primary research and policy interests currently are in the areas of payment reform, provider and plan pricing power, quality improvement, performance measurement, and delivery system reform. Dr. Berenson recently completed a 3-year term on the Medicare Payment Advisory Commission (MedPAC), the last 2 as vice chair. From 1998–2000, he was in charge of Medicare payment policy and private health plan contracting in the Centers for Medicare & Medicaid Services. Previously, he served as an assistant director of the Carter White House Domestic Policy Staff. Dr. Berenson is a board-certified internist who practiced for 20 years, the past 12 in a Washington, DC, group practice, and while practicing helped organize and manage a successful preferred provider organization serving the Washington, DC, metropolitan area. He was co-author, with Walter Zelman, of *The Managed Care Blues & How to Cure Them*, and, with Rick Mayes, *Medicare Prospective Payment and the Shaping of U.S. Health Care*. He is a graduate of the Mount Sinai School of Medicine, a Fellow of the American College of Physicians, and on the adjunct faculty of the George Washington University School of Public Health.

Pascale Carayon, Ph.D., is the Procter & Gamble Bascom Professor in Total Quality in the Department of Industrial and Systems Engineering and the director of the Center for Quality and Productivity Improvement at the University of Wisconsin–Madison. She leads the Systems Engineering Initiative for Patient Safety (SEIPS) at the University of Wisconsin–Madison (http://cqpi.engr.wisc.edu/seips_home). SEIPS is an internationally known interdisciplinary research program that brings together researchers from human factors and ergonomics with researchers from medicine, surgery, nursing, pharmacy, and health services research. Dr. Carayon received her engineer diploma from the Ecole Centrale de Paris, France, in 1984 and her Ph.D. in industrial engineering from the University of Wisconsin–Madison in 1988. Dr. Carayon's research belongs to the discipline of human factors engineering, in particular, macroergonomics. Her scholarly contributions aimed at modeling, assessing, and improving work systems (i.e., the systems of tasks performed by individuals using various technologies in a physical and organizational environment) in order to improve system performance and worker well-being. Her research has been funded by the Agency for Healthcare Research and Quality, the National Science Foundation, the National Institutes of Health, the National Institute for Occupational Safety and Health, the Department of Defense, various foundations, and private industry. She is a fellow of the Human Factors and Ergonomics Society and a fellow of the International Ergonomics Association. She is the recipient of the International Ergonomics Association Triennial Distinguished Service Award (2012) and is the first woman to receive this prestigious award. She has published more than 100 papers and more than 220 conference papers and 30 technical reports, and she is currently the co-editor-in-chief of *Applied Ergonomics*. She is the editor of the *Handbook of Human Factors and Ergonomics in Health Care and Patient Safety*. She is a member of the National Academies of Sciences, Engineering, and Medicine Board on Human-Systems Integration.

Christine K. Cassel, M.D., is president and chief executive officer of the National Quality Forum. Previously she served as president and chief executive officer of the American Board of Internal Medicine. Dr. Cassel is a member of the President's Council of Advisors on Science and Technology (PCAST). She is the co-chair and physician leader of PCAST working groups that have made recommendations to the President on issues relating to health information technology, scientific innovation in drug development, and systems engineering in health care delivery. She was a member of the Commonwealth Fund's Commission on a High Performance Health System and has served on Institute of Medicine committees that wrote the influential reports *To Err Is Human* and *Crossing the Quality Chasm*. She is an adjunct professor of medicine and a senior fellow in the Department of Medical Ethics and Health Policy at the University of Pennsylvania School of Medicine, a former dean of medicine at Oregon Health and Science University, the chair of geriatrics at Mount Sinai School of Medicine in New York, and the chief of general internal medicine at the University of Chicago. Dr. Cassel is a prolific scholar, having authored and edited 14 books and more than 200 published articles.

Carolyn M. Clancy, M.D., is the chief medical officer of the Veterans Health Administration. Previously, she was appointed the assistant deputy under secretary for health (ADUSH) for quality, safety, and value (QSV) for the Department of Veterans Affairs. Prior to her appointment as ADUSH for QSV, Dr. Clancy served as the director of the Agency for Healthcare Research and Quality (AHRQ) from February 2003 to August 2013. Dr. Clancy, a general internist and health services researcher, is a graduate of Boston College and the University of Massachusetts Medical School. Following clinical training in internal medicine, she was a Henry J. Kaiser Family Foundation Fellow at the University of Pennsylvania. Before joining AHRQ in 1990, she was also an assistant professor in the Department of Internal Medicine at the Medical College of Virginia. Dr. Clancy holds an academic appointment at the George Washington University School of Medicine (clinical associate professor, Department of Medicine) and serves as a senior associate editor at *Health Services Research*. She serves on multiple editorial boards, including those for *JAMA*, *Annals of Family Medicine*, *American Journal of Medical Quality*, and *Medical Care Research and Review*. She is a member of the National Academy of Medicine and was elected a Master of the American College of Physicians in 2004. In 2009 she was awarded the William B. Graham Prize for Health Services Research. Her major research interests include improving health care quality and patient safety and reducing disparities in care associated with patients' race, ethnicity, gender, income, and education. As director of AHRQ, she launched the first annual report to the Congress on health care disparities and health care quality.

Michael B. Cohen, M.D., is a medical director in the Anatomic Pathology and Oncology Division at ARUP Laboratories, a professor and vice chair for faculty and house staff development at the University of Utah School of Medicine, and the ombudsperson for the University of Utah Health Sciences Center. Dr. Cohen received his M.D. from Albany Medical College and completed his anatomic pathology residency at the University of California, San Francisco (UCSF). Dr. Cohen has been on the faculty at Columbia, UCSF, and the University of Iowa; he was chair of the Department of Pathology at Iowa for more than a dozen years. In addition, he has served on numerous editorial boards. He has been a National Institutes of Health–funded investigator and has published extensively in the field of prostate cancer and pathology. He is the recipient of multiple honors, including the Regents Award for Faculty Excellence at the University of Iowa and the Leonard Tow Humanism in Medicine Award. Dr. Cohen has been included in Castle Connolly American's Top Doctors since 2007 and America's Top Doctors for Cancer since 2005; Consumers' Research Council of America Guide to America's Top Pathologists since 2007; and Best Doctors in America list since 2005.

Patrick Croskerry, M.D., Ph.D., FRCP (Edin), is a professor in emergency medicine and in the Division of Medical Education at Dalhousie University, Halifax, Nova Scotia, Canada. He was appointed the director of the new Critical Thinking Program at Dalhousie Medical School in 2012. In addition to his medical training, he holds a doctorate in experimental psychology and a fellowship in clinical psychology. His research is principally concerned with clinical decision making, specifically on diagnostic error. He was on the organizing committee of the first national conference on diagnostic error in 2008 and the second one in 2009; he has contributed at each international conference since. He has published more than 80 journal articles and 30 book chapters in the area of patient safety, clinical decision making, and medical education reform. He was the senior editor on a major text, *Patient Safety in Emergency Medicine* (2009).

Thomas H. Gallagher, M.D., FACP, is a general internist who is professor and associate chair of the Department of Medicine at the University of Washington (UW), where is also professor in the Department of Bioethics and Humanities. Dr. Gallagher received his medical degree from Harvard University, completed his residency in Internal Medicine at Barnes Hospital, Washington University, St. Louis, and completed a fellowship in the Robert Wood Johnson Clinical Scholars Program, University of California, San Francisco. Dr. Gallagher's research addresses the interfaces between health care quality, communication, and transparency. Dr. Gallagher has published more than 95 articles and book chapters on patient safety and error disclosure, which have appeared in leading journals, including *JAMA*, *New England Journal of Medicine*, *Health Affairs*, *Surgery*, *Journal of Clinical Oncology*, *Archives of Internal Medicine*, *Archives of Pediatric and Adolescent Medicine*, and the *Joint Commission Journal*. His work in error disclosure received the 2004 Best Published Research Paper of the Year award from the Society of General Internal Medicine, as well as the 2012 Medically Induced Trauma Support Services Hope Award. He also received a Robert Wood Johnson Foundation Investigator Award in Health Policy Research. He has been principal investigator on multiple grants from the Agency for Healthcare Research and Quality, including a patient safety and medical liability demonstration project titled "Communication to Prevent and Respond to Medical Injuries: WA State Collaborative." He also was principal investigator on grants from the National Cancer Institute, the Robert Wood Johnson Foundation, and the Greenwall Foundation. He is senior author of *Talking with Patients and Families About Medical Errors: A Guide for Education and Practice*, published in 2011 by the Johns Hopkins University Press. At UW, he directs both the UW Medicine Center for Scholarship in Patient Care Quality and Safety and the UW Program in Hospital Medicine. He is an appointed Commissioner on the National Commission on Physician Payment Reform. Dr. Gallagher is an active member of many professional organizations, including the American College of Physicians (Fellow), the Society for General Internal Medicine, and the American Society of Bioethics and Humanities.

Christine A. Goeschel, Sc.D., M.P.A., M.P.S., R.N., F.A.A.N., is a health services researcher and the assistant vice president for quality at MedStar Health, a 10-hospital, $4.6 billion health system in the mid-Atlantic, where she oversees quality for both acute and non-acute health care services. She is a Fellow of the American Academy of Nursing, a National Baldrige Examiner, and associate faculty in the Johns Hopkins Bloomberg School of Public Health, where she teaches a required course in the Master of Hospital Administration program. Formerly the director of strategic research initiatives at the Johns Hopkins Armstrong Institute, Dr. Goeschel serves on the board of the Maryland Patient Safety Center and is the author of several book chapters and more than 65 peer-reviewed articles on topics ranging from implementation of large-scale clinical improvement projects to leadership for advancing the science of health care delivery and creating a culture of accountability in health care. Previous experience includes responsibility for quality, risk management, and service excellence in a Midwest teaching hospital and serving as an advisor to the World Health Organization Patient Safety Program. She served on the National Quality Forum (NQF) National Steering Committee for Serious Reportable Events and Healthcare Associated Conditions and currently serves on an NQF panel exploring linkages between cost and quality. She is increasingly interested in the study of diagnostic errors—both their etiology and understanding the relationship of diagnostic error with preventable morbidity, mortality, and costs of care.

Mark L. Graber, M.D., FACP, is a senior fellow at RTI International and professor emeritus of medicine at the State University of New York at Stony Brook. He retired as the chief of medicine at the Northport Veterans Affairs Medical Center in 2011. Dr. Graber has an extensive background in biomedical and health services research, with more than 80 peer-reviewed publications. He is a national leader in the field of patient safety and originated Patient Safety Awareness Week in 2002, an event now recognized internationally. Dr. Graber has also been a pioneer in efforts to address diagnostic errors in medicine. In 2008 he convened and chaired the Diagnostic Error in Medicine conference series, and in 2011 he founded the Society to Improve Diagnosis in Medicine (www.improvediagnosis. org). In 2014 he became the founding editor of a new journal, *Diagnosis*, devoted to improving the quality and safety of diagnosis, and he received the John M. Eisenberg Award for Individual Achievement in Advancing Patient Safety from the National Quality Forum and The Joint Commission.

Hedvig Hricak, M.D., Dr.Med.Sc. (Ph.D.), Dr.h.c., is the chair of the Department of Radiology at Memorial Sloan Kettering Cancer Center, a professor in the Gerstner Sloan Kettering Graduate School of Biomedical Sciences, and a professor of radiology at the Weill Medical College of Cornell University. She also holds a senior position within the Molecular Pharmacology and Chemistry Program of the Sloan Kettering Institute. Previously, she was chief of the uroradiology and abdominal imaging sections of the Department of Radiology, University of California, San Francisco. She earned her M.D. from the University of Zagreb in Croatia, and her Dr.Med.Sc. (Ph.D.) from the Karolinska Institute in Stockholm, Sweden. Her research and clinical expertise is in the use of diagnostic imaging, specifically for the detection and assessment of genitourinary and gynecological cancers. She has worked continuously to develop and promote the use of evidence-based imaging algorithms to assist in cancer management, focusing on the development and validation of biomarkers from cross-sectional (ultrasound, MRI, CT) and molecular (DCE-MRI, MR spectroscopy, PET/CT and PET/MRI) imaging. Over the last 20 years, while serving in administrative leadership positions, she has been actively engaged in continuous process improvement and quality assurance efforts. Dr. Hricak served on the National Institutes of Health Board of Scientific Counselors, the National Cancer Institute (NCI) board of scientific advisors, and the Advisory Council of the National Institute of Biomedical Imaging and Bioengineering. She is a member of the National Academy of Medicine. She served on the Institute of Medicine committee that produced the report *A National Cancer Clinical Trials System for the 21st Century: Reinvigorating the NCI Cooperative Group Program.* Since 2008 she has been a member of the Nuclear Radiation Studies Board of the National Academies of Sciences, Engineering, and Medicine. She chaired the Academies Committee on the State of the Science of Nuclear Medicine, which wrote the oft-cited report *Advancing Nuclear Medicine Through Innovation.* In addition, she chaired the 2009 Beebe symposium of the Academies, which focused on radiation exposures from imaging and image-guided interventions. The many leadership posts she has held in professional organizations include president of the California Academy of Medicine and president of the Radiological Society of North America board of directors. Over the course of her career, she has received numerous honors and awards, including foreign membership in both the Croatian Academy of Arts and Sciences and the Russian Academy of Medicine, and an honorary doctorate in medicine from Ludwig Maximilian University in Munich, Germany.

Anupam B. Jena, M.D., Ph.D., is an associate professor of health care policy and medicine at Harvard Medical School and an attending physician in the Department of Medicine at Massachusetts General Hospital, where he practices general inpatient medicine and teaches medical residents. He is also a faculty research fellow at the National Bureau of Economic Research. As an economist and a physician, Dr. Jena researches several areas of health economics and policy, including medical malpractice, the economics of medical innovation and cost effectiveness, the economics of physician behavior, and the effect on physician quality of reforms to medical education. Dr. Jena graduated Phi Beta Kappa from the Massachusetts Institute of Technology with majors in biology and economics. He received his M.D. and Ph.D. in economics from the University of Chicago. He completed his residency in internal medicine at Massachusetts General Hospital. In 2007 he was awarded the Eugene Garfield Award by Research America for his work demonstrating the economic value of medical innovation in HIV/AIDS. In 2013 he received the National Institutes of Health Director's Early Independence Award to fund research on the physician determinants of health care spending, quality, and patient outcomes.

Ashish K. Jha, M.D., M.P.H., is the K.T. Li Professor of International Health and director of the Harvard Global Health Institute at the Harvard T.H. Chan School of Public Health. He is also a practicing general internist with a clinical focus on hospital care. Over the past 6 years he has served as a senior advisor for quality and safety to the Department of Veterans Affairs (VA). Dr. Jha received his M.D. from Harvard Medical School in 1997 and trained in internal medicine at the University of California, San Francisco, where he also served as the chief medical resident. He completed his general medicine fellowship from Brigham and Women's Hospital and Harvard Medical School and received his M.P.H. in clinical effectiveness from the Harvard School of Public Health in 2004. He joined the faculty in July 2004. The major themes of his research include the impact of public policy on the health care delivery system with a focus on patient safety, clinical outcomes, and costs of care. Much of his work has focused on understanding how policy efforts such as public reporting, pay for performance, and the promotion of the use of health information technology affect clinical quality, patient safety, and health care costs. Dr. Jha's most recent work has focused on key levers for improvement, including organizational leadership and how it affects the delivery of safe, effective, and efficient care.

Michael Laposata, M.D., Ph.D., is the chair of the Department of Pathology at the University of Texas Medical Branch at Galveston. He received his M.D. and Ph.D. from Johns Hopkins University School of Medicine and completed a postdoctoral research fellowship and residency in Laboratory Medicine (Clinical Pathology) at the Washington University School of Medicine in St. Louis. He took his first faculty position at the University of Pennsylvania School of Medicine in Philadelphia in 1985, where he was an assistant professor and director of the hospital's coagulation laboratory. In 1989 he became the director of clinical laboratories at the Massachusetts General Hospital and was appointed to the faculty in pathology at Harvard Medical School, where he became a tenured full professor of pathology. His research program, with more than 160 peer-reviewed publications, has focused on fatty acids and their metabolites. His research group is currently focused on the study of fatty acid alterations in cystic fibrosis. Dr. Laposata's clinical expertise is in the field of blood coagulation, with a special expertise in the diagnosis of hypercoagulable states. Dr. Laposata implemented a system whereby the clinical laboratory data in coagulation and other areas of laboratory medicine are systematically interpreted with the generation of a patient-specific narrative paragraph by a physician with expertise in the area. This service is essentially identical to the service provided by physicians in radiology and anatomic pathology except that it involves clinical laboratory test results. In 2005 Dr. Laposata was recognized by the Institute of Quality in Laboratory Medicine of the Centers for Disease Control and Prevention for this innovation. Dr. Laposata is the recipient of 14 major teaching prizes at Harvard, the Massachusetts General Hospital, and the University of Pennsylvania School of Medicine. His recognitions include the 1989 Lindback award, a teaching prize with competition across the entire University of Pennsylvania system; the 1998 A. Clifford Barger mentorship award from Harvard Medical School; election to the Harvard Academy of Scholars in 2002 and to the Vanderbilt University School of Medicine Academy for Excellence in Teaching in 2009; and the highest award—by vote of the graduating class—for teaching in years 1 and 2 at Harvard Medical School in 1999, 2000, and 2005.

Kathryn McDonald, M.M., has more than 20 years of experience in health care, working in a variety of settings: industry, hospitals, and academia. She is the executive director of the Center for Health Policy and the Center for Primary Care and Outcomes Research (CHP/PCOR) at Stanford University, a senior scholar at the centers, and the associate director for the Stanford–University of California, San Francisco, Evidence-Based Practice Center (with RAND). Her research focuses on evidence-based health care quality measures and interventions, with an emphasis on organizational context and key health care stakeholders (patients/families, clinicians, systems administrators). Her research portfolio includes initial and ongoing development of the publicly released Agency for Healthcare Research and Quality (AHRQ) Patient Safety and Quality Indicators (www.qualityindicators.ahrq.gov), reviews of patient safety practices (*Making Healthcare Safer I* and *II*), and two series of evidence reports on quality improvement strategies (*Closing the Quality Gap, Quality Kaleidoscope*). She continues to lead a multi-institution measure development team for support of and expansions to the AHRQ Quality Indicators. She is the lead author of the *Care Coordination Measures Atlas* (www.ahrq.gov/qual/careatlas). She has published more than 100 peer-reviewed articles and evidence reports, presents regularly at national meetings, and collaborates with a wide network of investigators, health care practitioners, and patients and their families. Ms. McDonald has a strong service record, currently as the chair of the Patient Engagement Committee of the Society to Improve Diagnosis in Medicine and the associate editor of the journal *Diagnosis*. Previously, she was the president of the Society for Medical Decision Making and a member of the Institute of Medicine committee that issued the report *Child and Adolescent Health and Health Care Quality: Measuring What Matters*. She holds a master of management degree (M.B.A. equivalent) from Northwestern University's Kellogg School of Management, with an emphasis on the health care industry and organizational behavior, and a B.S. in chemical engineering from Stanford University.

Elizabeth A. McGlynn, Ph.D., is the director of Kaiser Permanente's Center for Effectiveness and Safety Research (CESR). She is responsible for the strategic direction and scientific oversight of CESR, a virtual center designed to improve the health and well-being of Kaiser's 9 million members and the public by conducting comparative effectiveness and safety research and implementing findings in policy and practice. Dr. McGlynn is an internationally known expert on methods for evaluating the appropriateness, quality, and efficiency of health care delivery. She has conducted research in the United States and in other countries. Dr. McGlynn has also led major initiatives to evaluate health reform options under consideration at the federal and state levels. Dr. McGlynn is a member of the National Academy of Medicine. She serves as the secretary and treasurer of the American Board of Internal Medicine Foundation board of trustees. She is on the board of AcademyHealth, the Institute of Medicine Board on Health Care Services of the National Academies of Sciences, Engineering, and Medicine, and the Reagan–Udall Foundation for the Food and Drug Administration. She chairs the scientific advisory group for the Institute for Healthcare Improvement. She co-chairs the coordinating committee for the National Quality Forum's Measures Application Partnership. She serves on the editorial boards for *Health Services Research* and *The Milbank Quarterly* and is a regular reviewer for many leading journals. Dr. McGlynn received her B.A. in international political economy from Colorado College, her M.P.P. from the University of Michigan's Gerald R. Ford School of Public Policy, and her Ph.D. in public policy analysis from the Pardee RAND Graduate School.

Michelle Rogers, Ph.D., is an associate professor in the College of Computing and Informatics at Drexel University. She has more than 10 years of experience using human factors engineering methods and sociotechnical systems theory to study the impact of health information technology (health IT) on clinical workflow and the usability of technology in order to support patient safety and reduce human error. Over her career, her projects focused on understanding the impact of health IT on clinical workflow and patient safety, as is demonstrated in her work with the Computerized Patient Record System, the Bar-Code Medication Administration system, and MyHealthVet (Veterans Affairs patient portal) in use at the Veterans Health Administration where she was a faculty research scientist. Her current work involves applying human factors engineering methods to study health care practices, information and data needs related to maternal/child care, as well as the implementation and use of electronic medical records at Makerere University in Uganda.

Urmimala Sarkar, M.D., M.P.H., is associate professor of medicine at the University of California, San Francisco (UCSF), in the Division of General Internal Medicine, a core faculty member of the UCSF Center for Vulnerable Populations, and a primary care physician at San Francisco General Hospital's Richard H. Fine People's Clinic. Dr. Sarkar's research focuses on patient safety in outpatient settings, including adverse drug events, missed and delayed diagnosis, failures of treatment monitoring, health information technology and social media to improve the safety and quality of outpatient care, and implementation of evidence-based innovations in real-world, safety-net care settings. She is the principal investigator of a Patient Safety Learning Laboratory, which applies design thinking and interdisciplinary, iterative approaches to characterize and address safety gaps in outpatient settings (Agency for Healthcare Research and Quality P30HS023558), and of an implementation and dissemination network to support innovations to improve the safety and quality of care in safety-net settings across California (Agency for Healthcare Research and Quality R24HS022047). Dr. Sarkar is an associate editor for Patient Safety Net (psnet.ahrq.gov), the most comprehensive national Web-based resource for patient safety, and a member of the editorial board of the *Joint Commission Journal of Quality and Patient Safety*. Dr. Sarkar completed clinical training in internal medicine and health services research fellowship training at UCSF, holds an M.P.H. in epidemiology from the University of California, Berkeley, an M.D. from the University of California, San Diego, and a B.S. with honors in biological sciences from Stanford University.

George E. Thibault, M.D., became the seventh president of the Josiah Macy Jr. Foundation in January 2008. Immediately prior to that, he served as the vice president of clinical affairs at Partners Healthcare System in Boston and the director of the Academy at Harvard Medical School (HMS). He was the first Daniel D. Federman Professor of Medicine and Medical Education at HMS and is now the Federman Professor, Emeritus. Dr. Thibault previously served as the chief medical officer at Brigham and Women's Hospital and as the chief of medicine at the Harvard-affiliated Brockton/West Roxbury Veterans Affairs Hospital. He was the associate chief of medicine and the director of the Internal Medical Residency Program at the Massachusetts General Hospital (MGH). At the MGH he also served as the director of the Medical Intensive Care Unit and the founding director of the Medical Practice Evaluation Unit. For nearly four decades at HMS, Dr. Thibault played leadership roles in many aspects of undergraduate and graduate medical education. He played a central role in the New Pathway curriculum reform and was a leader in the new integrated curriculum reform at HMS. He was the founding director of the Academy at HMS, which was created to recognize outstanding teachers and to promote innovations in medical education. Throughout his career he has been recognized for his roles in teaching and mentoring medical students, residents, fellows, and junior faculty. In addition to his teaching, his research has focused on the evaluation of practices and outcomes of medical intensive care and variations in the use of cardiac technologies. Dr. Thibault is chair of the board of the MGH Institute of Health Professions, and he serves on the boards of the New York Academy of Sciences, the New York Academy of Medicine, the Institute on Medicine as a Profession, the New York Academy of Medicine, and the Lebanese American University. He serves on the President's White House Fellows Commission, and for 12 years he chaired the Special Medical Advisory Group for the Department of Veterans Affairs. He is past president of the Harvard Medical Alumni Association and past chair of alumni relations at HMS. He is a member of the National Academy of Medicine. Dr. Thibault graduated summa cum laude from Georgetown University in 1965 and magna cum laude from HMS in 1969. He completed his internship and residency in medicine and fellowship in cardiology at MGH. He also trained in cardiology at the National Heart, Lung, and Blood Institute in Bethesda and at Guys Hospital in London, and he served as chief resident in medicine at MGH. Dr. Thibault has been the recipient of numerous awards and honors from Georgetown (Ryan Prize in Philosophy, Alumni Prize, and Cohongaroton Speaker) and Harvard (Alpha Omega Alpha, Henry Asbury Christian Award, and Society of Fellows). He has been a visiting scholar both at the Institute of Medicine and Harvard's Kennedy School of Government and a visiting professor of medicine at numerous medical schools in the United States and abroad.

John B. Wong, M.D., FACP, is a practicing general internist, the chief of the Division of Clinical Decision Making at Tufts Medical Center, the director of Comparative Effectiveness Research at Tufts Clinical Translational Science Institute, and a distinguished professor of medicine at Tufts University School of Medicine. A graduate of Haverford College, he received his M.D. from the University of Chicago followed by internal medicine residency and medical informatics fellowship in Clinical Decision Making at Tufts Medical Center. A past president of the Society for Medical Decision Making, he has participated in consensus conferences, guideline development and appropriateness use criteria assessment for the World Health Organization, National Institutes of Health, Centers for Disease Control and Prevention, Agency for Healthcare Research and Quality, American Association for the Study of Liver Diseases, American Heart Association, American College of Cardiology, European League Against Rheumatism, and OMERACT. Besides translating guidelines into quality improvement and performance measures in the American Medical Association Physician Consortium for Performance Improvement Work Groups, he has developed award-winning decision aids for shared decision making with the Informed Medical Decisions Foundation. Dr. Wong's research focuses on the application of decision analysis to help patients, physicians, and policy makers choose among alternative tests, treatments, and policies, thereby promoting rational evidence-based efficient and effective patient-centered care. A co-author of *Learning Clinical Reasoning* and *Decision Making in Health and Medicine* and more than 150 scientific publications and book chapters, including the *Reference Manual on Scientific Evidence* for the National Academy of Sciences, his research areas include clinical and diagnostic reasoning, decision sciences, test interpretation, Bayesian methods, quality and appropriateness of care, health economics, patient-centeredness, shared decision making, and evidence-based medicine.

STAFF BIOGRAPHIES

Erin Balogh, M.P.H., is a program officer for the Institute of Medicine's Board on Health Care Services and the National Cancer Policy Forum (NCPF) of the National Academies of Sciences, Engineering, and Medicine. She has directed NCPF workshops on patient-centered cancer treatment planning, affordable cancer care, precompetitive collaboration, combination cancer therapies, and reducing tobacco-related cancer incidence and mortality. She staffed consensus studies focusing on the quality of cancer care, omics-based test development, the national clinical trials system, and the evaluation of biomarkers and surrogate endpoints. She completed her M.P.H. in health management and policy at the University of Michigan School of Public Health, and she graduated summa cum laude from Arizona State University with bachelor's degrees in microbiology and psychology. Ms. Balogh interned with AcademyHealth in Washington, DC, and worked as a research site coordinator for the Urban Institute in Topeka, Kansas. Previously, Ms. Balogh was a management intern with the Arizona State University Office of University Initiatives, a strategic planning group for the university. She was the recipient of the Institute of Medicine Above and Beyond award (2014) and the staff team achievement award (2012).

Bryan Miller, Ph.D., is a research associate for the Institute of Medicine's Board on Health Care Services of the National Academies of Sciences, Engineering, and Medicine. He earned an M.A. from the Brains and Behavior program at Georgia State University in 2007, and he completed his Ph.D. in philosophy of science at Johns Hopkins University in the summer of 2014. He has performed research at the Berlin School of Mind and Brain and Charité University Hospital in Berlin and taught courses in the philosophy of science, the philosophy of psychology, and bioethics at several universities in the Baltimore–Washington, DC, area.

Sarah Naylor, Ph.D., completed a Ph.D. in developmental biology at Washington University in 2012 and earned a B.S. with distinction in bioengineering from the University of Illinois. She performed postdoctoral research at the National Institutes of Health and worked as an intern in the Office of Autism Research Coordination within the National Institute of Mental Health. She is currently a Science & Technology Policy Fellow with the American Association for the Advancement of Science in Evaluation and Assessment in the Office of the Assistant Director for Engineering.

Kathryn Garnham Ellett, M.P.P., is a policy analyst for the Assistant Secretary for Financial Resources at the Department of Health and Human Services (HHS), where she has been working on Centers for Medicare & Medicaid Services (CMS) policy since 2010. She was on detail as a research associate for the Institute of Medicine Board on Health Care Services of the National Academies of Sciences, Engineering, and Medicine from April through July 2015. At HHS her portfolio includes Medicare post-acute care and hospice, Medicare Quality Improvement Organizations, and CMS's survey and certification program. She completed her M.P.P. at the University of Toronto in 2010 and her B.S. at Queen's University in Kingston, Ontario. Prior to her time at HHS she worked in home health care. She also worked for a hospital system implementing an eldercare access strategy in emergency rooms and has researched nursing home staffing and palliative care.

Celynne Balatbat is the special assistant to the president of the National Academy of Medicine. Previously, she was a research assistant with the Institute of Medicine's Board on Health Care Services of the National Academies of Sciences, Engineering, and Medicine. She received her B.A. in neuroscience and behavior from Vassar College in 2013. Before coming to the Academies, she interned in the advocacy department at AARP California and worked as a laboratory assistant in a medical microbiology lab at the University of California, Davis.

Patrick Ross is a research assistant with the Institute of Medicine's Board on Health Care Services and National Cancer Policy Forum of the National Academies of Sciences, Engineering, and Medicine. Patrick graduated from Concordia College in Moorhead, Minnesota, in 2013 with a B.A. in psychology with minors in biology and chemistry, where his senior research project focused on bacteriocins in *Neisseria meningitidis*.

Before joining the Academies, Patrick worked in various health advocacy groups, including Families USA.

Laura Rosema, Ph.D., joined the Institute of Medicine's Board on Health Care Services of the National Academies of Sciences, Engineering, and Medicine as part of the Winter 2015 Christine Mirzayan Science and Technology Policy Fellowship class. Prior to the fellowship, she served as the scientific advisor for Bill Gates's Global Good Fund, a private initiative chartered to commercialize inventions in developing countries. At Global Good, Dr. Rosema advised on investment strategy and technical directions for the fund. She has led evaluations on topics that include using biometric signatures for health record tracking, implantable medical devices, and diagnostic development for malaria elimination programs. She received her Ph.D. in chemistry from the University of Washington and earned her master's and bachelor's degrees in inorganic chemistry from Bryn Mawr College. She is currently a Science & Technology Policy Fellow with the American Association for the Advancement of Science serving in the National Institutes of Health Office of Science Policy, in the Office of Science Management and Reporting.

Beatrice Kalisch, R.N., Ph.D., FAAN, is the 2013 Distinguished Nurse Scholar in residence at the Institute of Medicine and the Titus Professor at the University of Michigan in Ann Arbor. She has conducted numerous research studies on such subjects as nursing teamwork, missed nursing care (errors of omission), the image of the nurse, and the impact of U.S. federal funds on nursing education and practice. Dr. Kalisch has published extensively, authoring 10 books and more than 150 peer-reviewed articles. She has made more than 800 presentations of her research throughout the world. She serves on the editorial boards of several national and international journals. Dr. Kalisch has also served as a visiting professor at several institutions, including Huazhong University of Science and Technology, Tongji Medical College, Wuhan, China, and the University of Sao Paulo, Brazil. She is listed in numerous bibliographies, such as *Who's Who in America* and *Who's Who of American Women, Who's Who in the World, Foremost Women of the Twentieth Century*, and *Community Leaders of the World*. Dr. Kalisch is a Fellow in the American Academy of Nursing and a member of Phi Kappa Phi. She serves as a member as well as leader in numerous local, state, and national advisory committees addressing health policy and nursing issues. Dr. Kalisch has been the recipient of many awards, including distinguished alumna at both the University of Maryland and the University of Nebraska, the Shaw Medal from the President of Boston College, the Department of Labor research award, Joseph L. Andrews Bibliographic Award from the American Association of Law Libraries, book of the year awards, nurse researcher award from the American Organization of Nurse Executives, and the Sigma Theta Tau Award for Excellence in Nursing.

Roger Herdman, M.D., was the director of the Institute of Medicine's (IOM's) Board on Health Care Services of the National Academies of Sciences, Engineering, and Medicine until June 2014. He received his undergraduate and medical school degrees from Yale University. Following an internship at the University of Minnesota and a stint in the U.S. Navy, he returned to Minnesota, where he completed a residency in pediatrics and a fellowship in immunology and nephrology and also served on the faculty. He was a professor of pediatrics at Albany Medical College until 1979. In 1969 Dr. Herdman was appointed director of the New York State Kidney Disease Institute in Albany, New York, and shortly thereafter was appointed deputy commissioner of the New York State Department of Health, a position he held until 1977. That year he was named New York State's director of public health. From 1979 until joining the U.S. Congress Office of Technology Assessment (OTA), he served as a vice president of Memorial Sloan Kettering Cancer Center in New York City. In 1983 Dr. Herdman was named assistant director of OTA, where he subsequently served as director from 1993 to 1996. He later joined the IOM as a senior scholar and directed studies on graduate medical education, organ transplantation, silicone breast implants, and the Department of Veterans Affairs national formulary. Dr. Herdman was appointed director of the IOM/National Research Council National Cancer Policy Board from 2000 through 2005. From 2005 until 2009, Dr. Herdman directed the IOM National Cancer Policy Forum. In 2007 he was also appointed director of the IOM Board on Health Care Services. During his work at the IOM, Dr. Herdman worked closely with the U.S. Congress on a wide variety of health care policy issues.

Sharyl Nass, Ph.D., is director of the Board on Health Care Services and director of the National Cancer Policy Forum for the Institute of Medicine (IOM) of the National Academies of Sciences, Engineering, and Medicine. The Board addresses the organization, financing, effectiveness, workforce, and delivery of health care to ensure the best possible care for all patients. The Cancer Forum examines policy issues pertaining to the entire continuum of cancer research and care.

For more than 15 years at the IOM, Dr. Nass has worked on a broad range of topics that includes the quality of care, clinical trials, oversight of health research, development and assessment of medical technologies, and strategies for large-scale biomedical science. She has a Ph.D. in cell and tumor biology from Georgetown University and undertook postdoctoral training at the Johns Hopkins University School of Medicine. She also holds a B.S. in genetics from the University of Wisconsin–Madison, and she studied developmental genetics and molecular biology at the Max Planck Institute in Germany under a fellowship from the Heinrich Hertz-Stiftung Foundation. She was the 2007 recipient of the Cecil Award for Excellence in Health Policy Research, the 2010 recipient of a Distinguished Service Award from the Academies, and the 2012 recipient of the IOM staff team achievement award (as the team leader).

Appendix C

Previous Diagnostic Error Frameworks

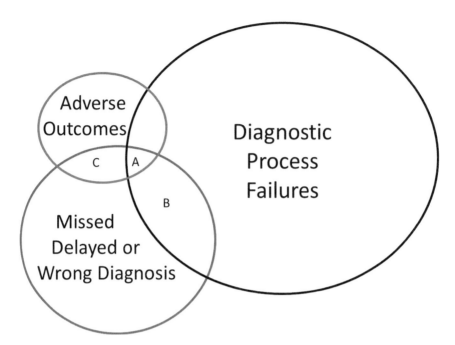

FIGURE C-1 Venn diagram illustrating relationships between errors in the diagnostic process; missed, delayed, or wrong diagnoses; and adverse patient outcomes. Group A represents adverse outcomes resulting from error-related misdiagnosis (pathology specimens erroneously mixed up [diagnostic process error], resulting in wrong patient being given diagnosis of cancer [misdiagnosis] who then undergoes surgery with adverse outcome [adverse event]). Group B represents delayed diagnoses or misdiagnoses due to process error (positive urine culture overlooked, thus a urinary tract infection is not diagnosed but patient has no symptoms or adverse consequences). Group C represents adverse events due to misdiagnoses but no identifiable process error (death from acute myocardial infarction but no chest pain or other symptoms that were missed).
SOURCES: Adapted from Schiff et al., 2005, and Schiff and Leape, 2012.

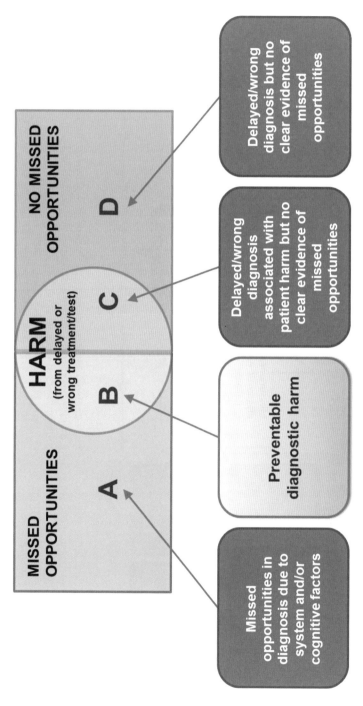

FIGURE C-2 Singh's diagnostic error framework, which employs the term "missed opportunity" to imply "that something different could have been done to make the correct diagnosis earlier."
SOURCE: Singh, 2014. © Joint Commission Resources: Joint Commission *Journal on Quality and Patient Safety*. Oakbrook Terrace, IL: Joint Commission on Accreditation of Healthcare Organizations (2014), 40(3), (100). Figure. Reprinted with permission.

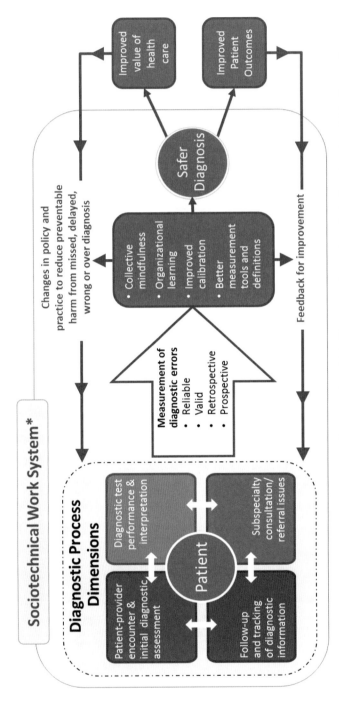

FIGURE C-3 Singh and Sittig's diagnostic error framework, which illustrates the sociotechnical system in which diagnosis occurs and opportunities to measure and learn from diagnostic errors to improve diagnosis and patient and system outcomes.

NOTE: * Includes eight technological and non-technological dimensions.

SOURCE: Reproduced from BMJ *Quality and Safety*, H. Singh and D. F. Sittig, 24(2), 103–110, 2015 with permission from BMJ Publishing Group Limited.

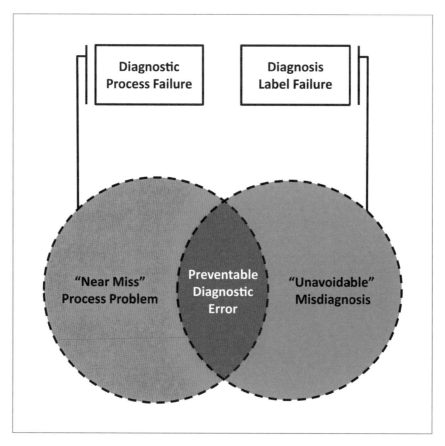

FIGURE C-4 Newman-Toker's diagnostic error framework, which defines preventable diagnostic error as the overlap between diagnostic process failures and diagnostic label failures.
SOURCE: Reprinted, with permission, from David Newman-Toker, A unified conceptual model for diagnostic errors: Underdiagnosis, overdiagnosis, and misdiagnosis; in *Diagnosis* 1(1), 2014, pp. 43–48.

434

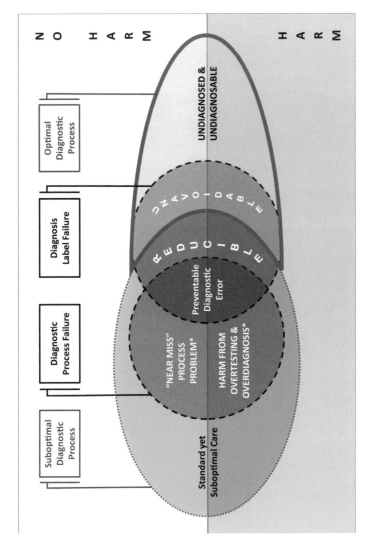

FIGURE C-5 Newman-Toker's diagnostic error framework, including suboptimal diagnostic process and optimal diagnostic process, as well as reducible and unavoidable diagnostic error.

NOTE: * "Near misses" and harm from overtesting and overdiagnosis also result from suboptimal diagnostic processes.

SOURCE: Reprinted, with permission, from David Newman-Toker, A unified conceptual model for diagnostic errors: Underdiagnosis, overdiagnosis, and misdiagnosis; in *Diagnosis* 1(1), 2014, pp. 43–48.

REFERENCES

Newman-Toker, D. E. 2014. A unified conceptual model for diagnostic errors: Under-diagnosis, overdiagnosis, and misdiagnosis. *Diagnosis* 1(1):43–48.

Schiff, G. D., and L. L. Leape. 2012. Commentary: How can we make diagnosis safer? *Academic Medicine* 87(2):135–138.

Schiff, G. D., S. Kim, R. Abrams, K. Cosby, B. Lambert, A. S. Elstein, S. Hasler, N. Krosnjar, R. Odwazny, M. F. Wisniewski, and R. A. McNutt. 2005. Diagnosing diagnosis errors: Lessons from a multi-institutional collaborative project. In K. Henriksen, J. B. Battles, E. S. Marks, and D. I. Lewin (eds.), *Advances in Patient Safety: From Research to Implementation (Volume 2: Concepts and Methodology)*. AHRQ Publication No. 05-0021-2. Rockville, MD: Agency for Healthcare Research and Quality. www.ncbi.nlm.nih.gov/books/NBK20492/pdf/Bookshelf_NBK20492.pdf (accessed Novembe 7, 2015).

Singh, H. 2014. Editorial: Helping health care organizations to define diagnostic errors as missed opportunities in diagnosis. *Joint Commission Journal on Quality and Patient Safety* 40(3):99–101.

Singh, H., and D. F. Sittig. 2015. Advancing the science of measurement of diagnostic errors in healthcare: The Safer Dx framework. *BMJ Quality and Safety* 24(2):103–110.

Appendix D

Examples of Diagnostic Error

Whereas the title of the Institute of Medicine (IOM) report *To Err Is Human: Building a Safer Health System* focused on human error, the primary focus of that report was describing the range of work system factors that can affect errors (IOM, 2000). The report emphasized the need to go beyond acute failure and the need to understand latent failures and the range of work system factors that contribute to errors over time. Consistent with the earlier IOM report, this report on diagnostic error in health care also emphasizes the need to look at errors in the diagnostic process, which is embedded in a larger work system.

The case studies presented in this appendix provide snapshots of various diagnostic errors. It is important to understand that a range of work system factors could have contributed to these diagnostic errors. As highlighted in the conceptual model (see Figures S-1 and S-2) and described in Chapters 2 and 3, the diagnostic process unfolds over time; various people and care settings are involved (e.g., outpatient care settings, hospitals, emergency departments, and long-term care settings), and multiple work systems factors (e.g., information flow and communication, the engagement of patients, culture, training and education, usable and useful technology) can contribute to diagnostic errors, including those briefly described in Box D-1.

437

BOX D-1
Examples of Diagnostic Error

Lack of appreciation for significant elements of the patient's history and physical exam led to a missed pulmonary embolism

A 33-year-old obese patient with remote history of asthma, and on oral contraceptives, presented to her primary care clinician with a three-day complaint of right thigh pain, swelling, and red streaking on her skin. On exam, her right inguinal lymph nodes were enlarged and antibiotics were prescribed. Three days later, she returned with complaint of new onset shortness of breath, chest pain, and rapid heart rate. The patient had diminished breath sounds. Her physician thought she was having an asthma flare and advised her to continue antibiotics and asthma medications. Later the same day, emergency personnel were called to the patient's home after she fell. She was brought to a local Emergency Department where she quickly decompensated and died. Autopsy revealed a large pulmonary thromboembolism.

SOURCE: CRICO, 2014. Reprinted with permission from CRICO/Risk Management Foundation of the Harvard Medical Institutions.

A misread X-ray of patient with pneumonia led to respiratory failure and death

A 55-year-old male was diagnosed by his primary care clinician with sinusitis and prescribed an antibiotic. Six days later, he was evaluated in an urgent care clinic for shortness of breath, labored breathing, extreme fatigue, and chest pain with cough. The patient had a temperature, a fast heart rate, and low oxygen saturation. After he was treated with an aerosolized nebulizer his oxygen saturation improved. Based on her negative interpretation of a chest X-ray, the urgent care clinician diagnosed a viral [upper respiratory infection] and instructed the patient to see his family doctor the next day. Two days later, the X-ray was read by a radiologist with impression of pneumonia. The clinic called the patient and instructed him to go to his local Emergency Department [ED] for evaluation and treatment. Before he could get to the ED, the patient died of respiratory failure associated with pneumonia.

SOURCE: CRICO, 2014. Reprinted with permission from CRICO/Risk Management Foundation of the Harvard Medical Institutions.

Multiple missteps in the referral process preceded patient's death from cardiac failure

A 51-year-old female with a history of attention deficit disorder and hyperlipidemia had been treated by her primary care physician for 14 years. Her high cholesterol was treated with medications and she was otherwise asymptomatic. Due to a family history of cardiac disease, the patient requested a cardiology referral for evaluation. Her [primary care provider] ordered the referral and a stress test. The office reports sending the referral information to the patient, however, the patient did not receive it. After the patient called the practice multiple times, a referral was scheduled (three months after initial request). On the day she was to have her cardiology appointment, the patient died. Her death was attributed to significant coronary artery disease, with hyperlipidemia noted.

SOURCE: CRICO, 2014. Reprinted with permission from CRICO/Risk Management Foundation of the Harvard Medical Institutions.

Radiology results not communicated

Mr. J, a patient with severe degenerative joint disease who is cared for by a rural physician, is referred to an orthopedist at an urban center. He receives a chest x-ray as part of the preoperative evaluation for knee replacement. The chest x-ray shows a mass, and his knee surgery is cancelled. The orthopedic surgeon is on vacation the following month, and the radiology report is never sent to the primary care physician. Mr. J follows up three months later with his primary care physician, who learns of the chest x-ray from Mr. J. He is found to have a primary lung cancer, which is successfully removed with surgery.

SOURCE: Sarkar et al., 2009. © Joint Commission Resources: *Joint Commission Journal on Quality and Patient Safety.* Oakbrook Terrace, IL: Joint Commission on Accreditation of Healthcare Organizations (2009), 35(7) (378). Case study. Reprinted with permission.

Poor care coordination and recognition of medication-related symptoms

Mr. F, who has diabetes, hypertension, and heart failure, sees a primary care physician, an endocrinologist, and a cardiologist. All three adjust his medications. When he presents for a scheduled primary care visit, he does not have his medicines, so the primary care physician does not have an accurate accounting of Mr. F's current drug regimen. Also, Mr. F did not submit to laboratory tests as requested at his prior primary care visit. His daughter, who cares for him, states that his endocrinologist had ordered laboratory tests the prior month, so she thought he did not need any more blood drawn. He reports feeling generally weak and unwell, so his primary care physician orders laboratory tests done the same day, and he is found to have dangerously low serum sodium.

SOURCE: Sarkar et al., 2009. © Joint Commission Resources: *Joint Commission Journal on Quality and Patient Safety.* Oakbrook Terrace, IL: Joint Commission on Accreditation of Healthcare Organizations (2009), 35(7) (378–379). Case study. Reprinted with permission.

Diagnostic failure due to intuitive biases

A 28-year-old female patient is sent to an emergency department from a nearby addictions treatment facility. Her chief complaints are anxiety and chest pain that have been going on for about a week. She is concerned that she may have a heart problem. An electrocardiogram is routinely done at triage. The emergency physician who signs up to see the patient is well known for his views on "addicts" and others with "self-inflicted" problems who tie up busy emergency departments. When he goes to see the patient, he is informed by the nurse that she has gone for a cigarette. He appears angry, and verbally expresses his irritation to the nurse. He reviews the patient's electrocardiogram, which is normal.

When the patient returns, he admonishes her for wasting his time and, after a cursory examination, informs her she has nothing wrong with her heart and discharges her with the advice that she should quit smoking. His discharge

continued

BOX D-1 Continued

diagnosis is "anxiety state." The patient is returned to the addictions centre, where she continues to complain of chest pain but is reassured that she has a normal cardiogram and has been "medically cleared" by the emergency department. Later in the evening, she suffers a cardiac arrest from which she cannot be resuscitated. At autopsy, multiple small emboli are evident in both lungs, with bilateral massive pulmonary saddle emboli.

SOURCE: Croskerry, 2012. Reprinted, with permission, from P. Croskerry 2012. Copyright 2012 by Longwoods Publishing.

Cognitive failures lead to insufficient search

A 21-year-old man is brought to a trauma center by ambulance. He has been stabbed multiple times in the arms, chest, and head. He is in no significant distress. He is inebriated but cooperative. He has no dyspnea or shortness of breath; air entry is equal in both lungs; oxygen saturation, blood pressure, and pulse are all within normal limits.

The chest laceration over his left scapula is deep but on exploration does not appear to penetrate the chest cavity. Nevertheless, there is concern that the chest cavity and major vessels may have been penetrated. Ultrasonography shows no free fluid in the chest; a chest film appears normal, with no pneumothorax; and an abdominal series is normal, with no free air. There is considerable discussion between the resident and the attending physician regarding the management of posterior chest stab wounds, but eventually agreement is reached that computed tomography (CT) of the chest is not indicated. The remaining lacerations are cleaned and sutured, and the patient is discharged home in the company of his friend.

Five days later, he presents to a different hospital reporting vomiting, blurred vision, and difficulty concentrating. A CT of his head reveals the track of a knife wound penetrating the skull and several inches into the brain.

SOURCE: Croskerry, 2013. From *New England Journal of Medicine*. P. Croskerry. From mindless to mindful practice—Cognitive bias and clinical decision making. 368(26):2445–2448. 2013. Massachusetts Medical Society. Reprinted with permission from Massachusetts Medical Society.

Incomplete patient history

A 45-year-old woman presents to the emergency department in an agitated state. She is holding a large empty bottle of aspirin and says that she has taken all of the pills a few hours ago to 'end it all'. Her breathing and heart rate are fast; she is nauseated and complains of ringing in her ears. Blood is drawn for testing that includes a toxic screen, intravenous lines are started and treatment is begun for salicylate poisoning. Within an hour, the laboratory reports that her salicylate level is at a toxic level.

Although her condition initially showed some marginal improvement, when she is reassessed by the emergency physician after two hours, the impression is that she is not progressing as well as expected. She now appears confused and her monitor shows a marked tachycardia. While the physician is reflecting on her condition, the patient's partner comes to the emergency department to enquire how she is doing. The physician tells him that she is not doing as well as expected but, given that she has taken a major overdose of salicylate, she may take a little time to stabilise. Her partner pulls an empty bottle of a tricyclic antidepressant out of his pocket and says that he found it on the bedroom floor when he got home from work. He wonders if this is important.

Shortly afterwards, the patient becomes hypotensive, with the monitor showing an intraventricular conduction delay with wide QRS, first-degree block and a prolonged QT interval; she then has seizures. She is intubated and transferred to the intensive care unit.

SOURCE: Croskerry and Nimmo, 2011. Reprinted, with permission, from Croskerry P, Nimmo G. *Journal of the Royal College of Physicians of Edinburgh* 2011; 41(2): 155–162. Copyright 2011 Journal of the Royal College of Physicians of Edinburgh.

Poor management plan and bias

A 32-year-old female presents to the emergency department with complaints of abdominal pain and vomiting. She is black, obese, schizophrenic and has poor personal hygiene. She does not communicate very well. She is treated with intravenous fluids, analgesics and anti-emetics. Her blood work-up and urinalysis are within normal limits.

A diagnosis of gastroenteritis is made and she is mobilised for discharge, but she begins to vomit again. It is getting late in the evening and the emergency physician decides to keep her overnight and arranges an ultrasound of her abdomen and repeat blood work for the morning.

The following morning, the ultrasound is reported as normal, but her white cell count has gone up to 13,000/mm3. Abdominal X-rays are done and appear normal. Her condition does not improve through the day and in the late afternoon a computed tomography exam of her abdomen reveals a four-inch-long metallic/plastic foreign body, a hair clasp, in her stomach. This is removed several hours later by endoscopy. There were four handovers during the course of 28 hours in the emergency department before the correct diagnosis was made.

SOURCE: Croskerry and Nimmo, 2011. Reprinted, with permission, from Croskerry P, Nimmo G. *Journal of the Royal College of Physicians of Edinburgh* 2011; 41(2): 155–162. Copyright 2011 Journal of the Royal College of Physicians of Edinburgh.

Rushed communication leads to error

The doctor informs the patient to refrain from aspirin ingestion prior to a particular laboratory test involving platelets. The consultation with the patient is rushed, and the physician fails to explain to the patient that aspirin is present in many medicines and that the patient should determine whether any over-the-counter product contains aspirin prior to using it. When the assay is performed, the result is incorrect. When the patient is asked about aspirin ingestion, she reports she has taken Alka-Seltzer within the past 24 hours, inadvertently ingesting an over-

continued

BOX D-1 Continued

the-counter product containing aspirin. This necessitates a repeat performance of a complicated assay.

SOURCE: Laposata, 2010. Republished with permission of Demos Medical Publishing, from *Coagulation disorders: Quality in laboratory diagnosis*, M. Laposata, 2010; permission conveyed through Copyright Clearance Center.

Poor emergency department diagnostic test tracking and reporting

A young woman with a complicated medical history, including systemic lupus erythematosis (lupus), presented to the ED with severe ankle pain, thought to be a partial Achilles tendon tear. She also had ulcerations of both of her palms. The physician performed an examination and ordered routine blood work and blood cultures. The gram stain showed gram + cocci in clusters; the final blood culture report revealed staphylococcus aureus. The CBC with differential and urinalysis were abnormal. The lab called the results to the ED, but a new charge nurse skipped the physician's review and the standard ED alert system. The patient went home, became septic, endured a prolonged hospital stay, and is now considered totally disabled.

SOURCE: MagMutual, 2014. Reprinted, with permission, from MagMutual Insurance Company, Atlanta, GA, 2015.

Diagnosis that is beyond current medical knowledge

Although alarmed at the sight of a red stream instead of straw-colored urine, Dunham Aurelius didn't realize that he needed to see a doctor. An endurance runner and triathlete in his early 20s, he brushed off the physical discomfort and reasoned that he may have pushed too hard on a long Sunday run. When the bleeding persisted, Aurelius made an appointment with a urologist, a specialist in diseases of the urinary tract and reproductive organs. The doctor diagnosed a kidney stone, the first of many that Aurelius would endure throughout his 20s and 30s. He became an all-too-frequent patient of urologists, as well as of endocrinologists and nephrologists, who specialize, respectively, in diseases of endocrine glands and kidneys.

Aurelius' kidneys formed stones at a size and frequency that surprised his doctors. He has passed more than 15 stones; one calcium phosphate mass in his kidney measured three centimeters. His doctors detected high vitamin D levels in his blood but they weren't sure of its significance or why he developed these stones.

Aurelius expelled many kidney stones without recourse to medical intervention. Once, he brought a bag of stones to his urologist, who hailed him as an ultimate fighter of the kidney stone world. Some stones, however, required painful and sometimes dangerous procedures. The problem worsened to the point that Aurelius was having multiple surgeries a year. He started to become desperate for a diagnosis at age 38, almost 20 years after his first stone.

In 2008, Aurelius' endocrinologist at the University of New Mexico Health Sciences Center learned about the Undiagnosed Diseases Program (UDP), a new NIH program. The UDP was recruiting patients whose conditions were unexplained despite doctors' best efforts to make a diagnosis. The new program would accept referrals if there were some clue for a multidisciplinary team of doctors at NIH to follow up. In Aurelius' case, the clue was his high vitamin D levels.

In 2009, he became the 37th of 75 patients evaluated in the first year of the UDP, during a week-long visit to the NIH Clinical Center. Through genomic analysis conducted in subsequent months, NIH doctors ultimately discovered that mutations in Aurelius' DNA caused loss in the function of an enzyme called CYP24A1, which results in high vitamin D levels. With his wife's help, Aurelius made dietary changes that have brought about vast improvements in his condition).

SOURCE: MacDougall, 2013.

REFERENCES

CRICO. 2014. 2014. *Annual benchmarking report (2014): Malpractice risks in the diagnostic process.* Cambridge, MA: CRICO Strategies. www.rmfstrategies.com/benchmarking (accessed June 11, 2015).

Croskerry, P. 2012. Perspectives on diagnostic failure and patient safety. *Healthcare Quarterly* 15(Special issue) April:50–56.

Croskerry, P. 2013. From mindless to mindful practice—Cognitive bias and clinical decision making. *New England Journal of Medicine* 368(26):2445–2448.

Croskerry, P., and G. Nimmo. 2011. Better clinical decision making and reducing diagnostic error. *Journal of the Royal College of Physicians of Edinburgh* 41(2):155–162.

IOM (Institute of Medicine). 2000. *To err is human: Building a safer health system.* Washington, DC: The National Academies Press.

Laposata, M. 2010. *Coagulation disorders: Quality in laboratory diagnosis.* New York: Demos Medical Publishing.

MacDougall, R. 2013. Expanding the limits of modern medicine: NIH Undiagnosed Diseases Network will address abundance of mystery cases. www.genome.gov/27552767 (accessed August 18, 2015).

MagMutual. 2014. Poor ED lab tracking and reporting system results in sepsis treatment delay. www.magmutual.com/sites/default/files/PoorEDLabTrack_SepsTreatmDelay.pdf (accessed July 23, 2015).

Sarkar, U., R. M. Wachter, S. A. Schroeder, and D. Schillinger. 2009. Refocusing the lens: Patient safety in ambulatory chronic disease care. *Joint Commission Journal on Quality and Patient Safety* 35(7):377–383, 341.